Sustainable Development Goals Series

The **Sustainable Development Goals Series** is Springer Nature's inaugural cross-imprint book series that addresses and supports the United Nations' seventeen Sustainable Development Goals. The series fosters comprehensive research focused on these global targets and endeavours to address some of society's greatest grand challenges. The SDGs are inherently multidisciplinary, and they bring people working across different fields together and working towards a common goal. In this spirit, the Sustainable Development Goals series is the first at Springer Nature to publish books under both the Springer and Palgrave Macmillan imprints, bringing the strengths of our imprints together.

The Sustainable Development Goals Series is organized into eighteen subseries: one subseries based around each of the seventeen respective Sustainable Development Goals, and an eighteenth subseries, "Connecting the Goals", which serves as a home for volumes addressing multiple goals or studying the SDGs as a whole. Each subseries is guided by an expert Subseries Advisor with years or decades of experience studying and addressing core components of their respective Goal.

The SDG Series has a remit as broad as the SDGs themselves, and contributions are welcome from scientists, academics, policymakers, and researchers working in fields related to any of the seventeen goals. If you are interested in contributing a monograph or curated volume to the series, please contact the Publishers: Zachary Romano [Springer; zachary.romano@springer.com] and Rachael Ballard [Palgrave Macmillan; rachael.ballard@palgrave.com].

Kassahun Dessie Gashu
Zeleke Abebaw Mekonnen
Moges Asressie Chanyalew
Habtamu Alganeh Guadie
Editors

Public Health Informatics

Implementation and Governance
in Resource-Limited Settings

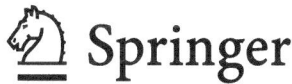 Springer

Editors
Kassahun Dessie Gashu
Institute of Public Health
University of Gondar
Gondar, Ethiopia

Moges Asressie Chanyalew
Planning, Monitoring and Evaluation
Amhara Region Health Bureau
Bahir Dar, Ethiopia

Zeleke Abebaw Mekonnen
Ministry of Health - Ethiopia
Addis Ababa, Ethiopia

Habtamu Alganeh Guadie
School of Public Health
Bahir Dar University
Bahir Dar, Ethiopia

ISSN 2523-3084   ISSN 2523-3092   (electronic)
Sustainable Development Goals Series
ISBN 978-3-031-71117-6   ISBN 978-3-031-71118-3   (eBook)
https://doi.org/10.1007/978-3-031-71118-3

Preface

Public health informatics is an evolving field that seeks to leverage the power of information and communication technologies to improve health outcomes and promote equity. In recent years, there has been growing recognition of the potential of informatics to support public health efforts, particularly in resource-limited settings where health systems face significant challenges.

This book, *Public Health Informatics: Implementation and Governance in Resource-Limited Settings*," was framed in seven sections. The first section provides an introduction to information communication technology (ICT) and its role in health development, which includes the evolution of ICT and its impact on strengthening the health system. The second section offers an overview of public health informatics, highlighting the concepts, rationales, and the role of public health informatics in the health system for readers. The third section examines about data analytics and public health. The fourth section covers the groundworks and major initiatives of public health informatics in resource-limited settings. The last three sections focus on implementation, leadership and governance, and ethics of public health informatics, particularly in resource-limited settings.

This book brought together experts with diverse experiences to explore the complex landscape of public health informatics implementations and governance in resource-limited settings. The authors provided a comprehensive overview of the foundational concepts, frameworks, and practices that underpin the implementation and governance of public health informatics in resource-limited settings. Throughout this book, the authors highlight the unique challenges and opportunities of working in resource-limited settings, where limited resources, infrastructure, and human capacity can pose significant obstacles to the implementation and governance of public health informatics. They also emphasized the importance of collaboration and partnership, both within and across sectors, to ensure the effective and equitable use of information and communication technologies to improve health outcomes.

This book offers insights for learners, instructors, practitioners, researchers, policymakers, and those who are interested in the field of digital health, aiming to promote access, quality and efficiency of health systems in resource-limited settings. We believe that the insights and perspectives shared in this book will inspire and inform new approaches to public health informatics, ultimately contributing to improved health and well-being of communities around the world.

Gondar, Ethiopia   Kassahun Dessie Gashu
Addis Ababa, Ethiopia   Zeleke Abebaw Mekonnen
Bahir Dar, Ethiopia   Moges Asressie Chanyalew
Bahir Dar, Ethiopia   Habtamu Alganeh Guadie

Acknowledgements

Writing a book is rarely a solitary endeavor, and we have been fortunate to have had the support and encouragement of many people along the way. First and foremost, we would like to thank SMART health, a powerful private firm that is making significant contributions to research and capacity building in the area of health informatics and public health in Ethiopia. We are grateful to SMART health for providing administrative support and facilitating our subsequent writing and evaluation workshops.

We would also like to thank our editor, Grant Weston (Executive Editor, Medicine and Life Sciences) and Anand Shanmugam (the books project coordinator) at Springer Nature for providing invaluable close follow-up, support, and guidance throughout the process. Their attention to detail and insightful suggestions have been instrumental in shaping this book into its final form.

We would like to extend our special recognitions to our families, colleagues, and friends, who have always been a source of our inspiration and motivation. We are always grateful for their support and encouragement.

Finally, we would like to express our gratitude to the readers of this book. Writing is a deeply rewarding yet often challenging pursuit, and it is the support and enthusiasm of readers that make it all worthwhile. Thank you for taking the time to read this book and for your continued support of our work.

Contents

ICT and Its Roles in Health Development

1

Kassahun Dessie Gashu

Abstract

The history of information technology goes further back from the period of pre-mechanical then followed by mechanical, electromechanical and electronic ages. Though, the efforts and shifting from analogue to digitalization were not smooth and immediate. It has now brought tremendous impacts in the global social and economic phenomena. But, still digital divide continues to be the major bottleneck in almost all domains of Information and Communication Technology (ICT) development index. The rapid and continuous advancement of the information technology has brought the concept of health informatics. This progressive use of the ubiquitous connected Information Technology (IT) helps to enhance efficiency, access and quality of health care.

Keywords

Information technology · Health informatics
Digital health · eHealth · Theoretical
frameworks

K. D. Gashu (✉)
Department of Health Informatics, Institute of Public Health, College of Medicine and Health Sciences, University of Gondar, Gondar, Ethiopia

SMART Health, Research and Publication Department, Bahir Dar, Ethiopia
e-mail: kassahun.dessie@uog.edu.et

1.1 Introduction

According to William H. Dutton [1], the era of computer development in 1950s and 1960s; microchip in 1970s; the age of superhighway internet and information society in 1980s and 1990s; and the e-everything enabled with internet in the twenty-first century were major milestones of revolution in information technology.

The debut of the personal computer and continuing advancement of information technology enhanced a free and fast flow of information and created a swift industrial revolution. The ICT has completely transformed towards the new global order of communication. Particularly, the rapid advancement of mobile technology is playing an important role in improving access to information and services in various ways. The digital revolution has enabled low-cost access to information and knowledge, which has sped up services and transactions while also lowering service costs, potentially benefiting customers and populations at large. Telecommunications and mass media streamlines information processing and distribution between humans and machines, as well as between humans and machines.

Despite the growing penetration and advancement of digital technologies, digital divide continues to be the major challenge particularly in resource-limited settings. With all the shortcomings, the use of ICT's potential that helping to facilitate and achieve the development goals (ICT4D).

The rapid and continuous advancement of the ICT has opened various windows of opportunity to strengthening the health system. It has brought the concept of health informatics (also referred as e-Health, digital health, and digital medicine) refers to the use of the potentials of ICT to improve health care.

This chapter aimed to outline the global digital revolution, and its impact in health care development. The contribution and advantages of ICT to the advancement of health care have been discussed. In-depth discussions are also had regarding the theoretical frameworks, domains, and trends in the development of digital health.

1.2   The Global Digital Revolution

Commonly, the history of information technology is divided in four main ages. Pre-mechanical age (3000 B.C. to 1450 A.D) as the earliest age followed by mechanical (1450 to 1840), electro-mechanical (1840 to 1940) and electronic age (from 1940's on) as the latest age of information technology. The efforts and then shifting from analogue to digitalization started in the 1950s, have now brought tremendous impacts in the global social and economic phenomena [2].

The transition, however, was not seamless and immediate as the new way of doing things often get resistance among other reasons. Research and innovation breakthroughs played significant roles in transforming and realizing the digital revolution. Particularly, in the era of internet, opportunities opened for everyone to create, contribute to a content and develop software applications. According to Moor's law, the computing power of a microchip keeps growing and as the chip size becomes smaller without significant price increases that was attributed to the improved accessibility of powerful PCs at relatively lower prices, known as the ref. [3]. Metcalfe's Law was on the demand side which indicated that the number of potential connections would increase faster as the networking grows in size [4].

The invention of Internet as an innovation commons has made transformation to the information age possible through sharing basic resources that facilitates the innovation and development of new contents and services [5]. Vannevar Bush, J.C.R. Licklider and Douglas Englebart were envisioned to create human communication through computer networks that vision had led to realize internet [6]. Later, the advancement of Internet technology became the main source and facilitator for further advancement of ICT. It happened as Internet is designed with the end-to-end (e2e) principle, the intelligence is at the ends of the network. Therefore, the network is mainly serving to transmit the data efficiently between the ends. The Internet age itself, has heightened the penetration and advancement of information technology as everyone can create new software applications, and engage in the global community of practice. Human beings from early history were striving to use technology to ease their communications, to enhance efficiency in their routine activities, and improve quality of life. The digital revolution was not just happened overnight and not yet ended. The process of innovation and advancement of ICT is inter-reliant. The invention of one piece of digital technology opens the door for the next invention that has been demonstrated in the last decade's trend of global penetration and advancement of ICT as indicated in Fig. 1.1.

The progressive growth and advancement of ICT has impacted lives through improving innovation, customer service, efficiency of the services, and market development. According to Lipsey [7], Economic, social and political growth have been periodically transformed by technological revolutions.

Lipsey identified the relationship between advancement of technologies and its effects on society that could:

- Slowdown initial productivity and delayed new technology's productivity payoff
- Technological unemployment
- Lead to destruction of human capital, since old skills are no longer wanted
- Widening disparities in the distribution of income

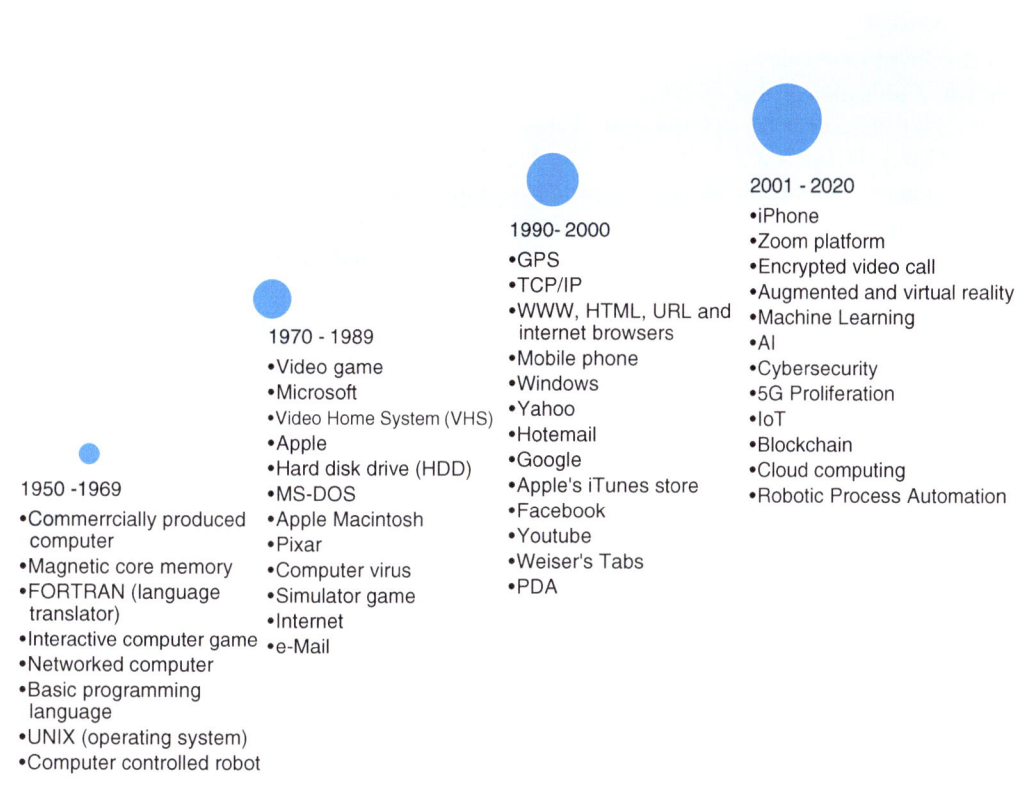

Fig. 1.1 History of ICT development

- Changes in required education
- Changes in regional patterns of industrial location
- Changes in infrastructure
- Changes in the way we live and interact
- Changes in rules and regulations such as intellectual property

The digital revolution has realized access to information and knowledge at low-cost that speed-up services, and transactions and as the same time reduces the cost related to the services that could finally resulted in benefiting the consumers and populations at large. Digitization of telecommunications and mass media streamlining information processing and dissemination between interpersonal and even people with machines and between machines [8].

Now a days, the ICT penetration and advancement is growing more than ever; despite, the existing challenge in the digital divide. Access to Internet connectivity and the bandwidth is now getting improvement including the resource-limited settings. Today, more people have access to a cell phone than to water supply, sewage, and electricity [9].

According to the ICT Development Index (IDI) Report (2018), which is based on data from the ITN showed a consistent growth in ICT development and use across the world [10]. In 2023, about 5.4 billion (67%) of the global population is using internet. But only 27% of the population is using internet in low-income countries. Access to basic communications services via mobile devices is still increasing. In 2023, mobile phone ownership reached 78% in the global population and 47% in low-income settings. The number of mobile phone subscribers already exceeds the number of people on the planet; however, this is not the case everywhere. The availability of broadband is still expanding. The number of fixed-broadband subscribers is steadily rising. Nowadays, almost everyone on the planet resides close to a mobile or cellular network connection. Furthermore, the majority of people have access to 3G or better networks for Internet access [10].

Nonetheless, one significant obstacle preventing people from using the Internet is a lack of ICT skills. Digital divide is still the key roadblock in practically every ICT development index domain, despite the increasing adoption and improvement of digital technology. Particularly, resource-limited countries are highly affected by the consequences related to digital divide which is clearly indicated in the ITU's information communication technology development [10]. Digital divide typically describes the difference in access to information technology, including computers and networks, between those who have it and those who do not [11]. With all the challenges, bridging the access-divide and closing the gap has now becoming an essential area of research and government's policy objectives. So that, fairly equal access to the technology needs to be ensured to get advantages of technology. Otherwise, digital divide could be a threat for widening inequity in all areas of development, as ensuring equal access would give equal opportunity for growth and development.

Technological revolution is often characterized by its nature of pervasiveness to penetrate all domains of human activities [12]. Information Technologies progressively utilize the ubiquitous connected devices to enhance personal and professional productivity and quality of life. According to Richard Heeks, Information and Communication Technology for Development (ICT4D) refers to the use of ICT's potential that helps to facilitate and achieve the development goals such as to reduce/end poverty, illiteracy, inequality, tyranny, climate change, hunger and others [13].

The explosion of ICT has brought the concept of health informatics (also referred as e-Health, digital health, and digital medicine). The ultimate purpose was to use the potentials of ICT tools such as, internet, computers, GIS, wearable devices, mobile phone, PDAs, Cameras, smartcards, Tablets, etc. to improve quality of care, safety, efficiencies and reduce costs related to health care [14–16]. Electronic health (e-Health) is an umbrella term that incorporates Telemedicine, Electronic Health Records (EHRs), and mobile health (mHealth). Telemedicine was relatively the oldest e-Health system first used in the 1920s and its history development even goes further back connected to the invention of telegraph [17].

The details on ICT's impact in healthcare development is mentioned in the next section of the book.

1.3   How ICT Impacting the Health Development?

Information communication technology refers to a family of technologies provided by and serving the institutional and business sectors as well as the general public, that are used to process, store, and disseminate information, facilitating the performance of information-related human activities [18].

It includes all forms of application software and communication devices including computers, networks, cell phones, PDAs, software Apps, internet, social media platforms, satellite systems, GIS, radio, television, video conference platforms, etc. ICT plays a pivotal role in social and economic developments via facilitating seamless information flow between entities.

According to Dutton 1999 [19], the four interrelated resources such as information, people, technology and services can be reconfigured through the social and technical choices of ICTs (Fig. 1.2).

The foundation and paradigm change for the development of health informatics as a field of study were established, among other reasons, by the inception of the Health Information Technology for Economic and Clinical Health Act (HITECH) Act of 2009 [20]. Now a days, incorporating different features of ICT in the health system is a springboard to jump high for better health outcomes. As a result, health informatics was emerged as a field of study.

Fig. 1.2 Social and technical choices of ICT

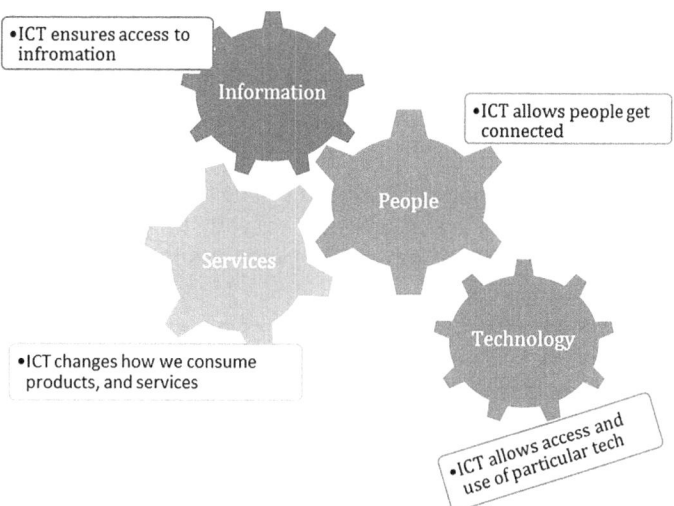

The rapid expansion and advancement of digital technology has created new opportunities for improving health and wellbeing. Tools such as smart phones, digital cameras, drones, and geolocation tools, as well as the use of machine learning and artificial intelligence, have transformed the flow of information within health systems. Use of digital technologies has now become a key concept in health promotion, prevention and control of diseases and other health problems [21].

Following that, many researchers attempted to define health informatics as a research and fled of study.

- Health informatics research refers to "a scientific endeavor that applies information science, computer technology, and statistical modeling techniques to develop decision support systems for improving both health service organizations' performance and patient care outcomes." *Wan* [22]
- Healthcare informatics as, "the integration of healthcare sciences, computer science, information science, and cognitive science to assist in the management of healthcare information." *Saba and McCormick* [23]
- Health informatics as "the interdisciplinary study of the design, development, adoption and application of IT-based innovations in healthcare services delivery, management and

planning." *The United States National Library of Medicine* [24]

However, information technology is a double sword that could be utilized both for good and bad. Therefore, appropriate use of technology is an essential concept. Appropriate use of digital technologies often consider ethical use, safety, cost-effectiveness, people-centeredness, evidence-based, effective, sustainable, inclusive, equitable and need to account contextual factors [25].

Overall, the introduction of health informatics as a field of study and research has contemplated the applications in health system including telemedicine, electronic health records, Clinical decision support systems, mHealth, data warehousing and eLearning tools. So that, the health informatics applications has been started to play important role in the health sector. It is difficult to clearly articulate the role of ICT in the health system improvement due to its multifunctioning and crosscutting nature of ICT that contributed in all section and levels of the health system. The major roles of ICT in the health sector includes:

1.3.1   Digitizing the Health System

According to WHO, Health System Strengthening (HSS) refers to "improving and combining six key health system strengthening building blocks in ways that achieve more equitable and sustained improvements across health services and outcomes" [26]. Health Information System (HIS) is one of the fundamental building-blocks of the health system, which also serve as a cross-cutting tool for other health system components [27]. Health Information System refers to the systems that capture, store, manage or transmit health data/information of individuals or the activities of the organizations. According to Anshari [28], HIS is the interplay of people, procedures, and technology to facilitate the delivery of critical information with the goal of raising the quality of healthcare services. In this concept, the purpose of ICT features is to make it easier to produce, share, and apply high-quality data to guide healthcare procedures [29].

The ultimate purpose of HIS is generally to strengthening the health system through enhancing data-informed decision-making and evidence-based healthcare practices. Sound and reliable information is essential for health system policy development and implementation, governance, research, human resources development, education and training, healthcare financing, and service delivery. The key functions of HIS includes, data generation, compilation, analysis and synthesis, and communication and use.

We categorized the role of digital health systems in the health sector in to three broad areas such as digitizing:

1.3.1.1 Automating the Health Administration

Digitalizing the health administrations allows all-in-one services that facilitate efficiency use of resources and seamless integration of the health system. Integrating ICT helps to facilitate evidence-based administrative strategic and operational decision-makings. Some of the major administrative areas that require digitization includes:

- Logistic management
- The human resource management
- Financial management including ordering and billing
- Quality assurance, etc.

1.3.1.2 Automating the Health Service Delivery

Data saves lives. A well-managed health information use is one of the essential components of public health practices. Clinical decisions, and practices in general requires timely and quality data to envisage efficiency, quality in health care. The complexity and volume data has surpassed the health system functioning. As a result, this challenge is affecting both the quality of data management and patient care as it is taking much time to manually manage both data management and patient care and management all together. Therefore, electronic ICT such as electronic medical recording system is becoming an essential and priority agenda in the health system [30, 31].

The role of ICT in managing healthcare records include:

- Electronic health/medical recording
- Clinical decision support systems
- Diagnostic imaging
- Use of mHealth for:
  - Patient/client education
  - Appointment and medication reminder system
  - Tracking system
  - Surveillance
  - Research data collection, etc.
- Remote health care service and remote diagnostic support using Tele-health
- Mapping of public health threats
- Data management and analysis
- Reporting, visualization and dissemination
- Applying cutting-edge tech such as hybrid operating rooms, as an assistive technology for the next generation of surgery. It integrates video recorded in EHR, patient clinic visits and operations.

1.3.1.3 Connecting the Consumers

According to Gibbons et al. [32], Consumer informatics refers to Any electronic device, technology, or application intended for direct consumer interaction—with or without the presence of a healthcare provider—that utilizes personal data to give the patient tailored support and helps them better manage their health or medical needs. The concept of consumer health informatics focused on preventive approaches and self-care. Some of the strategies employed to connect consumers are listed as follows:

The Quantified-Self

The quantified-self is about recording and reviewing daily-based personal activities and biometrics to improve personal health and life style. The advancement of ICT allows to individuals to measure the range of physiological parameters such as, vital signs (body temperature, respiration rate, pulse rate, and blood pressure), caloric intake, sleep quality; and environmental variables like, air quality, humidity, luminosity etc. [33].

Home-Based Telehealth

In addition to monitoring vital signs and symptoms of chronic conditions, patients and their families can use technology to access specialized educational resources, connect via video with home care providers, and transmit the data to a clinical facility.

The idea of telehealth encourages patient engagement, since it calls for patients and their families to actively monitor symptoms, educate themselves on the course of the disease, and record lifestyle decisions (such total activity or diet) [34].

Personal Health Record System

It is also a consumer-centric tools that is designed to facilitate recording, managing, tracking, and sharing personal health information [35].

Patient Portals

Patient portals, even though, do not often have consumers' data entry features, it can help to facilitate data sharing and allows the consumers to decide on their health matters [36].

Precision Medicine

Precision medicine refers to the "prevention and treatment strategies that take individual variability into account". Precision medicine is now an emerging and a priority agenda for research that could change the health care mode of service delivery.

Enormous biologic databases, sophisticated computational instruments for scrutinizing and evaluating vast datasets, and the application of proteomics, metabolomics, and genomics to enhance comprehension of patients and populations are all unleashing the possibility of customizing disease management and prevention, considering individual variations in genetics, surroundings, and way of life [37].

Social Media, and Online Health Communities

In general, the use of digital health helps to empower the community and patients that to facilitates to access to health care and service seeking behaviors at the point of care or remotely [38].

Others such as social media platforms and world of online health communities are also playing immense roles for creating awareness and improving knowledge about emerging and existing health conditions.

1.3.2 As a Health Data Management and Research Tool

The advancement of ICT had immense contribution for the current trend of health research development. It is due to the fact that ICT facilitates an easily access and management of electronic datasets for health services researches [39]. The major roles of information technology in research works include:

- Data collection using electronic tools such as: Google form, SurveyMonkey, KoboToolbox, etc.
- Data management and analysis tools
  - For quantitative data (*Epi Info™, SPSS®, Stata, SAS, R, etc.*)
  - For qualitative data (*OpenCode*, ATLAS.ti, MAXQDA, NVivo, etc.)
- Data presentation and visualization tools such as, *Charts, Graphs and Tables*
- Dissemination of research findings
  - e-Journals for research publications,
  - Virtual conferencing platforms, etc.

- Evidence archival and searching platforms databases such as: PubMed/MEDLINE, EMBASE, web of science, Cochrane Library (Wiley), CINAHL, PsycInfo, etc.

1.3.3 Serving as a Communication Platform

The heart of health information technology is all about communication. The carefully-selected, scalable and flexible digital communication tools enable connection and steady information sharing [38]. The communication is often between:

- Device-to-device (D2D) communications
- Team members to create common understanding, reporting and feedback
- Managers and providers: A real-time communications for updating treatment guideline, and reporting routine health services, etc.
- Providers and providers: For referrals, consultations, booking, discharging, second opinion, laboratory test requests and results reports, e-prescriptions etc.
- Patients/clients and providers: Using e-mail and web-based messaging for clinical counseling, disease monitoring, and appointment, symptom notifications, post-referral follow-up, etc.
- Different health facilities: Digital devices implemented to facilitate knowledge management, experience sharing and information sharing on possible outbreak and other natural and man-made disaster management
- Patients: Electronic networks can be used for disease specific clinical networking among patients aimed to share life skills, coping mechanisms and experiences of living with that particular disease
- Global and local communities: Mainstream and social medias enables to disseminate health information to the wider population

1.3.4 A Platform for Education and Continuous Professional Development

WHO has indicated the power of digital education systems to improve the health care workers' competencies and satisfaction; however, its effectiveness depends on how we implement the systems. Educational aids (guidelines, medical teaching) can be developed and implemented using digital platforms [40–42]. The selection of digital education modalities such as online digital education, virtual reality, mobile phones, gaming, etc. could influence the effectiveness of the technology. Similarly, the delivery modes (fully digital or blended); the instructional method (simulations or direct instruction); the assessment methods; learning pedagogies (problem-based or team-based); the target population; and the topic of interest intended for digital education could play significant role for the digital education system to be effective [42].

1.4 Benefits of Digitizing in the Health System

The use of ICTs brought new order of interaction between people, information, communities, and organizations. ICT has distinct benefits particularly in resource-limited settings where there are high demanding population, poor health infrastructure, and trained manpower.

Generally, the use of ICT is associated with an improved health outcome [43]. Integrating ICT in the health system creates a seamless collaboration, promoting patient-centered healthcare, reduces related costs, improves patient safety and quality of care, facilitates information sharing and use, assists a continuous professionals, minimizes travel time, and creates a platform for interaction between/within patients and health providers [44, 45]. The benefits of integrating ICT in the health system involves a wide range of areas ultimately intended to help the citizens [38, 46]. The major benefits include:

1.4.1 Improving Access and Exchange of Health Information

The importance of ICTs is not just about the technology, but its contribution to substantial functions for connecting people and increase in access to health information and communication. The growing penetration of Internet, mobile phones, radio, and other ICT applications helps people to find preventive measures, to eradicate and reduce the spread of the health problems [43].

Leveraging the potentials of ICT improves health information exchange through facilitating the navigation and management of the networks of HIS allows for the health care workers to access, and share vital medical information with enhanced speed, quality, security, safety, and cost of medical care. Therefore, information accessibility has been realized through the help of information and communication technology [47].

However, access to health information is limited in resource-limited settings [29]. The major challenges related to the relatively poor access to health information in resource-limited settings include poor digital literacy, digital divide, lack of information control, non-affordability of the tools, failure of equipment and security and privacy issues [48, 49].

1.4.2 Improving Access to Health Care Services

According to the Institute of Medicine (IOM) [50], access to health care is "having timely use of personal health services to achieve the best possible health outcome". Similarly, the National Academies of Sciences, Engineering, and Medicine [51], has defined access to health care as "People use healthcare services to diagnose, cure, or ameliorate disease or injury; to improve or maintain function; or to obtain information about their health status and prognosis". Generally, access to health care is about timely utilisation of health services to attain the best health outcomes.

However, achieving access to health care is not a simple task and remained unresolved challenges in the health system particularly in resource-limited settings due to many reasons such as, geographical distance, lack of information on service existence, physical or mental disability, restrictions, lockdown, internal and external displacement of people, etc.

Hence, the use of ICT could overcome the geographical, social and political and health related barriers that hinder access to healthcare services. According to WHO [52], "It has become increasingly clear that UHC cannot be achieved without the support of eHealth." Some of the digital tools that could improve access to health services include, Tele-health, Electronic Health Record, wearable devices, sensors, artificial intelligence, Block-chain, Internet of (medical) things, big data, etc. [38].

For instance the use of Telemedicine platforms can improve access to health care services mainly in rural, hard-to-reach areas and where there is scarcity of trained health manpower. The improvement in access to health care is attributed to the potentials of the Telemedicine technology that enables to overcome barriers related to geographical access and shortage of trained man power. Since, it helps to provide the required services without the patients/clients moving from where they are into the point of care. It does not required the patients/clients to be in the same place with the care provider. As a result, it improves access, and reduce cost of treatment [53, 54].

1.4.3 Improving Quality of Health Care

According to WHO [55], quality of care is "the degree to which health services for individuals and populations increase the likelihood of desired health outcomes". Quality health care was defined in various ways, but still there is agreement that quality of health care services that consists of six domains [56]:

- Effectiveness; Is providing evidence-based care
- Safety: Which is about avoiding harm during care
- People-centred: providing care based on individual preferences, needs and values
- Timely: Reducing delays
- Equitable: Providing same quality of care for all
- Efficient: maximizing the benefit with low cost

Generally, these domains indicate that high-quality health care service involves providing the right care, at the right time, with the right user's preferences, with minimum harm and waste of resource. Globally, progresses have been reported regarding the improvement of quality of healthcare, however the achievement was highly unequal. Particularly, in resource-limited settings improving the quality of health care remained a major challenge [57].

Above all, quality of care and patient safety are most important healthcare outcomes impacted by the appropriate use of ICT. Digital health is shaping the future of primary health care. Technology plays a vital role in facilitating an evidence-based medicine and a continuing of health care using digital health records from birth to death. It enables to keep records of patients' information, such as vaccinations, allergy reactions, diagnostic reports, medical history, treatment information, appointments, etc. which in turn tends to improve the health outcomes [58].

1.4.4 Reducing Medical Errors

According to the National Coordinating Council for Medication Error Reporting and Prevention (NCC MERP) [59], medical error refers to "any preventable event that may cause or lead to inappropriate medication use or patient harm while the medication is in the control of the health care professional, patient, or consumer. Such events may be related to professional practice, health care products, procedures, and systems, including prescribing; order communication; product labeling, packaging, and nomenclature; compounding;

dispensing; distribution; administration; education; monitoring; and use". Some of the errors are due to forgetfulness or inattention, errors of judgment in planning, and errors resulting from a lack of knowledge. Despite the fact that medical errors are preventable and related deaths are avoidable, the problem is globally growing in alarming rates. Previous studies indicated that the use of information technology such as EMR, e-Prescription, computerized provider order entry (CPOE), automated drug-dispensing, clinical bar code, and unit dosing systems, etc. could significantly reduce medication errors [60–62].

Using the potentials of digital technologies, for instance forgetfulness is inevitable in human beings, however, machines do not forget once, appropriately scheduled and used. Machines can compute quickly and free of error than humans do. These intrinsic potentials of digital technologies can support health providers' and patients' decisions in clinical care.

1.4.5 Improving Patient Empowerment

Nowadays, engagement of ICT in the health system is supporting patient's doubts to be cleared. The use of different digital platforms would enhance motivation and satisfaction in the health care services. It also enhance empowerment to decide and play a great role in their own treatment and care.

The use of ICT also helps towards the current patient-centered treatment approach that patients' preferences and values to be considered [63]. The use of digital systems often positively alter patient's behavior like: reducing forgetfulness, improving TB knowledge, attitude, reducing fear of stigma, and improve provider-patient relationship.

1.4.6 Improving Equitable Health Systems

Inequality contradicts the key principles of social justice, hence the protection in the Universal Declaration of Human Rights that "all human beings are born free and equal in dignity and rights" [64]. It is important to recognize that inequities within all health systems are also systemic [65]. According to the "inverse care law" [66], states that "the availability of good medical or social care tends to vary inversely with the needs of the population being served". In addition, shortage of skilled manpower is one of the challenges in achieving equitable health system. The WHO has estimated that ten million more health worker force are needed by 2030, mainly in low and lower-middle income countries [67].

The investment in health IT significantly eliminate health care disparities. So that minority and disadvantaged group of populations could benefit from the potentials of information technology that offer relatively equal opportunities for all [68, 69].

Previous studies indicated that engaging ICT in health system could also reduce racial disparities in accessing quality health care [70–72]. There are several ways that digital technologies can reduce inequalities in health care. Few major ways are listed below:

- Digital platforms allow to increase access to trusted, reliable health information so that all population in the network could assess and use the information. Democratizing the access through connecting the communities to trusted, reliable sources of health information [73].
- Digital tools such as electronic logistics management information systems (eLMIS) can ensure equitable supply chain management. Automated systems could be used to balance scarcity in one area and abundance in other areas which is a practical problem mainly in drug and vaccine distributions. As a result, disparities in access to medical logistics could be answered [74].
- ICT enables to reach and address gaps in hard-to-reach areas. For instance, using different Tele-health applications could minimize the current shortage of trained manpower, geographical inaccessibility of immediate and high-quality surgical care, cost of health care, potential complications, and long-distance

travel. Generally, ICTs have the potential to improve healthcare delivery Particularly, the potentials of Internet is overcoming geographical barriers—for instance using virtual conferencing that substitute face-to-face communication which results in reducing cost of travel and save time. As the same time, ICT reduces isolation of disadvantaged people behind. For instance: those who cannot afford physical presence can alternatively use virtual platforms so that disadvantage people can get opportunity to engage themselves in the global community [75–77].

- Use of digital technologies could reduce catastrophic health expenditure through improving access and reducing long-distance travel and stay related to health care [78].
- The use of digital technologies could improve representation mainly during data collections that would reduce under and over estimation of a certain health parameters. This would help to consider marginalized group of the community.

Rapidly developing technology, however, has the potential to worsen exclusion, create unanticipated biases, widen the digital divide, and keep some groups behind. Digital-divide (inequalities in the access and use of ICTs) would conversely widen the disparity of health services, if that is not well managed. People who owned and utilize ICT can be benefited and the technology-disadvantaged group of people would remain far behind accessing the services. Therefore, it requires to use alternative approaches (both digital and non-digital) to address inequalities in access and use of technology particularly in resource-limited settings [79].

1.4.7 Reduce Costs of Healthcare

The cost of health care has been addressed in one way or another. The use of ICT ensure organizational and health workers efficiency in many ways. For example: Automating health record system would avail basic information recorded at one point of care that significantly reduce repetition of the same tasks. Similarly, the use of decision support system could reduce of laboratory and radiology tests that would impact on patient's expense and organizations resource management at large [60, 80].

The use of Tele-health significantly reduce cost related to health care among other benefits. These technologies provide access to health information and health care services at remote (virtually) without expensing transportation and related costs required for accessing the health facility physically [75–77]. Generally, Integrating ICT in the health system improves efficient use of health care resources.

1.5 Trends of Digital Health Penetration

Health informatics as a field of study is relatively a recent phenomenon as indicated in the Table 1.1. Majority of the eHealth application areas are now undergoing development and many more innovations yet to come.

e-Health has now given recognition as one of the rapidly growing phenomena in the health sector today, following the WHO's series of World Health Assemblies delivered listed below the prominent resolutions and reports related to e-Health development.

1.5.1 Report EB101/INF.DOC./9

In December 1997, WHO had an international consultation convened to prepare inputs on "telematics" to achieve the WHO's health-for-all policy of the twenty-first century [92].

1.5.2 Resolution EB101.R3

In 1998, the WHO gave recognition the increasing impact of Internet in the global health development [93].

1.5.3 Resolution WHA58.28

In 2005 WHO gave recognition to the potential of e-Health in strengthening health systems through improving access, quality, and safety of health care. Hence, the WHO has defined e-Health as "the cost-effective and secure use of information and communications technology in support of health and health-related fields, including health services, health surveillance, health-related literature, education, knowledge and research". Following the deliberation, the WHO has recommended member states to incorporate e-Health into health systems and services [94].

Table 1.1 History of major inventions of ICT for health

Major inventions	Country	Year
Telemedicine first introduced [17]	Australia	1929
First attempt of medical informatics [15]	Russia	1961
Clinical decision support system initiated [81]	Canada	1961
Personalized medicine in pharmacogenomics began by Werner K. [82]	Canada	1962
Medical cyberneticists (medical informaticians) was introduced [15]	Russia	1973
Medical Informatics education started in the Free University [83]	Netherlands	1973
Electronic Health Record founded in the University of Manchester [84]	UK	1991
Professional development started in health informatics [85]	Belgium	1992
Big data first introduced by NASA researchers Cox and Ellsworth [86]	USA	1997
e-Health first initiated by John Mitchell [87]	Australia	1999
Digital medicine first coined by Shaffer, et' al in Harvard University [88]	USA	2002
mHealth was first defined by Istepanian, R.S. in Kingston University [89]	UK	2004
HIT for Economic and Clinical Health Act [20]	USA	2009
Use of tablet for healthcare record [90]	Canada	2014
Paperless (use only EHRs) for patient records [91]	UK	2018

1.5.4   Resolution WHA66.24

The World Health Assembly in 2013 acknowledged the need of data standardization in health as part of e-Health. The importance of proper governance and operation of Internet in the health sector [95].

1.5.5   Report EB139/8

In 2016 it has considered increasing importance of mHealth "as the use of mobile wireless technologies for public health" [96].

1.5.6   Report EB 142/20

In January 2018, updated the concept of mHealth use as the "use of appropriate digital technologies for public health". The report also included the use of other digital technologies for public health [97].

1.5.7   Resolution WHA71.7

The same year in 2018, the WHO has recognized potential of digital technologies in improving public health. This resolution urged the WHO Member States to give priority for the development and use of digital technologies in health sector as a tool to enhance Universal Health Coverage, the SDG [98].

According to a survey report in 2016 [99], by the WHO Global Observatory for e-Health (GOe) conducted in 125 WHO member countries have generally shown impressive progress in e-Health development and implementation.

The outstanding e-Health progresses listed below.

- More than half of WHO Member States have an e-Health strategy
- About 83% the countries reported at least one mHealth initiative
- Almost one quarter (24%) of responding countries (n = 120) reported a government-sponsored telehealth programme. Teleradiology was the most commonly (77%) used application.
- Over 84% of countries reported eLearning tools using for educating medical students
- National-based electronic health record systems were available in 47% of countries.
- About 78% of the countries reported legislation to protect privacy of personal information
- Nearly 80% of countries reported the use social media for promoting health messages in the health facilities.
- A national policy or strategy regulating "big data" reported in 17% of countries

According to ITU in 2019 [100], now a days, approximately more than 97% of the global population live within a reach of a mobile cellular network. The total number of mobile cellular subscriptions even overtaking the global population size, reaching 8.6 billion subscriptions in 2021. Despite this rapid growth, inequalities are still there. As shown the Fig. 1.3 (we presented the graph using the ITU's metadata, 2019), the status of mobile cellular subscription is far behind the average and the high income countries. This clearly indicates the need to see ways to reduce inequalities in ICT development, as its impact is more severe than simply the disparity in technology.

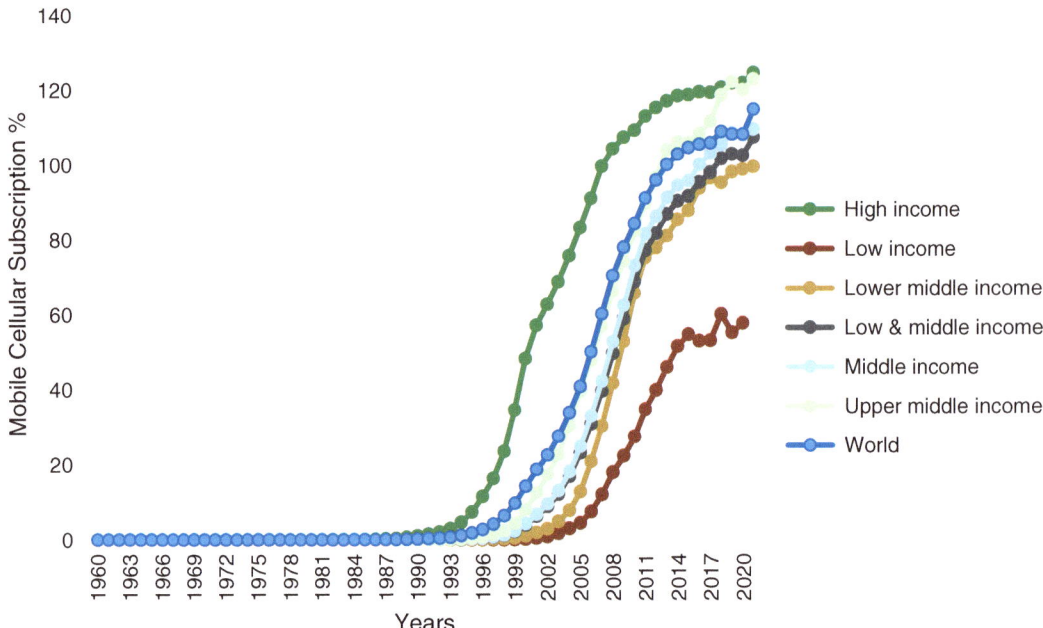

Fig. 1.3 Trends of mobile cellular subscription by national income category

1.6 Internet of Things and Health

E-everything in the twenty-first century has changed the global order of interaction. Internet of Things (IoT) is "a system of interrelated computing devices, mechanical and digital machines, objects, animals or people that are provided with unique identifiers (UIDs) and the ability to transfer data over a network without requiring human-to-human or human-to-computer interaction" [101].

A "thing" in the IoT can be a chronic patient with wearable medical devices, a person with a heart monitor implant, or it can be some other non-human entity with built-in sensors that can be assigned with Internet Protocol (IP) address that enables to transfer data over the network. The IoT is most common in transportation, living home (smart home), manufacturing, and utility organizations, that apply IoT devices and sensors toward digital transformation.

1.6.1 Internet of Medical Things

Now a days, IoT is becoming an essential component of e-Health that enables to automate the health system towards better access, efficiency and quality of health care. According to Joyia et al. [102], the Internet of Medical Thing (IoMT) is "playing a crucial role within the healthcare industry to increase the precision, consistency, and throughput of the electronic devices". The use of IoMT is evidenced to resolve quite a lot of troubles through connecting via remote monitoring, robotics, telemedicine, sensors, etc.

The IoMT system often works through the integration of different layers interconnected via network connections. Different layers involved in IoMT includes [103]:

(a) Perception layer: A sensor systems for data collection
(b) Gateway layer: Connectivity to the gateway established via networks such as:

- Personal Area Network (PAN) like, Bluetooth, ZigBee, and Ultra-Wideband
- Local Area Network (LAN), Ethernet and Wi-Fi
- Wide Area Network (WAN) such as global system for mobile communication (GSM) that do not require connectivity, and Wireless Sensor Networks (WSNs)
- High-frequency fourth-generation (4G) and evolving fifth generation (5G) cellular networks

The IoMT consists of different types of gateways that aimed to interconnect different devices to work together for the intended purposes like:

- Application Radio-Frequency Identification (RFID)
- Bluetooth
- Zigbee
- Near-Field Communication (NFC)
- Wireless Fidelity (Wi Fi)
- Satellite

(c) Application support layer data storage: It provides user management, data management and data analysis.

(d) Application/service layer: The AI component that interpretation of the data and delivery of application-specific service.

For example: during COVID-19, different types of technologies were integrated with IoMT to build a smart healthcare system [104].

(a) Virtual reality (VR), mixed reality (MR) and augmented reality (AR): Virtual, mixed and augmented reality technologies help to run activities in the related to healthcare including:
- Therapeutic procedures
- Healthcare facilities/industries
- Health education and training services

(b) Parallel computing-fog, edge and cloud computing: supports an easy keeping health records, classifying information, data mining and extraction, and modeling a prediction and decision systems.

(c) Big data visualization and analytics (BDVA): in support with cloud computing, it helps to predict risks and outcomes related to health.

(d) Block-chain: it is "a growing list of records (blocks) where records are connected to each other using a cryptographic method called hashing" [105]. The "CoviChain", a blockchain technology was used to transfer COVID-19 patient's data from one place to the other [106].

(e) Artificial intelligence (AI): Enhance accuracy of diagnosis, monitoring and mass screening.

(f) 5G networking: provides online reproducible information on real-time and as demanded.

There are different applications integrated with IoMT in the health system including [104]:

- Testing and tracing for disease spread
- Screening and monitoring health status at real-time using in-built sensors and monitoring devices such as:
  - Oxygen saturation monitoring devises
  - Blood glucose monitoring devises
  - Smart inhalers devises
  - Wearable smart devices including smart watches, implants, sleep trackers, loneliness detectors, etc.
  - Smart tooth brushes
  - Similarly, a non-invasive Oximeter [107], used to measure oxygen saturation in the blood, and pulse rate) that includes a wireless data transfer using Wi-Fi or Zigbee.
- Smart hospitals with the clinical and administrative processes are automated
- I-robotics: IoMT-aided robotic system that enables to interact patients with robots
- E-learning: Use of electronic devices and apps such as Zoom, Microsoft Teams and Google Classroom, etc. to support teaching and learning online.

1.7 Why Health Informatics?

The globe has been swept away by a quick wave of information technology revolution. The ICT has changed the global order of communication and the ways we look and approach thing. As a result, public services, organizations, and people becoming more modern. Some of the major driving factors for the realization of health informatics are listed below.

1.7.1 Driven by the Global Digital Revolution

The global digital revolution, among other driving factors, has played a significant role in the emergence of health informatics. The global explosion and day-to-day advancement of information technology have opened an enormous opportunity for health informatics to come as a field of study [12, 17]. Following the rapid expansion, urgent needs arise from ICT tools that can aggregate information from multiple sources, to give an overall understanding of the healthy human or to provide a clearer picture at the systems level.

These days, the use of Information technologies are no longer a luxury; they are a necessity [27]. Globally, nothing would substitute the potential impact of information technology that could play in advancing the health care delivery, public health, and health related research activities. The pervasive nature of ICT enables medical businesses to solve even more complex tasks related to the profile of a specific institution.

Now a days, it is unthinkable to advance the health system without the use of ICT. The invention of one component of a digital health solution would open the door for additional similar inventions in the domain.

1.7.2 High Healthcare Costs as a Driving Force

Health is a basic human right that needs an efficient and cost-effective pathways. But, health care is practically an expensive commodity. One of the most successful strategies for addressing stakeholder pressures, enhancing the caliber of healthcare services, and lowering costs was digital health transformation [108–110]. The need to provide healthcare to everyone, address the lack and unequal distribution of medical professionals, and take action about the rising expenses for health care is again another pushing factor for the health system to implement information technology.

The advances in information systems improve access to health care, enrich service delivery, and improve quality of service, and increase efficiency and coordination of care. Currently, use of ICT in the health system is a pathway towards achieving universal health coverage and the sustainable development goals, as the use of ICT in health care would improve the health care through various way.

Evidence from modern research, however, suggests that higher health care costs are now a result of better medical technology. For example, facilities for radiation oncology, computed tomography, cardiac and neonatal critical care units, angioplasty, positron emission tomography, and magnetic resonance imaging have been found to be more expensive despite their increased demand [111].

1.7.3 Driven by Unmet Health Needs

The high population growth is not being tempered by access to health services, especially in environments with limited resources. The WHO [52] has acknowledged that UHC cannot be realized without support from e-Health, as was covered in the book's previous section.

Digital technologies have also altered the way we manage our own health, driven by the widespread use of mobile phones worldwide. More health information, including false information, is available to us than at any other time in history. Most of us have Googled our symptoms before ever setting foot in a doctor's office and made our own, possibly incorrect, diagnoses. Similar to this, digital technologies are being employed to strengthen the education and performance of healthcare professionals as well as to address a variety of enduring flaws in health systems.

1.7.4 Global Health Crisis as a Driving Force to Digital Health Revolution

The ICTs played significant roles during global health crisis. Particularly Social Medias were crucial for addressing the public's wide range of information needs, demands for online consultation, and online enquiries.

For instance: The expansion of COVID-19 pandemic played as a significant catalyst for digital health revolution. According to a Deloitte report [112], following the development of the COVID19 pandemic, the healthcare institutions boosted their implementation of digital technologies to support working techniques and assist patients.

The use of ICT during the COVID-19 pandemic, as it had opportunities; there were also limitations, such as insufficient information, unreliable information, inaccessible information, and spread of misinformation.

1.8 Theoretical Frameworks in Health Informatics

Over the last decade, there has been an increased awareness of the necessity of developing implementation-facilitating tactics and theoretical underpinnings for implementation. The application of theories, models, and frameworks to understand the mechanisms underlying successful implementation is gaining popularity. These days, implementation studies incorporate theories, models, and frameworks produced within implementation science as well as theories derived from fields including sociology, psychology, and organizational theory [113].

According to Wacker [114], a theory refers to the collection of analytical principles or assertions intended to organize our perception, comprehension, and justification of the universe. Theory is an explanation for how certain phenomena occur. It starts with observing the specific phenomenon. People frequently resist change as an example of a phenomenon. But what causes this phenomenon and how does it happen? A theory based on this phenomenon would explain why people resist change and forecast when and how they will do so. A sound theory provides a clear explanation of how and why particular interactions result in particular outcomes. Theories can be described on a continuum of abstraction. Lower level abstraction theories are empirical generalizations with a restricted scope and applicability, whereas medium level

abstraction theories explain a restricted collection of phenomena. High abstraction level theories, also known as broad or grand theories, have an almost infinite scope.

Theoretical models often entail the purposeful simplification of a reality or a particular feature of a phenomenon [115]. For a model to be useful, it need not be a perfect replica of reality. Because theories and models are closely related, it is not always easy to distinguish between the two. Models are theories with a more limited scope of explanation; a theory is both explanatory and descriptive, whereas a model is descriptive only.

Frameworks are developed by academic fields to describe, guide, characterize, analyze, and evaluate events and processes [116]. The framework has the potential to enhance design technique by providing experts in the area with a helpful tool to remember the user throughout the entire design process, particularly in circumstances where the context is complex and unfamiliar to them [117]. The framework has the potential to enhance design technique by providing experts in the area with a helpful tool to remember the user throughout the entire design process, particularly in circumstances where the context is complex and unfamiliar to them [118].

Generally, numerous theories, models, and frameworks share similarities with one another. Even if, theories attempt to explain the causal mechanisms (i.e., how and why). Models are employed to explain or direct the process of putting research into application. While, frameworks identify factors found to influence implementation outcomes.

The application of theory, models and frameworks in health informatics can aid in the comprehension of phenomena, direct our analyses, and enhance our understanding of the significance, translating research findings into practice and identifying implementation barriers. It is now well acknowledged that the adoption of health information systems can significantly affect how healthcare is delivered and how well it works [119]. As a result, the necessity of making sure that health IT is thoroughly evaluated is given a lot of attention. Throughout the past few decades, many of the advancements in assessment research have paralleled the use of theory in health informatics. This is due to the fact that theory can offer a context for understanding the importance of evaluation results. To a higher understanding of the underlying causative mechanisms, health informatics is able to move beyond a simple "black box" evaluation that may indicate whether or not a health IT system is effective [113].

1.8.1 Prominent Theoretical Models in Health Informatics

In health informatics, several theoretical models were established. Each theoretical model was created to address particular disciplinary challenges. This section includes a few notable theoretical models that were chosen based on how frequently they were applied in studies. The theoretical models often intended to: Understand the process of health information management and use, Evaluate the design of health information systems, Evaluate new and emerging technologies, Understand IT use in health care, Evaluate success of a system and Provide empirical evidence for health IT decisions.

1.8.1.1 Understand the Process of Learning

The process of learning follows some models and theories including the Blum's Model information processing, or cognitive learning, theories and adult learning theory.

The Blum's Model

Bruce L. Blum categorized and defined programs based on the types of things they processed: data, information, or knowledge. Data is defined as a raw fact. Information as a collection of data that has been processed and displayed and knowledge results when data and information are identified and the relationships between the data and information are formalized [120].

Information Processing, or Cognitive Learning, Theories

Learning is divided into the four steps below by information processing theories or cognitive learning theories:

(a) How input is received by the system
(b) How information is processed
(c) What kind of learned behaviors are displayed as output
(d) The method for changing or improving behavior through system feedback

Information input as a result of senses of sight, hearing, smell, taste, touch, and position are used to enter data into the system. Many things could have an impact on the input procedure. As information enters the system, the learner organizes and interprets it to create useful information. The organization and interpretation of the facts are significantly influenced by prior learning [121].

Adult Learning Theory

According to adult learning theory, learning outcomes are influenced by one's learning setting. Thus, the context and culture in which formal learning activities, like training programs, are given, as well as the activities themselves, contribute to the evolution of knowledge [122].

1.8.1.2 Evaluate the Design of Health Information Systems

The life cycle models provide a framework for managing the development and evaluation of intricate health information systems. Conventional system development life cycles (SDLCs) presume that systems are developed in a series of predetermined stages, with the last stages being mostly devoted to system evaluation. These strategies have proven challenging to successfully apply in healthcare settings where identifying information needs can be challenging. Whereas, Evaluation in Life Cycle of Information Technology (ELICIT) framework focuses on all phases of the information technology development and deployment life cycle [123].

The most common models include Waterfall, Spiral, and Star models, relating to the order and arrangement of the various sub-stages [124]. Although in practice the more sequential Waterfall method is usually utilized, the Spiral and Star models are widely recommended because of their capacity to handle complexity and iteration [125].

All of these show how development and evaluation are interdependent, with the Spiral and Star models emphasizing iterative design. Software design and development techniques now almost always include user-developer interaction for requirements derivation, testing, and acceptance despite their gradual evolution; in fact, this is a key component of the Star Model.

1.8.1.3 Evaluate New and Emerging Technologies

Evaluating a new and emerging technology in health requires some framework that guides the process of evaluation at real world and complex contexts. Some of the frameworks are:

The Cheat's Framework

It is the comprehensive approach that involves medical, individual and organisational, educational, technical and social contacts between people to evaluate new and emerging technology in health informatics [126].

Consolidated Framework for Implementation Research (CFIR)

A meta-theoretical framework that offers an all-encompassing typology of implementation-related components, such as individual traits, outer and inner settings, and intervention features. The CFIR has updated and utilized in several implementation researches [127].

1.8.1.4 Understand IT Use in Health Care

Currently, various theories are employed to assess IT use in the healthcare. Some of the theories are listed below.

Behavioral Intention Theory

It is adopted to the health informatics field of research that focused on the behavioral intentions of individuals to predict the use of IT related technology in Health. The goal of this work is to uncover the factors that influence intentions, such as attitudes, social influences, and enabling circumstances [128].

Diffusion of Innovations (DOI) Theory

According to Rogers, people within a social system accept innovations sequentially rather than all at once. Innovators, early adopters, early majority, late majority, and laggards were the five adopter types he suggested. These classifications are based on the proportion of people (or groups) falling within each zone of the normal distribution, which is delineated by standard deviations from the mean. The communication process or the gathering and processing of information make up the majority of the dissemination process. Innovations contain unique traits including relative advantage, compatibility, complexity, trial ability, and observation ability that contribute to explain the variations in adoption rates [129].

Social-Cognitive Theory (SCT)

It helps describe patterns of IT usage. Reciprocal determinism and self-efficacy, which are ideas about one's capacity to carry out a particular behavior, are stressed in SCT [130].

The Task-Technology Fit Model (TTF)

It is also among the theories that describe patterns of IT usage. According to TTF, IT is more likely to be used if the features are useful for the user's tasks, and users will select the tools and approaches that give them the best overall results [131].

The Human, Organization and Technology-Fit (HOT-Fit) Framework

IT incorporates comprehensive dimensions and measures of HIS and provides a technological, human and organizational fit [118].

Institutional Theory

Posits that an organization's environment is capable of strongly influencing the development, acceptance, and use of e-Health interventions [132].

1.8.1.5 Evaluate Success of a System

Information systems success: The framework includes six dimensions or success factors: system quality, usage, information quality, individual impact, user satisfaction and organizational impact [133].

1.8.1.6 Provide Empirical Evidence for Health IT Decisions

Research works designed to generate empirical evidence for health IT decisions follow some framework like:

Comprehensive Health Technology Evaluation Framework

A framework to selecting health technologies, including information technologies. Its objective is to offer a platform for health technology decisions based on empirical research and evidence. The five main aspects in the conceptual framework includes people at risk, effect of population, economy, social situation (such as legal, political and ethical concerns), and technological evaluation. This multidisciplinary approach offers recommendations on how to use the right information to balance "stakeholder wishes" with "population needs" [134].

Identity Theory (IT)

Posits that the identity associated with a particular role is likely to drive individual decision making about e-Health interventions [135].

1.8.2 Frameworks Adopted in Resource-Limited Settings

Agnes et al. [136] reviewed that there were various digital health evaluation frameworks that have been widely adopted in resource-limited settings. Some of the frameworks listed below:

- Technology Acceptance Model
- Unified Theory of Acceptance and Use of Technology
- Organisation and Environment framework the Human Organisation Technology Fit
- Extended Technology Acceptance Model
- Diffusion Innovation Theory
- Logic model,
- Theory of Planned Behaviour
- Theory of Reasoned Act
- Fit between Individuals Task and Technology and Patient m-Health Adoption

- Technology Acceptance Model
- Unified Theory of Acceptance and Use of Technology, Organisation and Environment

They also proposed future researches in developing countries to include eight key dimensions such as, socio-demographic, sociocultural, technology, information, organization, governance, ethical and legal, and financial dimensions [136].

1.9 Health Informatics Domains and Sub-domains

The health informatics sub-domains include: clinical informatics, nursing informatics, imaging informatics, consumer health informatics, dental health informatics, clinical health research informatics, bioinformatics, pharmacy informatics and public health informatics [137].

1.9.1 Clinical Informatics

Clinical informatics a multidisciplinary field that consists of information science, computer science, and healthcare to manage and process medical data. The clinical informatics tools can be used to:

- Evaluate health care professionals and patient's need information and knowledge related to healthcare
- Develop, implement, and improve clinical decision support systems
- Develop health information systems for safe, efficient, effective, timely, patient-centered, and equitable medical care.

1.9.2 Nursing Informatics

It's a multidisciplinary field attempts to analyze, and modeling the process of data collect, manage, process into information and knowledge aimed for data-informed nursing practices and to facilitate research works.

1.9.3 Imaging Informatics

Imaging informatics combines knowledge and capabilities from medicine, medical imaging, biomedical informatics and Information Technology to digitize medical imaging. The commonly used areas of Imaging Informatics include Radiology Information Systems (RIS), Computer-Aided Detection and Diagnosis (CAD) and Picture Archiving and Communications Systems (PACS).

1.9.4 Consumer Health Informatics

Consumer health informatics is a subfield of medical informatics that investigates and implements strategies to make information accessible to consumers, models and incorporates consumers' preferences into medical information systems, and analyzes consumers' information demands.

1.9.5 Dental Informatics

Dental informatics refers to the knowledge, abilities, and resources that make it possible to share and use information in order to advance oral health and enhance dental management, practice, and research. It includes administrative data for all dental specialties, CAD/CAM technology, diagnostic digital imaging, and electronic health records.

1.9.6 Clinical Research Informatics

Clinical research informatics focuses on using informatics theory and techniques to plan, carry out, and enhance clinical research, as well as to communicate the discovered information. It shares a lot of similarities with the closely related but recently quickly emerging field of translational research informatics. According to the National Institutes of Health (NIH), clinical research includes investigations and tests on human beings that fit into one of three subcategories:

(a) Patient- oriented research that involves human subjects (or human-derived materials like tissues, specimens, and cognitive phenomena)
(b) Epidemiologic and behavioral studies
(c) Outcomes research; and health services

1.9.7 Translational Research Informatics

According to the NIH, there are two types of translation in translational research informatics. One is the process of incorporating new knowledge gained from laboratory and preclinical study development into the design of trials and human study. The second area of translation relates to studies intended to promote the adoption of excellent practices in the neighborhood. Translational science also emphasizes how cost-effective preventative and treatment methods are.

1.9.8 Bioinformatics

Bioinformatics and Computational Biology uses techniques such as applied mathematics, informatics, statistics, computer science, artificial intelligence, chemistry, and biochemistry to solve biological problems on the molecular level.

1.9.9 Pharmacy Informatics

Similarly, pharmacy Informatics is a field of study that enhances interfaces between people, healthcare processes and information systems to improve pharmaceutical care and patient safety.

1.9.10 Public Health Informatics

The systematic use of information, computer science, and technology in public health practice, research, and education is known as public health informatics. By focusing on population data rather than individual data, it differs from healthcare informatics. The gathering, storing, and analyzing of data pertaining to public health might be considered the main activities of public health informatics.

A recent study providing an agenda for the development of the field of public health informatics [138] argues for the necessity of building, putting into place, and integrating national and local public health surveillance systems to enable quick identification and reaction to disease hotspots.

Reminder systems using mHealth and other digital tools have been crucial in public health programs. One of the classical example was providing information for smokers on quitting smoking [139, 140]. Many more public health programs likely to benefit from the use of digital health such as improving timeliness and completeness of childhood immunization [141], supporting community-based Tuberculosis (TB) care and treatment in resource limited settings [142].

Using informatics tools to advance public health education, research, and practice through an interdisciplinary approach that incorporates the information sciences, public health sciences, such as epidemiology, and other fields such as gathering and storing vital statistics, disease surveillance, display disease statistics and trends, immunization, hospital statistics, etc. [143].

As the focus of this book is mainly on the evolution, principles, implementation and governance of public health informatics in resource-limited settings, the next chapters will address issues specific to the domain of public health informatics.

References

1. Dutton WH. The Internet and society. In: Internet, economic growth and globalization: perspectives on the new economy in Europe, Japan and the USA. Springer; 2003. p. 311–22.
2. Poslad S. Ubiquitous computing: smart devices, environments and interactions. John Wiley & Sons; 2011.
3. Yoo CS. Moore's Law, Metcalfe's Law, and the Theory of Optimal Interoperability. Faculty Scholarship at Penn Carey Law. 1651. 2015. https://scholarship.law.upenn.edu/faculty_scholarship/1651.
4. Metcalfe B. Metcalfe's law after 40 years of ethernet. Computer. 2013;46(12):26–31.
5. Keller D. The future of ideas: the fate of the commons in a connected world. Duke Law J. 2002;10:273.
6. Rogers EM, Malhotra S. Computers as communication: the rise of digital democracy. In: Digital democracy: Issues of theory and practice. Sage; 2000. p. 10–29.
7. Lipsey R, Carlaw KI, Bekar CT. Economic transformations: general purpose technologies and long-term economic growth. Oxford University Press; 2005.
8. Pavlik JV. New media technology: cultural and commercial perspectives. Allyn and Bacon; 1996.
9. Mitullah WV, Samson R, Wambua PM, Balongo S. Building on progress: infrastructure development still a major challenge in Africa. Afrobarometer; 2016.
10. Measuring digital development—ICT Development Index 2023. Dec 2023. https://www.itu.int/pub/D-IND-ICT_MDD-2023-2. Accessed 12 Apr 2024.
11. Van Dijk JA. Digital divide research, achievements and shortcomings. Poetics. 2006;34(4–5):221–35.
12. Castells M. The rise of the network society: the information age: economy, society, and culture. Wiley; 2010.
13. Heeks R. Information and communication technology for development (ICT4D). Taylor & Francis; 2017.
14. Elenko E, Underwood L, Zohar D. Defining digital medicine. Nat Biotechnol. 2015;33(5):456–61.
15. Hasman A, Mantas J, Zarubina T. An abridged history of medical informatics education in europe. Acta Inform Med. 2014;22(1):25–36.
16. Rooij T, Marsh S. eHealth: past and future perspectives. Pers Med. 2016;13(1):57–70.
17. Margolis SA, Ypinazar VA. Tele-pharmacy in remote medical practice: the Royal Flying Doctor Service Medical Chest Program. Rural Remote Health. 2008;8(2):937.
18. Salomon I, Cohen G, Nijkamp P. ICT and urban public policy: does knowledge meet policy, Research Memorandum No. 47. VU University Amsterdam; 1999.
19. Dutton W. Society on the Line. London: Information Politics in the Digital Age; 1999.
20. Jones E, Wittie M. Accelerated adoption of advanced health information technology in Beacon Community Health Centers. J Am Board Fam Med. 2015;28(5):565–75.
21. Bustreo, Flavia & Tanner, Marcel. (2020). How do we reimagine health in a digital age?. Bulletin of the World Health Organization, 98 (4), 232. World Health Organization. http://doi.org/10.2471/BLT.19.235358.
22. Wan TT. Healthcare informatics research: from data to evidence-based management. J Med Syst. 2006;30:3–7.

23. Saba VK, McCormick KA. Essentials of nursing informatics. McGraw Hill Education; 2015.

24. National Library of Medicine website. 2020. https://hsric.nlm.nih.gov/hsric_public/topic/informatics. Accessed 20 May 2020.

25. WHO. Global strategy on digital health 2020–2025. Geneva: WHO; 2021. https://www.who.int/docs/default-source/documents/gs4dhdaa2a9f352b-0445bafbc79ca799dce4d.pdf. Accessed 7 June 2021

26. World Health Organization. Strengthening health systems to improve health outcomes: WHO's framework for action. Geneva: WHO; 2007.

27. World Health Organization. WHO guideline: recommendations on digital interventions for health system strengthening: evidence and recommendations. Report No.: Contract No.: WHO/RHR/19.10. Geneva: World Health Organization; 2019.

28. Anshari M, Almunawar M, editors. Health Information Systems (HIS): concept and technology. International Conference Informatics Development: Yogyakarta; 2011.

29. Williamson L, Kaasbøll J, editors. Health information and managerial work: exploring the link. In: Proceedings of the international conference on social implications of computers in developing countries, Dubai; 2009.

30. Kwankam SY. What e-Health can offer. Bull World Health Organ. 2004;82(10):800–2.

31. Reidpath DD, Allotey P. Opening up public health: a strategy of information and communication technology to support population health. Lancet. 2009;373(9668):1050–1.

32. Gibbons MC, Wilson RF, Samal L, Lehmann CU, Dickersin K, Lehmann HP, et al. Consumer health informatics: results of a systematic evidence review and evidence based recommendations. Transl Behav Med. 2011;1(1):72–82.

33. Appelboom G, LoPresti M, Reginster JY, Sander Connolly E, Dumont EP. The quantified patient: a patient participatory culture. Curr Med Res Opin. 2014;30(12):2585–7.

34. Demiris G. Consumer health informatics: past, present, and future of a rapidly evolving domain. Yearb Med Inform. 2016;Suppl 1(Suppl 1):S42–7.

35. Kaelber DC, Jha AK, Johnston D, Middleton B, Bates DW. A research agenda for personal health records (PHRs). J Am Med Inform Assoc. 2008;15(6):729–36.

36. Halamka JD, Mandl KD, Tang PC. Early experiences with personal health records. J Am Med Inform Assoc. 2008;15(1):1–7.

37. Collins FS, Varmus H. A new initiative on precision medicine. N Engl J Med. 2015;372(9):793–5.

38. Najeeb A-S. Improving healthcare access through digital health: the use of information and communication technologies. In: Amit A, Srinivas K, editors. Healthcare access. Rijeka: IntechOpen; 2021.

39. Winter A, Funkat G, Haeber A, Mauz-Koerholz C, Pommerening K, Smers S, et al. Integrated information systems for translational medicine. Methods Inf Med. 2007;46(05):601–7.

40. Byungura JC, Nyiringango G, Fors U, Forsberg E, Tumusiime DK. Online learning for continuous professional development of healthcare workers: an exploratory study on perceptions of healthcare managers in Rwanda. BMC Med Educ. 2022;22(1):851.

41. Ramsden R, Colbran R, Christopher E, Edwards M. The role of digital technology in providing education, training, continuing professional development and support to the rural health workforce. Health Educ. 2022;122(2):126–49.

42. World Health Organization. Digital education for building health workforce capacity. World Health Organization; 2020.

43. Shao M, Fan J. The Impact of Information and Communication Technologies (ICTs) on health outcomes: a mediating effect analysis based on cross-national panel data. J Environ Public Health. 2022;2022:2225723.

44. Eysenbach G. What is e-health? J Med Internet Res. 2001;3(2):e833.

45. While A, Dewsbury G. Nursing and information and communication technology (ICT): a discussion of trends and future directions. Int J Nurs Stud. 2011;48(10):1302–10.

46. Dzenowagis J, Kernen G. Connecting for health: global vision, local insight: report for the World Summit on the Information Society. World Health Organization; 2005.

47. Ajuwon GA. Computer and internet use by first year clinical and nursing students in a Nigerian teaching hospital. BMC Med Inform Decis Mak. 2003;3:1–11.

48. Heron KE, Smyth JM. Ecological momentary interventions: incorporating mobile technology into psychosocial and health behaviour treatments. Br J Health Psychol. 2010;15(1):1–39.

49. Aderonke Ogungbade CLN, oluwatobi Abdul M. Information and Communication Technology Applications and use in Medical Records and Information Management in Selected Hospitals in Ijebu Ode Local Government Area, Ogun State. Library Philosophy & Practice; 2022.

50. Millman M. Access to health care in America. National Academies Press; 1993.

51. National Academies of Sciences, Engineering, and Medicine; Health and Medicine Division; Board on Health Care Services; Committee on Health Care Utilization and Adults with Disabilities. Health-care utilization as a proxy in disability determination. National Academies Press; 2018.

52. World Health Organization. Global tuberculosis report 2013. World Health Organization; 2013.

53. World Health Organization. Telemedicine: opportunities and developments in member states. Report on the second global survey on eHealth. World Health Organization; 2010.

54. Dixon BE, Hook JM, McGowan JJ. Using tele-health to improve quality and safety: Findings from the ahrq health it portfolio. Agency for Healthcare Research and Quality; 2008.

55. World Health Assembly. Quality of care: patient safety. Geneva: World Health Organization; 2002.

56. Baker A. Crossing the quality chasm: a new health system for the 21st century. Br Med J. 2001;323(7322):1192.

57. World Health Organization, OECD, and International Bank for Reconstruction and Development/The World Bank. Delivering quality health services: a global imperative for universal health coverage. Geneva: World Health Organization; 2018.

58. World Health Organization. Health Technology and Pharmaceuticals: 2000–2003 strategy. Geneva: World Health Organization; 2001.

59. Cousins DD, Heath WM. The National Coordinating Council for Medication Error Reporting and Prevention: promoting patient safety and quality through innovation and leadership. Jt Comm J Qual Patient Saf. 2008;34(12):700–2.

60. Bates DW, Leape LL, Cullen DJ, Laird N, Petersen LA, Teich JM, et al. Effect of computerized physician order entry and a team intervention on prevention of serious medication errors. JAMA. 1998;280(15):1311–6.

61. Evans RS, Pestotnik SL, Classen DC, Clemmer TP, Weaver LK, Orme JF Jr, et al. A computer-assisted management program for antibiotics and other antiinfective agents. N Engl J Med. 1998;338(4):232–8.

62. Potts AL, Barr FE, Gregory DF, Wright L, Patel NR. Computerized physician order entry and medication errors in a pediatric critical care unit. Pediatrics. 2004;113(1):59–63.

63. Barclay E. Text messages could hasten tuberculosis drug compliance. Lancet. 2009;373(9657):15–6.

64. UNAIDS. Universal declaration of human rights. UNAIDS; 1948.

65. Rasanathan K, Sivasankara Kurup A, Jaramillo E, Lonnroth K. The social determinants of health: key to global tuberculosis control. Int J Tuberc Lung Dis. 2011;15(Suppl 2):S30–6.

66. Hart JT. The inverse care law. Lancet. 1971;1(7696):405–12.

67. World Health Assembly. Human resources for health: global strategy on human resources for health: workforce 2030: report by the Director-General. Geneva: World Health Organization; 2019.

68. Nelson A. Unequal treatment: confronting racial and ethnic disparities in health care. J Natl Med Assoc. 2002;94(8):666.

69. Lee J. The impact of health information technology on disparity of process of care. Int J Equity Health. 2015;14(1):34.

70. Blumenthal D. Stimulating the adoption of health information technology. W V Med J. 2009;105(3):28–30.

71. DesRoches CM, Campbell EG, Vogeli C, Zheng J, Rao SR, Shields AE, Donelan K, Rosenbaum S, Bristol SJ, Jha AK. Electronic health records' limited successes suggest more targeted uses. Health Affairs. 2010;29(4):639–46.

72. Jha AK, DesRoches CM, Campbell EG, Donelan K, Rao SR, Ferris TG, et al. Use of electronic health records in U.S. hospitals. N Engl J Med. 2009;360(16):1628–38.

73. Wu D, Verhulst SG, Pentland A, Avila T, Finch K, Gupta A. How data governance technologies can democratize data sharing for community well-being. Data Policy. 2021;3:e14.

74. Gilbert SS, Bulula N, Yohana E, Thompson J, Beylerian E, Werner L, et al. The impact of an integrated electronic immunization registry and logistics management information system (EIR-eLMIS) on vaccine availability in three regions in Tanzania: a pre-post and time-series analysis. Vaccine. 2020;38(3):562–9.

75. Choi PJ, Oskouian RJ, Tubbs RS. Telesurgery: past, present, and future. Cureus. 2018;10(5):e2716.

76. Mohan A, Wara UU, Shaikh MTA, Rahman RM, Zaidi ZA. Telesurgery and robotics: an improved and efficient era. Cureus. 2021;13(3):e14124.

77. Hassibian MR, Hassibian S. Telemedicine acceptance and implementation in developing countries: benefits, categories, and barriers. Razavi Int J Med. 2016;4(3):e38332.

78. Meessen B. The role of digital strategies in financing health care for universal health coverage in low- and middle-income countries. Glob Health Sci Pract. 2018;6(Suppl 1):S29–s40.

79. López L, Green AR, Tan-McGrory A, King R, Betancourt JR. Bridging the digital divide in health care: the role of health information technology in addressing racial and ethnic disparities. Joint Commission journal on quality and patient safety. 2011;37(10):437–45. https://doi.org/10.1016/s1553-7250(11)37055-9.

80. Chaudhry B, Wang J, Wu S, Maglione M, Mojica W, Roth E, Morton SC, Shekelle PG. Systematic review: impact of health information technology on quality, efficiency, and costs of medical care. Ann Intern Med. 2006;144(10):742–52.

81. Warner HR, Toronto AF, Veasey LG, Stephenson R. A mathematical approach to medical diagnosis: application to congenital heart disease.1961. MD Comput Comput Med Pract. 1992;9(1):43–50.

82. Kalow W, Grant DM. Pharmacogenetics. Heredity and the response to drugs. London: Saunders Company. 1962;12.

83. van Bemmel JH. A comprehensive model for medical information processing. Methods Inf Med. 1983;22(3):124–30.

84. Rector AL, Nowlan WA, Kay S. Foundations for an electronic medical record. Methods Inf Med. 1991;30(3):179–86.

85. Ceusters W, De Moor G, Bonneu R, Schilders L. Training of health care personnel towards the

implementation and use of electronic health care records using integrated imaging technology. Med Inform. 1992;17(4):215–23.

86. Tiwari S, Wee HM, Daryanto Y. Big data analytics in supply chain management between 2010 and 2016: insights to industries. Comput Ind Eng. 2018;115:319–30.

87. Mitchell J. Increasing the cost-effectiveness of telemedicine by embracing e-health. J Telemed Telecare. 2000;6(1_suppl):16–9.

88. Shaffer DW, Kigin CM, Kaput JJ, Gazelle GS. What is digital medicine? Stud Health Technol Inform. 2002;80:195–204.

89. Istepanian RS, Jovanov E, Zhang Y. Guest editorial introduction to the special section on m-health: beyond seamless mobility and global wireless health-care connectivity. IEEE Trans Inf Technol Biomed. 2004;8(4):405–14.

90. Rooij TV, Marsh S. eHealth: past and future perspectives. Per Med. 2016;13(1):57–70.

91. McCluggage B. A paperless NHS by 2018 is possible. Health Serv J. 2013;123(6338):18–9.

92. Executive B. Health-for-all policy for the twenty-first century: "health telematics". Geneva: World Health Organization; 1998.

93. World Health Assembly. Cross-border advertising, promotion and sale of medical products using the internet. Geneva: World Health Organization; 1998.

94. World Health Assembly. eHealth. Geneva: World Health Organization; 2005.

95. World Health Assembly. eHealth standardization and interoperability. Geneva: World Health Organization; 2013.

96. WHO Global Observatory for eHealth. Building foundations for eHealth: progress of member states: report of the Global Observatory for eHealth. Geneva: World Health Organization; 2006.

97. Executive B. mHealth: use of appropriate digital technologies for public health: report by the Director-General. Geneva: World Health Organization; 2017.

98. World Health Organization. Digital health. Geneva: World Health Organization; 2018.

99. World Health Organization. Global diffusion of eHealth: making universal health coverage achievable: report of the third global survey on eHealth. Geneva: World Health Organization; 2016.

100. ITU. Measuring digital development: facts and figures 2019. ITU; 2019.

101. Sun Y, Lo FP-W, Lo B. Security and privacy for the internet of medical things enabled healthcare systems: a survey. IEEE Access. 2019;7:183339–55.

102. Joyia GJ, Liaqat RM, Farooq A, Rehman S. Internet of medical things (IoMT): applications, benefits and future challenges in healthcare domain. J Commun. 2017;12(4):240–7.

103. Lin YH. Novel smart home system architecture facilitated with distributed and embedded flexible edge analytics in demand-side management. Int Trans Electr Energy Syst. 2019;29(6):e12014.

104. Dwivedi R, Mehrotra D, Chandra S. Potential of Internet of Medical Things (IoMT) applications in building a smart healthcare system: a systematic review. J Oral Biol Craniofac Res. 2022;12(2):302–18.

105. Nørfeldt L, Bøtker J, Edinger M, Genina N, Rantanen J. Cryptopharmaceuticals: increasing the safety of medication by a blockchain of pharmaceutical products. J Pharm Sci. 2019;108(9):2838–41.

106. Vangipuram SLT, Mohanty SP. CoviChain: a blockchain based framework for nonrepudiable contact tracing in healthcare cyber-physical systems during pandemic outbreaks. SN Comput Sci. 2021;2(5):346.

107. Fu Y, Liu J. System design for wearable blood oxygen saturation and pulse measurement device. Proc Manufact. 2015;3:1187–94.

108. Locatelli P, Restifo N, Gastaldi L, Sini E, Torresani M. The evolution of hospital information systems and the role of electronic patient records: from the Italian scenario to a real case. Stud Health Technol Inform. 2010;160(Pt 1):247–51.

109. Locatelli P, Restifo N, Gastaldi L, Corso M. Health care information systems: architectural models and governance. In: Innovative information systems modelling and techniques. InTech; 2012. p. 71–96.

110. Secundo G, Toma A, Schiuma G, Passiante G. Knowledge transfer in open innovation: a classification framework for healthcare ecosystems. Bus Process Manag J. 2019;25(1):144–63.

111. Bodenheimer T. High and rising health care costs. Part 2: technologic innovation. Ann Intern Med. 2005;142(11):932–7.

112. Taylor K, Properzi F, Bhatti S, Ferris K. Digital transformation—shaping the future of European healthcare. Deloitte Centre for Health Solutions; 2020.

113. Chen HT. Theory-driven evaluations. Sage; 1990.

114. Wacker JG. A definition of theory: research guidelines for different theory-building research methods in operations management. J Oper Manag. 1998;16(4):361–85.

115. Carpiano RM, Daley DM. A guide and glossary on post-positivist theory building for population health. J Epidemiol Community Health. 2006;60(7):564–70.

116. Nilsen P. Making sense of implementation theories, models, and frameworks. In: Albers B, Shlonsky A, Mildon R, editors. Implementation science 30. Cham: Springer International Publishing; 2020. p. 53–79.

117. Esser PE, Goossens RH. A framework for the design of user-centred teleconsulting systems. J Telemed Telecare. 2009;15(1):32–9.

118. Yusof MM, Kuljis J, Papazafeiropoulou A, Stergioulas LK. An evaluation framework for health information systems: human, organization and technology-fit factors (HOT-fit). Int J Med Inform. 2008;77(6):386–98.

119. Ammenwerth E, Brender J, Nykänen P, Prokosch H-U, Rigby M, Talmon J. Visions and strategies to improve evaluation of health information systems: reflections and lessons based on the HIS-EVAL workshop in Innsbruck. Int J Med Inform. 2004;73(6):479–91.

120. Blum BI. Clinical information systems—a review. West J Med. 1986;145(6):791–7.

121. Ariel S. An information processing theory of family dysfunction. Psychotherapy. 1987;24(3S):477.

122. McAlearney AS, Robbins J, Kowalczyk N, Chisolm DJ, Song PH. The role of cognitive and learning theories in supporting successful EHR system implementation training: a qualitative study. Med Care Res Rev. 2012;69(3):294–315.

123. Kukhareva PV, Weir C, Del Fiol G, Aarons GA, Taft TY, Schlechter CR, et al. Evaluation in Life Cycle of Information Technology (ELICIT) framework: supporting the innovation life cycle from business case assessment to summative evaluation. J Biomed Inform. 2022;127:104014.

124. Royce WW, editor. Managing the development of large software systems: concepts and techniques. In: Proceedings of the 9th international conference on Software Engineering; 1987.

125. Laplante PA, Neill CJ. The demise of the waterfall model is imminent, and other urban myths: rumors of the demise of the waterfall life-cycle model are greatly exaggerated. Queue. 2004;1(10):10–5.

126. Shaw NT. 'CHEATS': a generic information communication technology (ICT) evaluation framework. Comput Biol Med. 2002;32(3):209–20.

127. Damschroder LJ, Aron DC, Keith RE, Kirsh SR, Alexander JA, Lowery JC. Fostering implementation of health services research findings into practice: a consolidated framework for advancing implementation science. Implement Sci. 2009;4(1):50.

128. Davis FD. Perceived usefulness, perceived ease of use, and user acceptance of information technology. MIS Q. 1989;13:319–40.

129. Rogers EM. Diffusion of innovations. Simon and Schuster; 2010.

130. Bandura A, Walters RH. Social learning theory. Englewood Cliffs, NJ: Prentice Hall; 1977.

131. Dishaw MT, Strong DM. Extending the technology acceptance model with task–technology fit constructs. Inf Manag. 1999;36(1):9–21.

132. Sherer SA, Meyerhoefer CD, Peng L. Applying institutional theory to the adoption of electronic health records in the U.S. Inf Manag. 2016;53(5):570–80.

133. DeLone WH, McLean ER. Information systems success: the quest for the dependent variable. Inf Syst Res. 1992;3(1):60–95.

134. Kazanjian A, Green CJ. Beyond effectiveness: the evaluation of information systems using a comprehensive health technology assessment framework. Comput Biol Med. 2002;32(3):165–77.

135. Mishra AN, Anderson C, Angst CM, Agarwal R. Electronic health records assimilation and physician identity evolution: an identity theory perspective. Inform Syst Res. 2012;23(3-part-1):738–60.

136. Semwanga AR, Namatovu HK, Kyanda S, Kaawaase M, Magumba A. An ehealth adoption framework for developing countries: a systematic review. Health Inform Int J. 2021;10(3):1–16. https://doi.org/10.5121/hiij.2021.10301.

137. Kashyap V. Taxonomy: biomedical health informatics. In: Liu L, Özsu MT, editors. Encyclopedia of database systems. New York: Springer; 2016. p. 1–4.

138. Yasnoff WA, O'Carroll PW, Koo D, Linkins RW, Kilbourne EM. Public health informatics: improving and transforming public health in the information age. J Public Health Manag Pract. 2000;6:67–75.

139. Wyatt JC, Liu JL. Basic concepts in medical informatics. J Epidemiol Community Health. 2002;56(11):808–12.

140. Law M, Tang JL. An analysis of the effectiveness of interventions intended to help people stop smoking. Arch Intern Med. 1995;155(18):1933–41.

141. Mekonnen ZA, Gelaye KA. Effect of mobile phone text message reminders on the completion and timely receipt of routine childhood vaccinations: superiority randomized controlled trial in Northwest Ethiopia. JMIR Mhealth Uhealth. 2021;9(6):e27603.

142. Gashu KD, Gelaye KA, Lester R, Tilahun B. Effect of a phone reminder system on patient-centered tuberculosis treatment adherence among adults in Northwest Ethiopia: a randomised controlled trial. BMJ Health Care Inform. 2021;28(1):e100268.

143. Greenes RA, Shortliffe EH. Medical informatics: an emerging academic discipline and institutional priority. JAMA. 1990;263(8):1114–20.

Zeleke Abebaw Mekonnen

Abstract

Public health informatics (PHI) is a specialized area that is emerging within the broader field of health informatics. In simple terms, PHI refers to the use of informatics in the public health to focus on preventing and promoting health at a population level. Public health informatics plays a crucial role in improving population health outcomes by providing information that aids in decision-making.

Public health informatics benefits healthcare seekers, providers, and health institutions as digitizing the health system improves efficiency and quality of care. The use of information systems in public health contributes to enhancing population health outcomes through improving the access, quality, and safety of public health services. It also helps to reduce health disparities and lowers the cost of healthcare. It supports early preparedness and response for public health surveillance, helps to develop resilient, efficient, and responsive health systems.

Public health informatics is more helpful in developing countries where resources and infrastructure are limited. Thus, the development and adoption of public health information systems require careful and rigorous approaches to ensure sustainability.

This chapter consists of the concepts, scope, role and impact of public health informatics in advancing the health system to respond public health challenges.

Keywords

Health informatics · Public health informatics Resource limited setting

2.1 Concepts of Public Health Informatics

2.1.1 Concepts of Public Health

Public health encompasses the scientific and creative methods to prevent illness, extend life span, and enhance overall wellbeing through collaborative endeavors and informed choices made by various stakeholders at different levels. Unlike focusing solely on the health of an individual patient, public health concentrates on the health of the entire community. The primary emphasis in public health is placed on preventing illness and harm, rather than simply reacting to problems once they have already occurred.

Public health initiatives are not limited to the clinical setting alone. Instead, they consider fac-

Z. A. Mekonnen (✉)
Policy, Strategy and Research Lead Executive Office, Federal Ministry of Health, Addis Ababa, Ethiopia

SMART Health, Research and Publication Department, Bahir Dar, Ethiopia
e-mail: Zeleke.abebaw@moh.gov.et

tors such as cost, efficiency, and social acceptability when determining effective points of intervention throughout the chain of events leading to disease, harm, or disability. This approach prioritizes the overall impact of interventions on public health rather than the specific expertise of an intervention designer [1].

There are core responsibilities of public health including assessment, policy creation, and assurance.

2.1.1.1 Assessment

It includes spotting and containing epidemics and disease outbreaks on population health. It is feasible to create and evaluate theories about the genesis, transmission, and risk factors that contribute to health problems by correlating health status with a number of demographic, regional, environmental, and other factors.

2.1.1.2 Policy Creation

The second essential role of public health is the creation of policies. It makes recommendations for interventions and public policies that promote health status using the findings of assessment activities and etiologic research in conjunction with contextual values and culture.

2.1.1.3 Assurance

The assurance in public health includes evaluating, ensuring competent workforce, linking to care and enforcement of public health and related laws.

2.1.2 Why Informatics in Public Health?

It is evident that the conventional paper-based information systems are ineffective at promptly supplying data necessary for public health intervention. Thus, the provision, use, and availability of a current, reliable information system is essential to public health practice. In keeping with this, traditional public health practices have long benefited from the application of computers and Information Technology (IT). However, there are also special issues for privacy and confidentiality, security, data integrity, and availability when low- and middle-income countries switch from paper-based to digital systems, which may outweigh the advantages. Even with the apparent need for a new paradigm in record-keeping, most healthcare facilities have encountered difficulties in attempting to transition to computer-based, paperless systems.

A strong and growing interest in gathering more and more health-related data electronically is being driven by the ongoing changes in the healthcare system, the growing emphasis on standardizing healthcare transactions, the introduction of the internet, and other information technology advancements. Therefore, in an effort to capitalize on these opportunities, public health organizations are shifting from independent systems that are programmatic or disease-based to a more comprehensive approach that involves capturing data that is already electronic, particularly from the healthcare system [2]. This is why the extraordinary public health challenges we are facing today have led to a recent surge in interest in health informatics applications.

According to the United States National Library of Medicine, Health informatics is an "interdisciplinary study of the design, development, adoption and application of IT-based innovations in healthcare services delivery, management and planning". It is an interdisciplinary study that consists of health care, computer science, and information science [3]. Inspiring the same analogy, we modified the health informatics model of multidisciplinary interaction specific to public health informatics that comprises of computer science, information science and public health as shown in Fig. 2.1.

The use of IT to support the provision of healthcare services, including coordination, communication, logistics, and other business operations, as well as relevant procedures and practices surrounding IT use in healthcare, are all included in under health informatics domain. IT systems and health informatics offer revolutionary tools to guarantee effective information flow and access. Health informatics has improved client-provider relationships and given people more autonomy over their medical care throughout

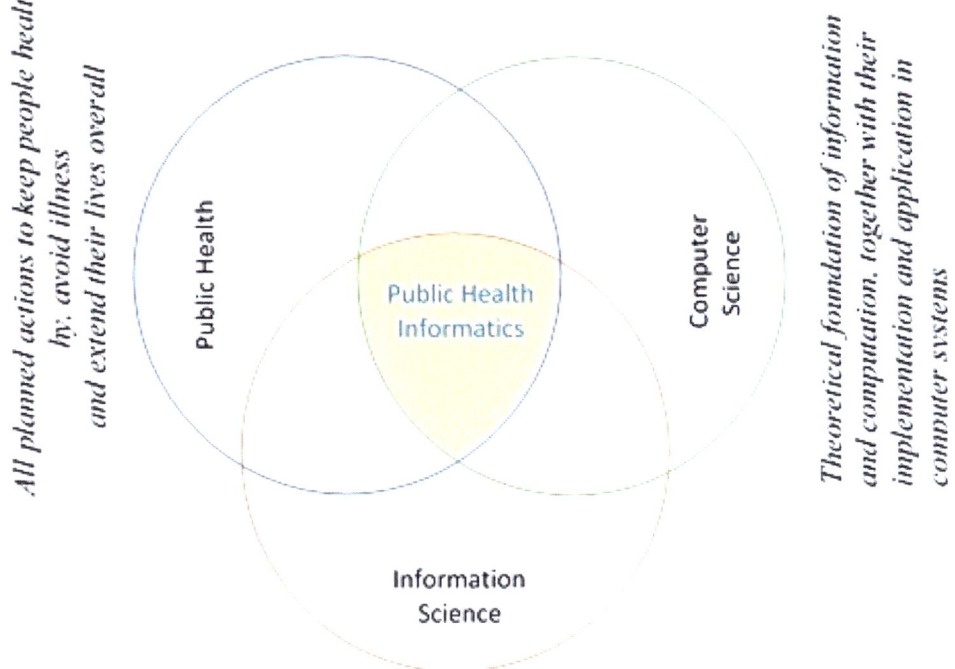

Fig. 2.1 Interaction of information science, computer science and public health to form PHI

time. The rise of component-driven technologies and the significance of mobile communications are the two most promising developments that could have a significant impact on the advancement of healthcare IT systems.

The medical and public health sectors have made significant investments in IT and communication technologies throughout the past 20 years. As a result, it becomes inevitable that information technology be used to public health practice, giving rise to the idea of PHI which is the subfield of the broader area of health informatics [4].

The scientific application of information, computer science, and technology to public health practice is known as Public Health Informatics, or PHI [5, 6]. Put simply, it refers to the application of informatics to public health practice, with an emphasis on population-level promotive and preventive health.

Throughout the last 20 years, the convergence of information technology and public health, which started to take shape in the mid to late 1990s, has been referred to as public health informatics. Since then, PHI has developed into a specialist field within the field of public health, with an emphasis on using IT and informatics to encourage communities and individuals to make changes to their environmental, social, and behavioral habits in order to improve their overall health and well-being.

Furthermore, a growing number of informatics and IT systems are being adopted in order to deliver population-centered public health services faster and more effectively. This drive has also made it necessary for public health to provide top attention to the creation and implementation of new technologies in order to enable the delivery of evidence-based public health together with the successful and efficient administration of health initiatives [7].

There are three categories into which public health informatics falls as outlined below.

- Explaining intricate systems (like public health work flow or models of disease transmission).
- Finding ways to use information or collect data in novel ways to increase the efficacy and efficiency of public health systems.
- Putting methods and procedures into place and keeping them up to date in order to accomplish such gains.

Public health informatics is distinct from other informatics specialty areas, albeit sharing many similarities with them [2, 4, 6]. Among them are:

- Pay attention to technological applications that advance population health rather than individual health.
- Prioritize illness prevention over diagnosis and treatment. It is not just restricted to medical and surgical procedures; it encompasses interventions carried out outside of the healthcare system.
- Prioritize preventative measures at every susceptible juncture along the causal chains that result in illness, trauma, or disability.
- Operating inside governmental platforms since government entities are almost always involved in public health initiatives rather than private ones.

2.1.3 The Principles of Public Health Informatics

Within the larger field of informatics, public health informatics is a unique specialty area that is governed by a certain set of rules. Four such concepts, which stem directly from the nature and scope of public health, set public health informatics apart from other informatics specialty areas. The sorts of tasks and difficulties that make up this emerging field are defined, directed, and contextualized by these four guiding concepts [2, 4] described below.

2.1.3.1 PHI to Advance the Health of Populations Rather Than the Health of Particular Individuals

Public health is a discipline that places more emphasis on community and population health than it does on the health of a single patient. The patient, who appears with a particular sickness or condition that has to be diagnosed and treated, is the main focus of attention in the healthcare setting. In contrast, populations are the main focus of concern in public health. The community as a whole can be viewed as the patient. In addition, variables that impact the health risk of entire populations as opposed to individuals must be taken into consideration in public health practice.

2.1.3.2 PHI as a Main Tool to Avoid Public Health Issues That Put Large Groups of People at Risk

Traditional health care primarily treats people who already have an illness or high-risk condition, but there are few significant exceptions. In contrast, public health practice aims to prevent the conditions that first caused the sickness. This shift in emphasis directly affects the potential applications of information technology. PHI changes the circumstances or environment that put populations of people at risk in order to prevent the occurrence of public health issues including illness and injuries.

2.1.3.3 PHI as a Tool to Investigate the Possibilities for Disease, Damage, and Disability Prevention at All Susceptible Points in the Causal Chains

In public health, a preventive interventions character is determined by its efficacy, expediency, cost, and social acceptability at different potentially susceptible stages in a causal chain. These applications are not limited to specific social, behavioral, or environmental contexts. Public health activity is not restricted to the clinical contact, even though some of these interactions with the healthcare system are legitimately classified as public health interventions (such as immunization).

2.1.3.4 PHI as a Governmental Framework in Which Public Health Is Practiced Is Reflected in the Field of Public Health Informatics

A large portion of public health is carried out by government organizations, which are required to balance conflicting goals, respond directly to legislative, regulatory, and policy mandates, and disclose all actions in an open and transparent manner. Furthermore, in certain public health initiatives, authority is required to implement particular and occasionally coercive measures to safeguard the population during an emergency.

2.1.4 Fundamentals of Data, Information, Knowledge and Wisdom

Data, information, knowledge, and wisdom are the core ideas that guide the study of public health informatics and aid in the comprehension of the nature of information and communication systems in the field. These components are placed in a hierarchy, with the data at the models base serving as the foundation for information establishment and, subsequently, the possibility of knowledge and wisdom development as shown in Fig. 2.2.

In everyday routines, these phrases are frequently used interchangeably. In public health informatics, however, each of these phrases has a very specific and unique definition. The following definitions of these terms apply to public health informatics.

Data consists of a collection of observations and facts. In a certain context, data are interpreted to create information. An ordered body of information makes up knowledge, and it is these information patterns that serve as the foundation for the kinds of conclusions and insights that we refer to as wisdom. The following figure describes the fundamental distinctions between data, information, knowledge and wisdom (Fig. 2.3).

Fig. 2.2 Fundamental concepts in public health informatics

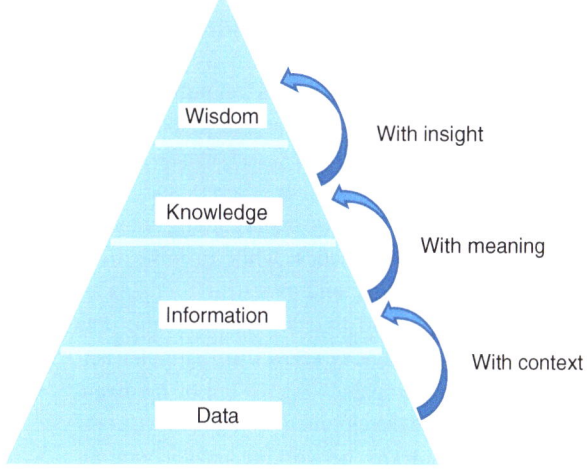

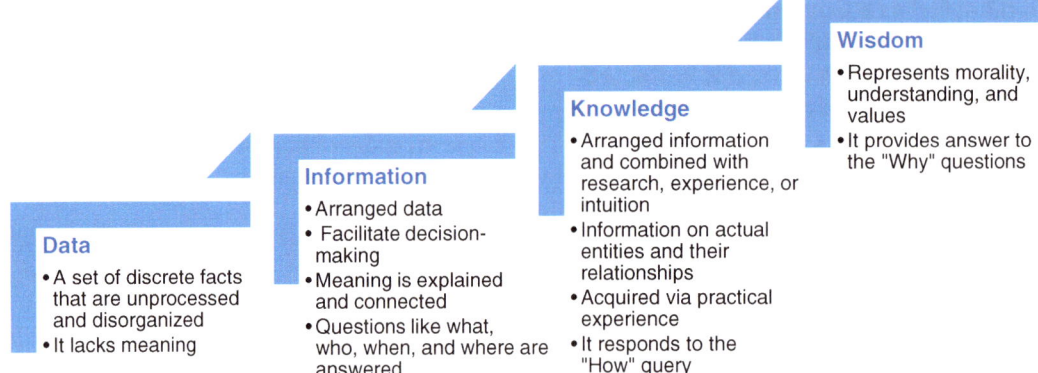

Fig. 2.3 Difference between data, information, knowledge and wisdom

2.2 Scope of Public Health Informatics

The conception, design, development, implementation, optimization and assessment of communication, surveillance, and information systems pertinent to public health are all included in the field of public health informatics [6].

2.2.1 Potential Areas of Application

The application of informatics to public health domains such as health promotion, preparedness, prevention, and surveillance is known as public health informatics. Computer science and informatics science are the key underpinning sciences of public health informatics, while it draws from many other scientific and practical domains as well. The theory and practice of automatic data processing equipment is known as computer science, and it encompasses the design of hardware and software, the development of algorithms, computational complexity, networking and telecommunications, artificial intelligence, and pattern recognition. The study of information's organization, composition, and storage and retrieval is also included in informatics science [4].

The expanded range of public health informatics application domain includes:

- Risk assessment for epidemics and outbreaks, epidemiological disease surveillance

- Preparedness, mitigation, and response in disaster management
- Giving the public access to health information and education
- Remote health care delivery and illness screening
- Electronic health records/electronic medical records and its connections
- Education and training: health care practitioners receive ongoing medical education
- The creation of Clinical Decision Support Systems (CDSS)
- Improving public health governance by making health services highly accessible
- Research on public health

Similarly, public health informatics interventions also apply at different levels. According to the WHO digital health services are also divided as follows [8]:

- Client-centered interventions
- Provider-focused interventions and
- Health system focused interventions

2.2.2 Goals of Public Health Informatics

Public health informatics relies on the utilization of information technology for data collection, data management, analysis, and disseminate information, forming an essential capability within the field. Consistent application of technology in public health information systems is crucial to monitor and enhance the implementation of health service delivery [4].

Given the multidisciplinary and interdisciplinary character of public health informatics, it is inevitable that the field will absorb knowledge from other fields into its own and knowledge from a wide range of academic fields, including information science, computer science, management and organizational theory must be applied to the field of public health informatics. Its practice must also take into account information from other disciplines that support public health, such as statistics, microbiology, and epidemiology [2].

Accessing real-time data is critical for public health decision-makers, and informatics is at the core of supporting access and dissemination of information, especially for health care workers, healthcare program managers and decision makers. Creating and utilizing interoperable health information systems is a major priority and there are several uses for these systems in public health including population-focused health promotion, illness prevention, bio-surveillance, and outbreak control. Essentially, the goals are to use data analytics, information systems, technical tools, gadgets, and innovative technologies to improve overall health, provide better health outcomes, and generally raise the quality of life for huge population groups worldwide.

In nutshell, PHI is primarily used for two purposes:

- Improving population health, which in turn improves individual health; and
- Preventing illnesses and injuries by modifying factors that raise population risk. PHI essentially uses informatics to gather, analyze, and act upon public health data.

Aspects that distinguish PHI from other fields of informatics include its focus on population-level illness prevention, use of a wide range of interventions to achieve its goals, and work in governmental contexts [9]. The following list provides a summary of common purposes of public health informatics.

- For recording accurate public health data
- To have public health data available in a timely manner
- To inform public health managers for better decisions
- Resource allocation and planning
- Public health risk management
- Training for public health workers
- Support for shared public health care
- Staff coordination
- Stock management
- Research

PHI facilitates use information communication technology and other machine interfaced technologies in health care delivery for planning and management related issues associated with decision making process. Along this, priorities for public health should include digital health and transparency, accessibility, scalability, replicability, interoperability, privacy, security, and secrecy should all be considered during its development [10].

The ICT applications that form the basis for public health care setup in resource limited setting includes: remote service provision through telecommunications (Telehealth/Telemedicine), GIS, applications for health practice for mobile health (m-Health), Electronic Health Records (EMR), electronic learning, decision support, social media and big data [11]. The following list of items outline the major innovations in digital-based healthcare today will also have an impact on public health practices [4, 12].

2.2.2.1 Personal Health Record (PHR)/ Electronic Health Record (EHR)

Unlike the Electronic Health Record (EHR) that is kept by an institution; a patient health record (PHR) is kept by the patient or the client. In order to improve public participation and promote the avoidance of harmful health disorders, public health systems should devise and implement strategies to enhance EHRs/PHRs in particular for resource limited settings.

2.2.2.2 Mobile Technology

Public health workers can employ mobile technologies for tracking and surveillance, including using GPS to map disease outbreaks

2.2.2.3 Tele-Health

Telehealth can be used to deliver public health services to rural and hard to reach settings. The benefits include: less travel time for residents of rural areas to visit a super-specialty health facilities; lower treatment and follow-up costs; prompt and convenient access to expert medical services; improved prognosis due to standard treatment availability; and faster response times for managing epidemics and outbreaks.

2.2.2.4 GIS (Geographic Information System)

Remote sensing, geographical modeling, and geographic solutions make up GIS. GIS allows users to access information on social infrastructure, healthcare facilities, demographics, and patients geo-positioned places all in one view. Given that it can support information demands, GIS can also contribute to the study of population-based public health.

2.3   Roles of Public Health Informatics

Every facet of public health is being challenged by the information technology revolution. As we transform public health through the adoption of new information systems, use of electronic tools for disease surveillance, and reformation of antiquated processes, individuals, care providers, and public health agencies can all benefit. However, it will not be simple or affordable to realize the advantages [2].

The goal of public health informatics is to apply informatics and solve public health issues with new technological solutions. In our contemporary healthcare system, informatics plays a crucial role that cannot be overstated, especially in situations where resources are scarce. Public health informatics has significant links across the public health spectrum, with the main goal of

PHI being the information-based prevention of illness, damage, or disability in populations that are at risk.

In order to develop tactics including surveillance, prevention, preparedness, outbreak management, predictive modeling, and health promotion, public health informatics makes use of technology and information systems. The main roles of public health informatics are outlined below.

2.3.1   Early Warning, Preparedness and Response System

The amount of data on public health is growing exponentially in the twenty-first century, and population health monitoring is a crucial part of any public health practice. Monitoring trends and patterns, spotting epidemics, creating and assessing interventions, determining the focus of future research, keeping the standard of care and health outcomes, pinpointing marginalized communities, and organizing services all require data.

Population health is the focus of public health, and paper-based reporting is no longer practical for studying huge populations and tracking health trends. Therefore, case detection and reporting for early warning, preparedness, and response systems are nowadays being automated along with the improvements in ICT. The main goal of recent ICT advancements is to move the burden of case detection and reporting from manual to automated methods. ICT advancements improve, enable, and empower both passive and active health care data management.

Essential public health functions (i.e., detection, analyses, reporting, feedback and response) can be enabled, enhanced, and empowered when public health informatics is used for public health monitoring. ICT is showing promise in the areas of analytics, predictive surveillance, push notifications, laboratory reporting, prevention, detection, and response, as well as the use of new data sources to execute public health solutions [13]. The following lists the key responsibilities of public health and the part that ICT plays in each domain.

2.3.1.1 Detection of Outbreaks

When coupled with the increasing number of individuals accessing the internet technology, ICT has the potential to enhance outbreak detection and management.

2.3.1.2 Predictive Surveillance of Public Health

Early disease outbreak detection is possible with predictive public health surveillance with computer algorithms that are verified by past data and real-time data analysis. Predictive analytics is unique in that it looks for and tests correlations in the data, particularly between environmental and human health data, to predict risk, rather of the one-dimensional perspective that descriptive analytics offers.

2.3.1.3 Reporting on Cases Automatically

The main goal of recent ICT advancements is to replace manual, clinical, and laboratory reporting for public health cases by automating the process. Active public health monitoring typically entails searching Electronic Medical Records for information while doing contact tracing and case investigations.

Even in environments with limited resources, global public health readiness and response are essential for the detection and prevention of newly and reemerging diseases. It should promptly deliver health information so that countries have the knowledge they require to combat epidemics immediately or make long-term plans. Development and upkeep of monitoring systems have proven beneficial in addressing a number of public health issues [14].

Geographic information systems are now commonplace to correlate public health epidemiology data with geography to produce dramatic visual representation of a variety of public health conditions such as outbreaks. It helps to strengthen digital technology supported disease prevention, surveillance, detection, response, reporting, and control at all levels of the health system especially in resource limited settings [12, 15].

Because GIS can support information demands, it has a great deal of potential to contribute to the study of population-based public health. Public health professionals can use GIS to manage vast amounts of data, map the prevalence of diseases in the population and health care resources, examine the connections between socioeconomic and environmental factors, and disease outcomes, choose the best location for new medical facilities, and even make decisions regarding the creation or application of health policies. Evidence also showed that there is growing evidence of the positive effects of using GIS globally, even in environments with low resources [11].

The potential for enhancing the healthcare system has also been demonstrated by the introduction of computerized clinical decision support systems, telemedicine, mobile health, and electronic medical and health records [16]. The diagnosis and management of disease outbreaks can be accelerated by mobile devices and computer-based applications [17]. During the COVID-19 pandemic, telehealth became viable, practical, and crucial [18].

Time-sensitive data on public health issues are becoming more widely collected, allowing clients and healthcare providers to make decisions more quickly. Applications for mobile health are being tested in a variety of contexts, including enhancing prompt access to emergency and general public health services and information.

The goal of mHealth initiatives in this field is to take advantage of mobile phones rapid, affordable, and effective data collection and transmission capabilities. Information concerning the location and levels of specific diseases (such as Malaria, HIV/AIDS, TB) can help health systems identify outbreaks and better target resources to areas of greatest need. Such mHealth programs can be particularly useful during emergencies, in order to identify where the greatest public health needs are within a country [19].

With its capacity to promptly record and send data on disease incidence, mobile device deployment can play a critical role in both containing and preventing epidemics. Evidence also suggests that the implementation of digital health can contribute to advancements in disease identification and management.

In the midst of the Ebola and SARS outbreaks, digital health was proved to be effective in identifying and combating international health crises. A review revealed that data-driven disease surveillance, screening, triage, diagnosis, and monitoring can all be done with digital technologies at various stages of the COVID-19 outbreak [20].

In developing countries like Ethiopia, there are electronic systems for data collection, compilation, analysis, dissemination of information on reportable diseases and other events that present a potential threat to public health security. The COVID-19 Response Application that has been developed and used by MOH and EPHI is a typical example [21].

2.3.2 Disease Surveillance

Public health surveillance entails the continuous and organized gathering, elucidation and dissemination of information pertaining to health status and potential health risks. It is closely tied to prevention and control efforts and plays a vital role in the planning, implementation, and evaluation of public health practices [7]. Public health surveillance is among the earliest established and essential operations within the public health sector, serving as a foundational component for various key services, including the fundamental function of assessment. Surveillance data is a primary tool used to determine the priorities in public health interventions.

Monitoring illness patterns, directing fast public health interventions and disease prevention strategies, proposing epidemiological theories, and identifying emerging public health issues are among the goals of public health surveillance. A number of characteristics, including timeliness, sensitivity and specificity, completeness, and utility of the data obtained, can be used to assess the success of public health monitoring. In low-resource settings, public health surveillance assumes a crucial toward achieving population health outcomes.

While identifying disease outbreaks including any public health catastrophes, it is a must to utilize surveillance data. The data are uti-

lized to project the extent and scale of a problem, including epidemiology of health problem in the area. Understanding the geographical and demographic occurrence and distribution helps to facilitates effective planning and management.

Furthermore, the data helps to track the alterations in environmental and infectious agents, identify shifts in health behaviors, evaluate control strategies, and provide insights into the natural progression of a health event within a community. These applications can generate hypotheses and stimulate applied research. In summary, public health monitoring serves as the foundation for informed decision-making in public health by providing relevant and timely data to lead and manage more effectively.

With the rapid advancements in information technology, surveillance techniques have evolved alongside the issues they address. Electronic health records offer the potential to enhance the efficiency and timeliness of surveillance; however, there are significant challenges to overcome in realizing this potential. It is crucial for the public health community to receive information from these records regarding the health of the populations they serve. Those responsible for public health monitoring have a duty to ensure that the data is utilized for the benefit of the general public while safeguarding the privacy of individuals whose identities are included.

The advancement of information technology has opened up new ways of effectively addressing public health issues. The value of surveillance lies in the efficient and successful dissemination of relevant information. A delayed information may result in missed opportunities for timely action, particularly in the context of significant community events. Incomplete information may hinder the identification of threats to public health. If surveillance systems are unable to adapt to changing information needs, it becomes challenging to assess the impact of novel preventive treatments across different population subgroups. Ineffective surveillance systems ultimately serve no purpose.

The increasing availability of databases and data sources, coupled with advancements in information sciences and technology, present opportunities for the advancement of public health surveillance. Utilization of digital health platforms such as, electronic-based data capturing, reporting, sharing, and processing is an indication of the potential of ICT to advance public health. These sources enable a more comprehensive understanding of public health events in terms of their timing, location, and affected individuals.

To meet the needs of decision-makers and guide future prevention and control efforts, public health surveillance must embrace innovation. Despite the significant growth of ICT in the last few decades, its integration into the realm of public health remains limited in many countries, particularly in resource-limited settings. While, leveraging ICT was big opportunity that potentially advance public health even in resource-limited settings. Regrettably, the coordination necessary to effectively identify, adopt and scale-up of best available evidence and innovations regarding public health informatics is lacking.

The potential for improving public health exists through the use of innovative digital health technologies [22]. With the emergence of new technologies, it is crucial to adopt a systematic and transparent approach to identifying and curating the most effective practices. Additionally, there is a need to actively pursue a tailored approach of adopting technology according to the specific contexts for low-resource settings [23].

Informatics encompasses also different perspective of public health as well. Some of the essential components of these aspects include [3].

2.3.2.1 System Designing
PHI facilitates the identification of the most suitable data and sources to support surveillance objectives. It also helps determine the appropriate access, methods, and conditions for data usage. Furthermore, public health informatics enhances the analysis and action by fostering improved communication between surveillance systems and other data systems.

2.3.2.2 Data Management and Collation
Public health informatics simplifies the process of sharing data within diverse digital platforms. It enables the seamless connection of data across different systems and facilitates the identification and resolution of issues related to data quality, all while ensuring data security and privacy.

2.3.2.3 Data Analysis
ICT gives an opportunity to provide relevant statistical and visual aids, algorisms used to data analysis including big data sets.

2.3.2.4 Interpretation
Public health informatics enables the comparison of information from different surveillance programs with diverse data sets, allowing for the generation of new insights and the integration of data from multiple sources and quality standards. It facilitates an interpretive framework to enhance understanding and analysis.

2.3.2.5 Information Dissemination
Public health informatics plays a role in presenting pertinent data to users and identifying the most effective methods to reach the intended audience. It simplifies information retrieval and highlights the benefits for data producers.

2.3.2.6 Data-Informed Initiatives
It facilitates the assessment of the benefits derived from the direct integration of data into information systems that support interventions, evaluating performances, informing any administrative decisions and plans.

Public health surveillance plays a vital role in implementing targeted preventive measures and swiftly detecting outbreaks to prevent the escalation of epidemics. The rise in international travel, urbanization, and mass gatherings has accelerated the transmission of human diseases, underscoring the importance of effective surveillance.

During global pandemics like Ebola and COVID-19, electronic surveillance platforms facilitated efficient information sharing and access, leading to the rapid containment of these epidemics. Ongoing developments in public health informatics continue to enable, enhance, and empower the essential functions of surveillance, promising a promising future for the field.

However, the full potential of these advancements can only be realized if healthcare providers, decision-makers, and stakeholders in public health demonstrate willingness to adapt to the evolving landscape and embrace the changes brought about by public health informatics.

2.3.3 Prevention and Control of Diseases and Health Related Problems

The information that forms the foundation of knowledge in the field of public health is produced through the gathering and processing of population health data. The demand for up-to-date information regarding the health of nations and communities is constantly growing. Understanding the trends in diseases and other aspects of community health can help with decision-making, program design, and the provision of care.

With the use of information technology, it is now possible to integrate and analyze many data sources in a spatially-temporal context, supporting the creation of predictive models and prompt interventions for the prevention and treatment of illnesses and other health-related issues [24]. Using a range of information and communications technologies, public health informatics promotes both disease prevention and population well-being maintenance. Public health organizations employ a variety of information systems to assist stop and slow the spread of disease. However, there are still a lot of issues that, if resolved, would improve the public health system and assist governments in becoming ready for the next wave of new and reemerging illnesses.

It is becoming increasingly clear that the future of public health will be driven by technology, which highlights the extraordinary importance of public health informatics and its role in keeping society safe, healthy and informed. Public health efforts play a major role to respond to new threats and crisis, such as Ebola, COVID-19, heart disease, cancer, stroke and diabetes. As the world-wide COVID-19 pandemic continues to affect our daily lives, the importance of protecting our families and communities through public health has likely never been greater.

Internet-enabled applications for chronic diseases also have the potential to significantly impact patient treatment in the future. They can empower citizens to make decisions that support their own health maintenance and well-being. Typically, the purpose of diagnostic and treatment support systems is to give medical personnel in remote locations guidance on patient diagnosis and care. In these situations, termed as telemedicine, patients may snap a picture of a wound or sickness and allow a health worker to diagnose and treat the condition from a distance.

There are new options for determining needs and providing health care (from preventive and health promotion to curative interventions and self-management). Among these, mHealth interventions have been proposed as a promising means of supporting the health system, especially in countries where resources are limited [8, 25]. In developing nations, mobile phones are a suitable and promising instrument for interventions aimed at controlling diseases [26].

Considering the widespread usage of mobile phones worldwide and the benefits of mobile phone technology, such as its wide reach, affordability, and ease of use, it holds immense promise for resolving health system problems. Because of this benefit, mHealth technologies present chances to improve healthcare delivery for disease surveillance, behavior modification, prevention, and control of a range of health issues, as well as increasing patient attendance for medical services [27, 28].

Optimizing care for individuals with chronic illnesses, such as through remote monitoring for managing chronic diseases, is another area where public health informatics may be useful. Treatment monitoring models and strategies to increase treatment adherence show the most promise for effectiveness.

In underdeveloped nations with limited access to healthcare institutions, remote monitoring presents new opportunities for outpatient patient treatment. Virtual monitoring and management enables to increase engagement in the ongoing care of patients. In resource-constrained settings, it offers care providers with improved capabilities to monitor patient progress, ensure adherence to treatment and appoint for follow-up visits.

In times of public health emergency, evidence-based health informatics is extremely important. It is crucial to have access to precise, evidence-based information regarding the safety and efficacy of health informatics technology in supporting public health measures during a public health emergency. The new coronavirus disease 2019 (COVID-19) pandemic, a serious public health emergency, highlights the pressing need for safe, efficient, and evidence-based digital health implementations. The global COVID-19 pandemic is having an unparalleled impact on health care systems worldwide, impacting not only the containment and handling of the COVID-19 crisis but also the overall provision of healthcare services. When developing and implementing digital health tools that have been quickly deployed in response to the pandemic, it is critical to use a multidisciplinary approach that takes into account human factors, ethics, data privacy, and the variety of contexts at the local, national, and international levels [29].

Public health authorities require data collecting, analysis, and distribution systems, just like they do for all health care data, in order to give precise, dependable, consistent, and comprehensive information for assessing current resources, making future plans, and implementing preventative actions. Informatics systems also aid in the maintenance of data that gives medical professionals instant access to client records and other medical data, facilitating crucial decision-making to deliver the best possible public health care.

Preventive care can be advanced by automated data sorting, which makes it easier for health care workers to identify patients who are more likely to have health problems and to treat them before more serious issues arise. Governments and health systems are able to promptly conduct public health interventions when they detect the spread of illness during an epidemic. Additionally, public health informatics offers a direct, reliable, and easily accessible source of information that can be very helpful in the early diagnosis and containment of pandemics. A study and synthesis of the literature demonstrates that PHI has been utilized to address a wide range of pandemic-related public health challenges [22].

Innovations in health technology are revolutionizing the identification, creation, and provision of medical services and goods. They are also profoundly altering the diagnosis, management, and prevention of medical disorders. Wearable technology, web-based platforms, and smartphone apps are examples of digital health technologies that are quickly becoming recognized as promising therapies for illness management. In order to reduce infectious and chronic diseases, this endeavor will address the need for digitalized screenings, patient follow-up procedures, and population health surveillance made possible by technology [30–32]. However, many low-income countries are unable to support locally sustainable initiatives for the prevention and screening of communicable and non-communicable diseases, as well as new therapeutic treatment plans that have the potential to save millions of lives due to critical deficiencies in their health information technology systems.

Digital health interventions are primarily an empowerment method for managing one's own health and illness, as well as for health facilities service delivery to improve NCD management in primary health care, according to the conclusions of a scoping review [33, 34]. Additionally, digital health interventions can promote primary prevention (e.g., completion of required screens), secondary (e.g., timely receipt of immunizations), tertiary (e.g., routine monitoring of chronic illnesses) and quaternary (e.g., avoidance of over medicalization) [35].

2.3.4 Elimination and Eradication of Diseases and Health Related Problems

In settings with limited resources, public health informatics may be one of the most helpful tools for managing disease monitoring, epidemics, and natural catastrophes. The monitoring of populations could be aided by the deployment of computerized global surveillance and data collection systems. Analysis and prediction of infectious diseases using AI-based surveillance systems are among the new advancements in disease prevention, elimination and eradication [9].

Applications of digital public health technology could be highly helpful in understanding and mapping illness cluster identification, population growth, health service provider mapping, and geographic access to healthcare. Improving early warning alerts, documenting efficient surveillance indicators for prompt preparedness, and responding to the elimination and eradication of diseases and health-related issues that arise at the population level are all made possible by utilizing digital public health surveillance and monitoring response to current infectious disease approaches and interventions [36].

In an increasingly technologically driven healthcare environment, digital health solutions that enable the convergence of primary care and public health will be critical for quick and efficient responses to health and healthcare concerns [35]. By offering automatic and real-time mapping, generating new data sources, and assisting in the detection of pathogens, digital technology can enhance the capacity to both detect and respond to developing infectious illnesses while also lowering costs.

The following essential public health tasks for the eradication and elimination of disease are supported by public health informatics.

- Diagnostics and screening: diagnosing infectious diseases in people
- Surveillance and monitoring: keeping an eye on population trends and patterns of infectious diseases
- Predicting infectious disease outbreaks (e.g., for outbreak prediction) is known as forecasting
- Identification and validation of signal outbreaks: identifying and verifying epidemics of infectious diseases
- Outbreak response: handling sudden increases in infectious diseases
- Collaboration and communication: Communication uses digital tools (such as social media) to inform, educate, and empower people about infectious diseases [24].

Digital technologies explosive growth and development have opened up new avenues for enhancing health and wellness [37]. The way information moves through health systems has changed dramatically as a result of technologies like smartphones, digital cameras, drones, and geolocation tools, in addition to the application of artificial intelligence and machine learning. For example, the development of big data, field responses, and reporting with digital support are useful instruments for enhancing malaria control efforts [38]. In settings with limited resources, digital intervention in malaria control efforts, such as bolstering medicine compliance, boosting surveillance, and improving policy and governance, access, and service delivery, may help eradicate malaria. The quality and quantity (real-time reporting) of malaria surveillance data may be improved by using smartphones, digital portable tablets, and web application software to record clinical signs and symptoms, diagnosis, treatment, and medication compliance [39].

Further, strong mechanisms for case reporting, investigation, and response will be necessary to eradicate malaria in LMICs and stop the disease from spreading. Malaria surveillance could be enhanced by mobile health (mHealth), but to achieve this, applications must be well-designed to consider contextual factors (such as current workflows), be rooted in national eHealth strategies, scalable, sustainable, and enable formal monitoring and evaluation [40].

Similarly, in settings with limited resources, the use of digital technologies has emerged as a critical idea in the fight against communicable diseases like Tuberculosis (TB). mHealth systems are emerging as a viable global tool to aid in the elimination of tuberculosis. According to an interventional TB study, phone reminder systems may be very important in patient-centered TB treatment programs in environments with limited resources [41]. An analysis of NTDs also showed that, in hard-to-reach and poorly accessible health service locations, the use or intervention of electronic technologies improves disease management, case identification, treatment outcome, and illness diagnosis of neglected tropical diseases [42].

One potential way to change the way healthcare is provided in resource-constrained settings during the COVID-19 pandemic is by digitizing the healthcare system [43]. According to a review, it was possible to identify patients, treat and diagnose them through contact with medical professionals and teleconsultations, and support better health service delivery at the community health system for managing the disease by utilizing digital public health technology applications like mHealth, eHealth, EMR, and Telehealth [42].

In addition to granting access to vital medical treatments, telemedicine and telehealth have decreased the risks of COVID-19 infections for both the patient and the healthcare provider. Telehealth can help with speedy information availability and distant care triage during infectious disease epidemics. Through video discussions with medical professionals, telehealth can also help with disease diagnosis. Furthermore, during an infectious disease outbreak, telehealth can help people receive normal care and navigate the healthcare system [44].

2.3.5 Health Promotion and Communication

Ensuring healthy behavior through access to relevant health information, education, and communication using digital technologies is very crucial. The public should be aware of the importance, usage, and mechanisms for communication of health information and citizens have a right to receive relevant information about health conditions and services.

In the multidisciplinary field of public health informatics, people are empowered to practice self-care and collaborative decisionmaking by using information technology accessible via the internet, smartphones, or wearables [22].

Rapid technological advancements have altered many facets of human experience, and one area where significant gains in terms of enhancing health and encouraging healthy lifestyle choices are feasible is health promotion. Health promotion and education using technology has the ability to reach more people while yet being user-friendly. Technology's ability to adapt and respond can increase the effectiveness of health promotion and education by delivering messages at a comprehension level that may encourage behavioral change. The ability to reach a wider audience has made technology-based health promotions an effective means of disseminating health messages and health interventions. Technology is far-reaching and linked, which makes it easier to reach more individuals with crucial information, direction, and counseling [45].

The proliferation of mobile phone networks has revolutionized global communications. Mobile technologies can be extremely useful for reaching out to, educating, and connecting with highly mobile population [46]. Today mobile phones with text messaging capabilities are nearly ubiquitous enabling SMS reminders to be considered as one of the many tools used to strengthen the health system [47, 48]. According to the WHO, mHealth can transform the delivery of health care and bring a paradigm shift in healthcare delivery processes [19].

The use of mobile phones has surged in low and middle-income countries, and it presents a significant opportunity to promptly support health systems that are underfunded. Digital communications through text messaging or social networking sites offer an opportunity to improve reach of health information and services to diverse and remote population in the context of Universal Health Coverage, which is arguably a priority for many low-resource regions [49]. To stop avoidable fatalities, behavior change at the population level is required. Communication and media platforms have been used to promote change in health behaviors for decades [50].

PHI is also important for provision of education and awareness activities at population level. In the realm of digital health, education and awareness campaigns mostly focus on using short messaging services to disseminate mass information from source to recipient. SMS messages are delivered straight to users' phones in education and awareness applications, providing information on a range of topics such as disease management, testing and treatment options, and the accessibility of healthcare facilities. Furthermore, SMS offer a means of reaching remote locations, such rural areas, where access to healthcare workers, facilities, and public health education may be limited.

Coordinated communication between providers and clients ultimately leads to better public health care management. The public should be aware of the importance, usage, and mechanisms for communication of health information. For the public health community to function at its best, data from a wide range of sources, both inside and outside the field, must be accessible to be used, and information must be quickly distributed to those who must take action to safeguard the public's health [2]. With this regard, PHI enhances behavior change communication and client education [51]. Research conducted in environments with low resources revealed that the quality of health communication between patients, treatment supports, and clinicians has increased with the advent of SMS-based reminder systems [52–54].

Through digital health, individuals can access information about their own health as well as have a stronger relationship with their public health care provider. For example, many health facilities have digital health portals where individuals can message their providers and receive answers back relatively quickly, rather than needing to wait for their next appointment. With digital health portals, individuals can also meet with the health workers via video chat, which is especially important during the COVID-19 pandemic. For instance, government organizations used social media to encourage citizen participation during the COVID-19 pandemic [22].

PHI also significantly improves attendance to different health service appointments. mHealth services have garnered extensive attention worldwide with a growing trend in harnessing the technology for different health services including behavior change [50]. An RCT study revealed that patients' adherence to TB treatment was greatly increased by a web-based approach that combined weekly refill reminders with daily drug reminders. Additionally, the system has strengthened the bond between health workers and clients [41].

SMS reminders may also contribute to higher vaccination rates and a more favorable public perception of immunization programs. An SMS vaccine reminder system has been suggested as a practical and easily scalable way to reassure caregivers about the value of immunization, address any concerns about vaccine safety, and remind them of vaccination schedules and campaigns as mobile phones become more widely available in Africa. Additionally, SMS can be used to alert caretakers to problems at the medical institution, like stock shortages and lengthy wait times, and advise them to attend another facility or return on a different day [55].

Further, PHI improves access to information and promotes lifestyle changes among the population. The amount of education individuals have access to because of digital health is immense and can lead to lifestyle modifications for individuals who may be at risk for common diseases, such as heart disease or diabetes. Using digital health technologies, individuals can actively manage their own health and monitor any irregularities that they may experience.

PHI also enhances provider-to-provider communication [54]. In order to increase service demand and increase access to health information, digital health interventions could be utilized, for instance, to enable targeted communications to people via reminders and health promotion messaging. Health professionals may also be the target of digital health initiatives, which provide them with faster access to clinical procedures through telemedicine consultations with other health professionals or decision-support tools [56]. Client clinical data may be transmitted asynchronously or synchronously using two-way video conferencing in real time. Apart from conversation, telemedicine can offer health data that is gathered remotely from personal mobile devices or medical equipment. This data could be utilized to follow, observe, or modify the behavior of clients [57].

PHI also leverages digital tools to enhance communication and training for healthcare workers in resource limited settings. Enabling health workers to access information through mobile technology is a solid foundation for empowerment since it gives them the assistance they require to carry out their duties efficiently and independently. Enhancing communication across various health units is also crucial in order to enable more effective patient care. Connecting healthcare professionals to information sources via their mobile phones is a component of mHealth interventions, which fall under the subgroup of communication and training for healthcare workers. Increased information transfer among healthcare professionals and better public health service results are the goals of improved communication.

PHI advances made it possible to detect health hazards more quickly and to communicate health information more fully and effectively, which led to breakthroughs in public health and increased the value of interventions. With the significant rise in information technology invested in healthcare and the key trends toward electronic medical records and personal health records, PHI is now well-positioned to accelerate.

According to a scoping assessment, using digital health promotion and prevention in settings with limited resources can help improve population health, reach particular target groups, and cut implementation costs. Information from digital media is the most essential source, especially for younger people [58]. Additionally, social media is becoming a more powerful tool for health promotion since it provides direct access to pre-existing online social networks. This is made possible by digitalization. Social media allows for the targeting of populations that are frequently difficult to reach through traditional health promotion [59].

Particularly in environments with low resources, the digitization and abundance of digital technologies provide significant promise for health promotion and prevention. To achieve adequate continuity of public health care, a continuous flow of health information is required between systems, healthcare organizations, and even countries. Data gathering, clinical management, administrative procedures, and the care process are all hampered by the information's widespread dispersion and high fragmentation across numerous sources that often operate as silos. No country is immune to this reality, which affects both developed and developing countries [58].

In order to employ digital health systems as a helpful instrument for the successful and efficient delivery of public health services, health care organizations must invest a significant amount of resources in this area. The digital health architecture must also ensure that health information is consistent, accessible and used cost-effectively for improvement of public health services.

2.3.6 Health System Strengthening

The goal of the field of public health informatics is to assist the public health enterprise, which is to enhance population health and well-being. In order to support coordinated health management, enable informed decision-making, empower clients to participate actively in their care decisions, and enhance population health overall, it is imperative that all individuals, their families, and their healthcare providers have appropriate access to health information.

Global health care delivery has changed and improved because of the health information technology. Digital health technologies have the potential to enhance the whole health system's functionality and inter-system interactions [15]. Public health organizations can employ information and communications technologies to gather, store, manage, analyze, use, and communicate data and information. Public health organizations should ideally be able to use the data and information they manage and employ to create policies or carry out initiatives that enhance population health outcomes. Information technology and communications has great role in strengthening healthcare:

- It can reduces overall health care cost
- It improves access of healthcare
- It improves quality of healthcare

A collaborative, people-centered strategy for ongoing health and wellness is made possible by digital health technologies. In contrast to the largely fragmented, reactive health care system that currently exists, it is now possible to envision a system that is more holistic, centers on the needs of the client and their support structure, and embraces a longitudinal view of health, wellness, and social equity that has been resulted from the evolving digital foundation of a person-centered health care system [8]. The success of digital health applications deployed at the level of healthcare organization, service provider, and service user will be enhanced by a supporting health system. Advantages for the healthcare system consist of:

- Better emergency response with instant access to clinical and service data
- A better comprehension of the population's demands for health and service delivery
- Better public health information distribution and encouragement of public dialogue and readiness for significant public health risks
- Increased capacity to track quality and performance metrics for the health system and to spot disparities and relative discrepancy and
- Priorities and insights in health budget allocation supported by data

Digital health services have a significant impact on client health and wellbeing as well as the efficiency of the healthcare system. The implementation of digital health technologies and applications will unavoidably alter the ways in which services are provided. In order to encourage a wider usage of technology in the health system, policies and strategies must be in place. This includes collaborations and engagement with key stakeholders, workforce capability, appropriate governance arrangements, and national digital health policies and initiatives.

Telemedicine is one area of public health informatics that supports the health system [57].The convergence of continuous technological advancements in multimedia, images, computers, information systems, and telecommunications has made telemedicine more feasible today. Telemedicine has demonstrated benefits for public health, including: lessening the burden and distance to access health facilities; lowering health care costs and time; improved outcomes. Additionally, telemedicine facilitates remote training of health care providers by experts in the field; providing clients and healthcare workers with updated health information; and reducing response times for managing epidemics, outbreaks and disasters.

Digitalization of a persons or client's health and medical records is another benefit of an electronic medical record or electronic health record. Even in highly developed nations, there is vari-

ance in the use of EHR in healthcare systems around the world. EMR solutions simplify data systems and improve the provision of healthcare [60]. The health care system is thought to benefit from EMRs in the following ways:

- Safety by lowering medical errors
- Coordination of care
- Communication
- Timely access to medical information
- Improvement of efficiency and effectiveness of care [61].

Improving population accessibility and health service consumption is critical to strengthening the health system in settings with limited resources and delivering faster and longer-lasting improvements in health status [57, 62]. Health decision-makers will be receptive to messages that portray mHealth technology as instruments that can improve the delivery of life-saving therapies through enhancements in health systems performance, such as coverage, quality, equity or efficiency [54].

Applications utilizing mobile phones and other telecommunication technology have a plethora of prospects in developing nations due to declining costs and expanding network coverage. In Africa, mHealth represents a novel method of providing public health services. Particularly in nations where the number of mobile phone subscriptions is rapidly increasing, mHealth may be able to provide answers for healthcare systems in developing nations that are beset by a lack of funding, subpar health information systems, restricted resources, and a shortage of skilled medical personnel [63]. Hence, closing the digital divide and bolstering the delivery of healthcare services will need developing digital leadership abilities and raising the digital literacy of customers and providers [64].

The digital transformation of public health care systems can be disruptive. However, there is evidence that technologies like wearables, artificial intelligence, virtual care, remote monitoring, wearable data capture, tools for data exchange and storage, and tools for sharing pertinent information across the health ecosystem to create a continuum of care can improve health outcomes. This can be accomplished through enhancing medical diagnosis, data-driven treatment choices, patient-centered care, self-management, and person-centered care, as well as by equipping public health personnel with greater evidence-based knowledge, abilities and competence to support healthcare.

Future health care may be more mobile and accurate due to the increasing number of gadgets and equipment becoming smaller and more portable, as well as the likelihood of more targeted treatments. Instead of using paper-based surveys that need to be turned in in person and manually input into the central health database, surveys can be completed more quickly and reliably using smartphones, PDAs or mobile phones. Additionally, there is proof that using IT in primary healthcare can save costs, guarantee service accountability, and assist in changing beneficiaries behaviors in settings with limited resources.

For public health informatics to strengthen the health system, there is a need to:

- Enhance the leadership capacity to execute the digital health strategy initiatives that improves health system responsiveness
- Improve digital health governance for better coordination, implementation and monitoring of digital health initiatives

- Enhance digital health research and innovation to improve clinical practices, decision support and program designs

Enabling people, families, and communities to maintain and enhance their health through timely access to high-quality services provided in a courteous and effective manner is the ultimate goal of any health system. The way the country responds to health risks will be completely transformed by modern, integrated, real-time public health data systems at every level of the health system.

A national ecosystem for public health data is obviously needed, one that can scale and adapt easily to meet evolving public health needs. Using the right technological breakthroughs in public health is essential for the safety, security, and general health of the country [65]. At all health care levels, digital health investment is necessary for long-term improvements in service delivery.

The following (Fig. 2.4) illustrates how the use of public health informatics contributes to improvements in the cost, quality and accessibility of public health services [7].

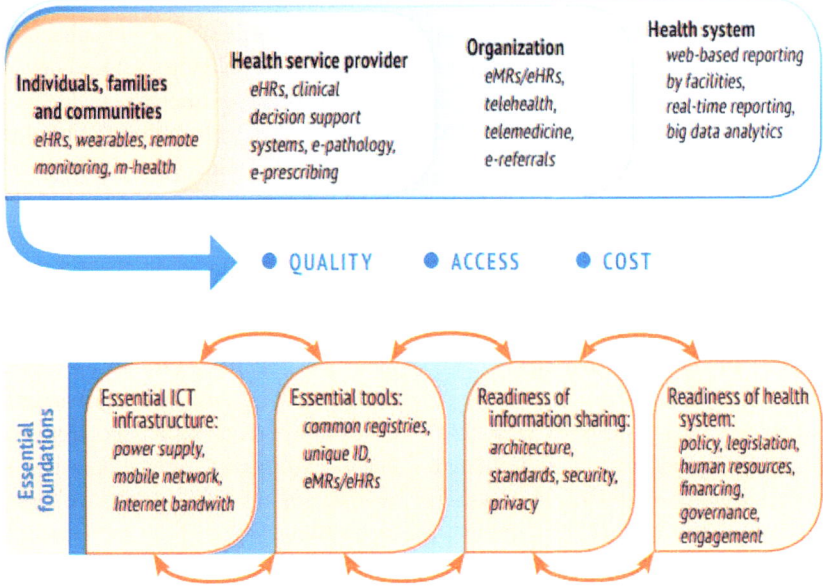

Fig. 2.4 Framework of digital health for improved health service delivery

2.4 Impacts of Public Health Informatics

Improved diagnosis and outcome accuracy, greater client involvement in their care, enhanced care coordination, and enhanced health system efficiency are all made possible by public health informatics. The availability of health information is the main way in which it can enhance the quality and accessibility of health services. PHI makes it possible to exchange and use trustworthy data in an effective and integrated way, even though there are few large-scale sustainable implementations in developing nations.

Technology's use in preventive health showed informatics' capacity to raise the standard and timeliness of preventive care while keeping costs down. PHI provides information to make decisions that leads to better health outcomes of the population.

It helps to:

- Permit greater access to care
- Improve quality and safety of public health services
- Drive down the cost of health care
- Minimize health inequalities
- Involve clients and their families
- Enhance care coordination
- Maintain privacy & security of client information
- Greater accountability and effectiveness
- More reliable information about health systems

The major impacts of public health informatics are discussed below.

2.4.1 Quality of Health Services

Interactions between the client, other stakeholders, and the interdisciplinary team of healthcare experts are necessary in the extremely transaction-intensive healthcare area. To enable continuity of care, high-quality healthcare necessitates efficient teamwork and the capacity to exchange crucial information among all parties involved.

Hence, the field of health informatics has great promise for optimizing clinical workflow by augmenting and broadening the health worker's capacity to handle public health care data and information.

It guarantees that trustworthy and high-quality data are accessible when needed and that sharing that data among healthcare professionals is simple. Public health care may suffer if pertinent discussions, information, and guidelines are not coordinately shared. PHI paves the way by streamlining the collaboration required to deliver high-quality public health services. ICT has the ability to completely change the way healthcare is delivered by making it more easily accessible, reasonably priced, and efficient in providing high-quality medical treatment [19].

Furthermore, client rights, present work practices, and legal obligations of healthcare providers may all be impacted by the secure administration of electronic medical information. If medical professionals have access to all pertinent patient medical history, they can make the best judgments regarding patient care. Lack of access to data could negatively affect patient care by delaying clinical treatment choices. Therefore, enhancing the safety culture in public health care is crucial to preventing or minimizing errors and raising the standard of quality care generally.

PHI primarily focuses on enhancing the use of digital health technology by clients and healthcare providers to improve health service supply procedures, as well as the quality of services and citizens' well-being, by facilitating easy access to data for decision-making by all stakeholders. PHI can also be thought of as a way to guarantee that, in order to maximize accessibility and quality of health care delivery, the appropriate health information is given to the right person at the right time in a secure electronic format. PHI should also be seen as a major enabler and driver of better health outcomes for a population, as well as the vital infrastructure supporting information sharing amongst all parties involved in a healthcare system.

The enhancement of healthcare and the health system as a whole depends critically on having access to timely and high-quality health information at all decision-making stages. PHI guarantees data quality for clinical and public health practices that are grounded in evidence. It gives health workers in practice optimism for better access to client-specific data and should have a significant positive impact on both the standard of care and their own well-being.

The EMR, is a fundamental tool for utilizing ICT to enhance the quality and continuity of healthcare services. It facilitates the gathering, sharing, and tracking of health-related data. It is generally acknowledged as a vital health IT tool for raising the standard of healthcare [60]. Additionally, research demonstrates that EMRs can enhance data quality by capturing patient data and carrying out medical tasks [66]. Health professionals may examine client histories more rapidly using the EHR systems, which enhances the responsiveness and quality of public health care by making it easier to obtain health data [28]. Additionally, PHI enhances the delivery of high-quality healthcare, for instance by enabling remote monitoring, consultation, diagnosis, and treatment. One way to enhance the delivery of public health care in settings with limited resources is to use PHI in telemedicine and telehealth.

Additionally, new avenues for addressing health system issues are presented by digital technologies, which provide an opportunity to improve the accessibility and caliber of medical procedures and services [56]. One benefit of digital health is the enhancement of the caliber of medical services through electronic decision assistance. By urging frontline healthcare providers to adhere to predetermined criteria, mHealth projects that integrate point-of-care decision support tools with automated algorithm- or rule-based instructions can ensure quality of treatment in these task-shifting scenarios. In situations where resources are scarce, electronic decision support technologies can also be used to identify and rank high-risk clients for medical attention [54].

Better overall healthcare management, higher-quality care, more focused and efficient workflows leading to increased productivity, more administrative efficiency, fewer medical errors, improved client communication, and reduced health care costs are some of the common advantages of PHI. Below is a summary of how PHI can improve the quality of care.

2.4.1.1 Record Keeping
Using informatics technology to store public health data increases security. Data and files stored on paper are more prone to being forgotten or lost. PHI successfully addresses this since access to computer-based records can be regulated and monitored, and they are more secure than paper-based records. Better administration of client records has been made possible by the transformation of client record keeping through the usage of EHR.

2.4.1.2 Record Retrieval
Health record retrieval is improved with informatics. Recognizing the existence of a patient's medical records is crucial to providing high-quality care that addresses each patient's unique needs.

2.4.1.3 Sharing Health Information
Optimizing information storage and retrieval is the goal of PHI, allowing health workers to exchange pertinent information more securely and effectively while also improving patient care. Health information exchange is a significant application of PHI. PHI facilitates better patient information standards, which facilitates practice streamlining for aspiring medical professionals. This raises the standard of care by enabling them to make decisions in concert.

2.4.1.4 Avoiding Errors
Clinical judgments and care that are not optimal are caused by missing knowledge. EHR, for example, helps prevent mistakes. For example, automated patient dosage calculation systems may potentially help to improve the standard of healthcare delivery by preventing mistakes in this domain.

2.4.1.5 Client & Community Participation
Clients have self-access to their medical records at any time, which empowers them to take control of their own health and comprehend their

situation. In addition to providing a better path to receiving the necessary medical care, comprehensive health tracking allows clients to take part in the decision-making process. Patients who have electronic access to their personal health records and recommendations are better able to take charge of their own health, which raises standards of care.

2.4.2   Equity in Health Services

Disparities are systematic inequalities that are determined by one's social place, which is controlled by broader systems of power, rather than just variances in health practices and outcomes across some groups [67].

Since a big portion of the current data on health inequalities is gathered at the population level, it frequently takes a long time for the data to be genuinely distributed in the field. How to effectively use this data in the community healthcare sector is still a gap in the healthcare field.

In order to achieve fairness in healthcare, health facilities must prioritize the elimination of unnecessary obstacles that hinder access to medical services. It is crucial to thoroughly examine and pinpoint the particular inequalities that prevent specific groups of clients from receiving timely and suitable care. Subsequently, exploring digital solutions becomes essential to address these disparities effectively.

The discipline of health informatics has the potential to make a significant contribution by providing extra knowledge that will aid in better assessing and comprehending the inequities that various demographic groups encounter. In particular, population healthcare delivery systems and public health organizations can function as knowledge hubs for information regarding the factors that contribute to health disparities if they are planned and executed in a an organized manner. To promote equitable healthcare delivery and address health inequalities more effectively, the utilization of this extensive flow of data becomes imperative.

It is crucial to integrate social evaluation into information systems, including Electronic Medical Record (EMR). This integration will enable the identification of potential risks and determinant factors that may disproportionately impact risk groups of the population, leading to increased health related risks and unfavorable health and health related outcomes. Healthcare management, health workers, clients, and policymakers may find it easier to discover health inequalities with the gathering and analysis of this data on health behaviors and outcomes. It may also be possible to determine what variables may be linked to or potentially cause these disparities [67].

Multiple reports have indicated the potential contribution of public health informatics to the reduction of health disparities in underprivileged groups. Public health informatics have the potential to capture social determinants of health to bring in-depth understanding of the factors affecting health and well-being.

Addressing structural power as it affects both individual health and the gathering, usage, administration, storage, and exchange of data within the healthcare system is necessary for achieving equity in digital health. Digital health emphasizes technological access and digital knowledge, which changes the already unequal landscape of health determinants. Significant changes must be made to all facets of healthcare and health in order to address health disparities [68].

The discipline of health informatics has the potential to make a significant contribution by providing extra knowledge that will aid in better assessing and comprehending the inequities that various demographic groups encounter. The abundance of data, expertise, and information may then be applied to more effectively address health inequities and deliver healthcare that is more equitable [67]. Moreover, healthcare systems use electronic health records (EHRs) to gather information on the socioeconomic determinants of health [46, 69].

Furthermore, health care ecosystems and public health organizations should use population health informatics tools to identify the factors exacerbating health disparities that impact socially disadvantaged populations [70]. It is crucial to understand, too, that not all communities have easy access to high-quality demographic data or the means to gather, share, or analyze data in order to spot or keep track of health disparities among marginalized or minority groups. The implementation of PHI may also make it easier to create and monitor over time established quality metrics of health equality that health systems can employ to lessen inequities, cut costs associated with medical care, and ultimately improve patient outcomes [46, 69].

By expanding access to healthcare, meeting unmet needs, individualized patient care, and taking into account the historical background of the communities they serve, digital tools can enhance equity. Digital technology can reduce the disparity in access to healthcare in a number of ways, including by expediting complex medical bureaucracy procedures and removing travel and transportation barriers. By lowering the time it takes to get care, the expense of delivering care, and the requirement that patients and clinicians share a physical location, telehealth may result in greater accessibility to healthcare. However, by restricting access for individuals with impairments and others with limited access to high-bandwidth technology or digital literacy, there is also a chance that this could exacerbate health disparities. Telehealth could result in care for existing medically marginalized areas missing important examinations on a regular basis if it is the primary tactic used to lower access barriers [68].

Participating in the community fosters innovation and offers chances to support technology developments aimed at preventing health disparities. More effective interventions result from their insightful viewpoints on addressing population health within the framework of their social and physical settings. The following are recommended best practices for the strategic planning and execution of health informatics interventions in underserved populations [70]:

- In order to examine how different technologies respond to and produce varied outcomes, and to counteract privileged access to certain population segments, it is important to increase the recruitment.
- Make use of reliable social networks and well-established stakeholders to learn about the assets and strengths of marginalized populations.
- Recognize the social context of target audiences and possible end users in order to comprehend the social determinants of health and how they are entwined with systems of inequality in marginalized areas.
- Incorporate community involvement through participatory or user-centered design to better understand the needs and preferences of potential end users in order to create treatments that are meaningful and culturally appropriate.
- Acquire knowledge of the technological infrastructure of community partners in order to develop capacity and enhance community-based health informatics interventions.

One of the promises of digital health is that it will increase health care equity, but there is also a real risk that it could widen the divide between the "haves" and the "have-nots". Effective computer use is impossible for those without the resources, know-how, or access to computers and networks. Further, despite the potential benefits of digital health in closing gaps in health equity, there are valid concerns about how these exciting technical advancements could have unforeseen implications, such as maintaining health and health care disparities for underserved people. If health equity considerations are not given particular attention during the design, implementation, and assessment stages, the rapid spread of digital health techniques poses a risk of exacerbating rather than mitigating pre-existing health inequities.

In order to mitigate this possible pitfall, it is essential for the health informatics scientific communities to understand the difficulties faced by marginalized groups that hinder their ability to achieve ideal health. In order to truly achieve health equity for all, evidence also suggests that community participation is integrated into the development of data-driven, updated solutions for every sector of society [70].

Unless political measures secure equitable access for all, these populations which would really benefit the most from health information are the least likely to profit from developments in information technology. It appears that UHC and digital health are closely related. Therefore, reducing public health disparities requires enhancing health care delivery for all people, everywhere by speeding up the creation and uptake of suitable, cheap, scalable, and sustainable digital health solutions.

2.4.3   Access to Health Care

A large portion of the population in many developing countries, particularly in rural regions, lacks access to the public health care system as a result of a lack of resources, inefficiencies in the system, and a lack of knowledge about the services that are available. People in settings with low resources are unable to receive basic health care because they lack the resources to pay for it, it is too distant from their homes, or there is a paucity of trained health personnel, supplies, or medication.

One of the main obstacles to reaching the aim of UHC is the absence of access for populations that are difficult to reach. Besides, a lot of programs continue to address particular health issues in a "silo" or vertical manner, ignoring the advantages of more comprehensive, people-centered, cross-sectoral collaboration for better service delivery. Moreover, low middle income countries are facing issues like rising healthcare costs, shifting demographics, aging populations, shifting disease burdens, maintaining a health workforce, and rising community expectations.

Effective service delivery is the cornerstone of UHC. One of the main obstacles to reaching UHC is expanding access to high-quality services for both individuals and the general public. As the population ages and non-communicable diseases become more prevalent, there is a growing demand for primary and secondary prevention strategies, seamless care coordination across various levels of services, and a comprehensive approach that involves relevant stakeholders in collaborative healthcare delivery.

PHI could enhance the provision of healthcare services and promote universal access to care.

PHI helps to improve equitable access to health services through the state-of-the-art and remotely accessible technology solutions. It also enhances access and quality of health services through digitally enabled, client centered and community based tracking, service delivery and management of referral in the continuum of care. As the public face of UHC, ICT has a great deal of potential to improve healthcare delivery.

Numerous advances, such as the electronic health record, artificial intelligence, wearable technology, mobile health, sensors, wearable devices, Internet of things, big data, and other applications, have affected access to healthcare services [28]. EHRs and telemedicine are two fundamental digital health tools that have been widely adopted by wildly disparate nations in an effort to lower access barriers and raise service quality. Underserved or previously unreached areas are covered by telemedicine. Advancements in mobile collaboration technologies can also facilitate information sharing and in-person discussions about client concerns between healthcare professionals who work in different places [7].

Using public health informatics, more people can obtain care. Because many nations have implemented lockdowns and physical segregation, COVID-19 has brought about new realities when it comes to receiving healthcare services through telehealth and telemedicine services. Rapid surveillance systems and telemedicine are utilized to enhance community well-being, healthcare quality, and access to services. Today, clients can consult with physicians more easily, no matter where they are in the world, thanks to data-driven telemedicine systems, virtual health care systems, and linked vital sign monitoring technology.

People in general and clients in particular have benefited from the use of digital health by being able to access healthcare services remotely or at the point of care. The medical and public health communities have also shown a great deal of interest in digital health, particularly in low- and middle-income nations where mobile connectivity has created a new avenue for addressing the geographic inaccessibility of healthcare [56].

One of the main obstacles to promoting UHC is expanding equitable access to high-quality care. As nations move closer to UHC, digital health is revolutionizing the quality and accessibility of health services while also keeping costs under control. Ensuring access to high-quality healthcare services, particularly for marginalized populations, is vital for every country striving towards UHC. Information and communications technology (ICT), which includes e-health, has the potential to enhance preventive health care, raise the standard of care, lower costs for service providers and patients alike, and increase the accessibility of health services for the underprivileged, the vulnerable, the poor, and those residing in remote areas.

Digital health plays a significant role in enhancing the delivery of health services and can also be used to prevent health issues, enhance care quality and lower family health expenditures. Ethiopia has adopted the Electronic Community Health Information System (eCHIS) to enhance access to public health services and reach a large number of households [71].

Governments are working harder to improve health systems so that care is more accessible to those who need it. Most mHealth interventions in Africa, especially those aimed at the general public rather than health or data professionals, have relied on comparatively basic mobile technology and equipment [28]. Similarly, mobile health technology and other digital health efforts were created to provide low- and middle-income areas with improved access. The field of global health research is increasingly focusing on mobile health (mHealth) interventions due to their ability to reach remote populations and underprivileged communities through novel means [72].

In places where the infrastructure for traditional health services or the internet (or other technologies) is lacking but mobile communications technology infrastructure has been given priority, it can be leveraged to improve access to and delivery of health care. It is less expensive to supply the mobile communications technology than it is to provide in-person services.

Mobile health interventions that aim to enhance the processes involved in the delivery of health care services have been applied to target consumer-provider communication. By enabling the exchange of patient and service data through mechanisms and bringing services to underprivileged communities and rural populations, mHealth can help achieve universal health coverage (UHC).

In general, reaching UHC will depend heavily on the application of digital health. The swift advancement of digital health technologies and applications is contributing to the revolution of services. In order to improve services and address national health priorities, governments should choose the right digital health applications at the individual, service provider, health-care organization, and health-system levels. This will maximize the benefits of digital health for service delivery. Moreover, new or piloted digital health applications should have their worth evaluated before being scaled up, with an emphasis on lower unit costs of healthcare and improved quality and access, through an evaluation of measurable outcomes at various levels.

2.4.4   Health Service Coverage

Digital health solutions should facilitate the transition from disease silos to resilient health systems that can provide universal access to people-centered health care [28]. As countries work toward achieving universal health coverage, digital health solutions as a critical facilitator of health information across the range of data, analytics, and knowledge strengthen health systems. Integrated digital solutions, when fully functioning and optimized, have the potential to favorably influence sustainable health outcomes, including agreed-upon sustainable development goals and targets in settings with limited resources [73]. The Agenda for Sustainable Development also emphasizes how global interconnectedness and the growth of ICTs have the potential to significantly speed up human progress, close the digital divide, and expand access to and coverage of public health services in settings with limited resources [74].

The global community increasingly recognizes the importance of leveraging innovative digital technologies as a vital catalyst for achieving broader access to universal health coverage, enhancing protection against health emergency, and promoting improved health and well-being in a resource limited setting.

Nevertheless, other obstacles hamper in our way of achieving the UHC, the major among them being the substantial financial and operational expenditures associated with providing health care to a large number of people while simultaneously upholding a respectable standard of care. It has now become clear that we may not be able to deliver on universal health coverage unless we change the ways we deliver care and manage our health care systems. Therefore, creative methods of providing critical services in today's social and economic contexts that can guarantee universal coverage are empirical. The world has recently come to acknowledge digital health as a tool for innovation to address these issues and progress the SDGs and UHC's achievement.

In the near future, digital technologies have the potential to revolutionize how people interact with digital health services and solutions. As a result, PHI is essential to the cause of universal health coverage in many different ways. For example, it assists in providing Telehealth or mHealth services to underprivileged communities and rural people. By using electronic health records to provide precise and fast patient information, it improves diagnosis and treatment. Additionally, by strategically utilizing ICT, health care systems operational and financial efficiency are enhanced, improving health service coverage in environments with limited resources [75].

Public health informatics can be used to detect and address sociocultural, physical, and financial barriers to equitable access and improved health service coverage. It can also be applied to the delivery of remote health care services, which improves access to health care services, particularly for those in hard-to-reach areas.

The WHO's third global study on eHealth states that digital health technologies are essential to achieving UHC, particularly in settings with limited resources. It seems that the rise in UHC, HIS, and eHealth are closely related. The evaluation also showed that countries are becoming more interested in eHealth and its expanding importance in healthcare [28].

Effective digital health interventions contributed to improving health service coverage [76]. An RCT study validated the beneficial impact of an SMS-based mobile phone intervention on the majority of the chosen MCH service indicators, such as improvements in the percentage of ANC visits that are advised, the percentage of deliveries that are attended by health professionals, and the provision of PNC services in rural areas [77].

Additionally, a review emphasizes the potential advantages of using mobile text message reminders to enhance the management of childhood vaccination schedules and healthcare appointment attendance, particularly in low- and middle-income nations [72, 78, 79]. Interventions using mobile phones can help increase vaccination service acceptance. Text message reminders can be used to augment the routine vaccination program in resource-constrained situations. An RCT study in a resource limited setting found that mobile phone text message reminders significantly enhanced complete and timely receipt of all recommended vaccines [80].

2.4.5 Efficiency of Health Services

Public health infrastructures are built by societies to monitor and safeguard communities. Strong ICT systems, competent public health workers, and efficient organizations are characteristics of a prepared, competent public health infrastructure. However, public health organizations that aim to modernize and develop the public health infrastructure face many obstacles, such as the quickly advancing ICT and the growing workload of public health personnel. Organizations must put in place a technology architecture that permits integration across public health information silos in order to address the issues facing the field. In order to accommodate the evolving work patterns in public health, organizations must also restructure their work processes and system interfaces for better efficiency [4].

The fields of technology, information, and health are all evolving quickly. There are exciting chances to stay up to date with this transition and find innovative informatics solutions to ensure universal health care. If public health informatics is supported by enough funding for institutional, workforce, and governance capacity to enable changes in digital systems and data use training, planning, and management that are necessary as health systems and services become more digitally connected, it has the potential to drastically alter health outcomes. Digital health can increase the effectiveness and cost-effectiveness of care by making this crucial investment in people and procedures, in keeping with national strategies that outline a vision for the digitalization of the health sector. This will open the door to new business models for the provision of public health services [10].

The utilization of digital health technologies facilitates fair and inclusive access to basic healthcare, while simultaneously enhancing the sustainability and efficiency of health care system in delivering affordable and better quality care. Along with technological advancements, the confluence of substantial investments in health technology, is shaping the landscape of digital health information systems.

Healthcare costs continue to rise and public health informatics reduces healthcare costs. The potential for cost savings in healthcare through increased efficiency is one of the promises of public health informatics. Avoiding redundant or needless preventative or promotional actions, improving opportunities for communication amongst healthcare practitioners, and involving the public and community are a few potential ways to cut expenses. Hence, strengthening availability & efficiency of health information systems can avail high-quality data and enable health managers to plan, administer and monitor health systems effectively.

For instance, by lowering the cost of travel to see a specialist, telemedicine lowers the opportunity costs for individuals seeking care. It reduces the need for travel and promotes resource effi-

ciency. Further, data suggested that provider-to-provider telemedicine could enhance the effectiveness of health workers, shorten the time it takes for clients to receive follow-up or appropriate treatment, and shorten the duration of stay for clients and communities in low- and middle-income countries [56, 81, 82].

The capacity to collect large amounts of data in safe cloud storage has shown to be economical and beneficial in reducing healthcare expenses. Furthermore, fraud, errors, and financial losses from things like missed appointments and delayed medical care are reduced with the use of health informatics.

Role of public health informatics on improving efficiency of public health services includes:

- Enhancing the availability of public health information (from any location and at any time)
- Merging data from various external & internal sources, and
- Facilitating coordination of public health care delivery

Due to its ability to allocate scarce health resources to the most critical areas, digital technology holds great promise for closing gaps in the delivery of healthcare. People can receive the care they require more promptly with the use of informatics. By greatly expanding access to health data and granting individuals more control over their health, digital tools also provide healthcare providers with a comprehensive picture of the health of their clients. Better medical outcomes and greater efficiency are the end results. Additionally, evidence suggests that the benefits of digitalizing health care outweigh the expenses involved.

Although the incorporation of digital health has shown advantages for population health and increased effectiveness in the provision of treatment, it has also occasionally revealed and intensified a number of long-standing disparities in healthcare systems and society at large. The field of digital health is growing quickly and contributing to increased healthcare efficiency. Many healthcare organizations and providers adopted digital health even before the COVID-19 pandemic in an effort to reduce costs, enhance access to care, and boost productivity [46].

2.4.6 Safety Health Services

As a subset of healthcare, client safety is the avoidance, prevention, and mitigation of unfavorable consequences or injuries resulting from medical procedures [83]. Enhancing the safety culture in the medical field is crucial to lowering or eliminating errors and raising the standard of care generally. It is vital and essential to monitor and manage the safety of public health services.

In order to meet the needs of the population, healthcare requirements are increasingly becoming demand-driven. Healthcare organization's top priority is patient safety. Moreover, clients want to control when and how they interact with their healthcare system. It will be a struggle for governments, health authorities, and the medical community to give clients the knowledge and resources they need to make informed healthcare decisions.

In order for health care providers to deliver exceptional care, enhance patient outcomes, lower infection rates, avoid major adverse events, manage near misses, and standardize treatments using evidence-based public health, it is essential to be able to record and measure patient safety. By reporting patient safety incidents and preventive events, it is possible to make sure that the knowledge gleaned from a client's experience is applied to lower the likelihood that future clients would encounter a similar situation.

Numerous opportunities exist for healthcare improvement and transformation through the use of health information technology, including the reduction of human error, enhancement of clinical outcomes, facilitation of care coordination, improvement of practice efficiencies, and long-term data tracking.

By increasing adherence to recommended practices, health information technology also improves the safety of healthcare. Without a doubt, health information technology plays a significant role in enhancing the quality and safety of healthcare, but healthcare companies must exercise caution when deciding which technologies to invest in [83].

Health workers require high-quality data from numerous sources to make evidence-based decision, which can only be achieved through digital systems such as electronic health records. Based on a review, there is strong evidence that using an electronic medical record increases patient safety and lowers medical errors. Decision support systems are the best health information technology available for enhancing patient safety. Health care professionals receive knowledge and patient-specific data from clinical decision support.

Clinical decision support encompasses a range of tools aimed at enhancing clinical decision and health system process [57]. Clinical decision assistance, complete patient data availability, clinical flags and reminders, improved recording and reporting of consultations and diagnostic testing, and medication alarms all have the potential to increase patient safety. It has been shown that data acquired via health IT can be utilized to assess the effectiveness of therapeutic interventions and enhance medical practice. Alerts have the potential to improve evidence-based care and standards adherence. In order to minimize practice variances, optimize evidence-based care for common conditions, and conduct systematic audits for quality assurance, record consistency might be designed.

Patient safety and quality should remain top priorities as more health IT systems are implemented and used. All aspects of health IT require improvement, particularly in terms of platform integration, design, and implementation inside the workplace. For safe care, robust system interoperability is essential.

By streamlining communication between healthcare professionals, enhancing drug safety, tracking, and reporting, and fostering quality of care through optimal access to and adherence to guidelines, public health informatics enhances the safety of public health services [57]. Prescription errors and dangerous treatments can be avoided with the aid of informatics.

Utilizing informatics technology ensures the security of patient data. Electronic health record systems provide encrypted and secure patient data storage through the use of cutting-edge computing technologies. Not only is the data stored securely, but patients and healthcare professionals also have more reliable access to it, which cuts down on any delays that may otherwise prevent the provision of efficient, patient-centered treatment. The results of patient care improve in tandem with advances in health science and technology.

In order to identify the best patterns of care, major healthcare companies and governmental organizations are realizing the importance of information found in digital technology. The development of adaptable, component-based technological architecture will enable patients to take a more active and proactive part in their own health, making future health care more accurate and mobile. Privacy and information security are becoming more and more important challenges in the healthcare industry. However, there are still significant barriers to its adoption, including growing concerns about healthcare coverage, privacy, and particularly the security of EHRs.

Healthcare facilities, providers, and patients all still want guarantees that these documents are kept safe. As a result, as the usage of EHRs has grown over time, procedural, professional, social, political, and particularly ethical issues, as well as the requirement for information security and standard compliance, have continued to take precedence over technical issues. Health businesses can protect patient privacy by strictly adhering to encryption protocols, privacy and security regulations, audit trails, and access limits.

Research revealed that enhancing clinical decision-making and patient information security and privacy requires the use of electronic medical records [61]. While maintaining patient privacy and confidentiality, electronic medical records encompass various health service units. According to a study assessing community-based remote patient monitoring, or Telemonitoring, patients with a number of chronic illnesses, such as heart failure, stroke, COPD, asthma, and hypertension, have better patient outcomes [57].

2.4.7 Responsiveness of the Health System

In order to fulfill the demands of the twenty-first century and beyond, public health service must be reengineered. The creation of systems that can gather, process, and transform data into forms that are meaningful has been a basic challenge of public health practice from the earliest days of traditional machines to the most advanced public health systems of today. Modern public health information and data management systems have, for the most part, developed in tandem with the science behind public health practice.

The complexity of the information systems required for gathering and comprehending higher volumes of data, as well as the analytical systems required for processing those data, has increased. The systems that are currently necessary for the practice of public health can now be automated by applying the technological advancements [4].

For the purpose of making decisions, all aspects of the health system depend on the fast, reliable, and accurate availability of information. It has also been demonstrated that, in an environment with limited resources, it is possible to use a wide range of IT solutions to improve the health system [28].

Significant changes are occurring in the field of public health, including the quickening pace of technological advancements, the growing adoption of electronic health records, and health reform. It takes expertise to manage and operate within the adaptive complexity of the underlying societal structures and functions in order to improve population health. Technology advancements and significant modifications to existing structures and functions present a plethora of potential for improving efficiency and developing responsive health systems.

In order to solve complicated health problems and find informatics solutions, multidisciplinary practice, research, and teaching are needed. The WHO survey indicates that governments in low- and middle-income nations are showing interest in digital health as an additional tactic for bolstering health systems and accomplishing the SDGs related to health [19].

The health sector must transition from outdated, custom-based technology to more contemporary technology because ICTs completely changed the way information is managed. This progress is accelerated even further by the degree of technological innovation in the industry. This force can be understood as the technology environment's stimulant and the health systems response to capitalize on its advantages. The community is also empowered to work toward realizing the goal of health for all through the use of digital health technology by the consumers and healthcare providers [10].

For public health officials, embracing the information technology revolution and integrating it into various facets of healthcare has become imperative. Adopting new information systems, using electronic techniques for disease surveillance, and revamping outdated procedures are all ways that clients, healthcare providers, and public health officials can contribute to the transformation of public health.

In summary, PHI improves various aspects of public health systems responsiveness by:

- Encouraging evidence-based practice and error reduction
- Supporting the delivery of public health services tailored to communities
- Encouraging community empowerment and participation in health decision-making
- Decreasing waiting times and waste, optimizing procedures, and increasing cost-efficiency
- Improving communication between providers (e.g., EHR facilitate the exchange of information between collaborating providers)
- Improving data/information aggregation by supporting the creation of groups and summaries from big volumes of public health data
- Improving access to knowledge bases: Public health informatics provide contextual access to knowledge bases when providers need it
- Integration with clinical decision support system (CDSS): one of the main reasons for collecting public health data in a controlled manner is to offer support for health care decisions in the form of reminders and alerts
- Improved data integrity: better organized, accurate, complete data will be obtained with PHI

- Improved productivity: access data whenever, wherever for timely decision
- Increased quality of public health services
- Increased satisfaction for the community: easy access to client data and related public health services

The role of public health informatics for public healthcare organizations, healthcare providers, and the community/clients is described below.

2.4.7.1 For Healthcare Organization
- Enhances accountability and openness of health care processes across institutional and geographical borders
- Enhances cost-effectiveness and resource distribution via streamlined procedures, shorter wait times and fewer mistakes
- Enhances oversight of referral system operations
- Better record security
- Fewer lost records
- Instant notice of eligibility or procedure authorization
- Decreases need and cost for record storage of public health data or information
- Decreases length of stay due to waiting
- Increases compliance with regulatory requirements

2.4.7.2 For Public Health Care Provider
- Improved documentation and reporting
- Decreased redundant data collection
- Allowed data comparison from prior visits
- Ongoing access and update of public health record
- Improved documentation and quality of care
- Supported timely decision
- Better/faster/simultaneous data access
- Prompted to ensure administration of public health interventions
- Supported automation of critical pathways/ workflows
- Improved efficiency: eligibility, early warning of status changes
- Early warning and prediction of public health problems
- Capacity to deliver personalized healthcare tailored to an individual's health status, needs,

and choices by utilizing extensive and ongoing data for that individual
- Increases precision in diagnosis and treatment, for instance, via the use of decision support systems that issue alarms and prompts and through risk or health status screening of individuals

2.4.7.3 For Community/Clients
- Increases access to information and health education program
- Reduces treatment waiting times
- Enhances access to and management of health information
- Enhances application of best practices and decision assistance
- Enhances capacity to pose well-informed inquiries
- Increases responsibility for own public health service
- Reminds and alerts regarding scheduled exams and appointments
- Enhances contentment and comprehension of options

2.4.8 Health System Resilience

The field of public health is charged with safeguarding and enhancing community health via the delivery of efficient and effective education, promotion of healthy lifestyles, and illness and injury prevention. These include longer life expectancies, lower rates of chronic illnesses, and maternal and newborn deaths. But in order to tackle public health issues in an efficient manner, researchers and practitioners demand fast and accurate information that supports evidence-based decision-making.

In underprivileged areas or when human and health system resources are limited, public health service delivery procedures and health worker mobilization might be difficult. To address these issues, digital health approaches and capacity building have been widely used in low- and middle-income countries [76]. This is required because, in addition to facilitating the flow of products and services more quickly, globaliza-

tion has opened up new avenues for the spread of illness and other dangers to public health. It is essential to prepare adequately for these threats and occurrences in order to prevent panic and ensure public safety. Making a resilient health system through the use of technology and informatics in public health delivery is one of the methods to realize this [7].

Inadequate response or adaptation of healthcare systems to unfavorable occurrences such as pandemics, particularly in resource-constrained environments, is another obstacle in the delivery of healthcare. Additionally, to track and analyze epidemics or dangers and speed up response times for early warning systems, better information management resources and technologies as well as improved communication are needed.

In the digital health era, when public health services are being disrupted by multifaceted factors, countries need to have a way of tapping the potential of digital health technologies. Informatics and information technology usage have increased dramatically in this information-driven era due to the mounting demands for population-centered, evidence-based public health and real-time response [84].

Information technology has been adopted by the public health and medical care systems as a potent, revolutionary tool for improving outcomes and fostering change in the delivery of public health services. This can eventually improve the equity, quality, and accessibility of healthcare delivery at all levels. In an environment with limited resources, public health informatics generates durable, cost-effective, and benefit-driven solutions that have the capacity to grow in the future. Application of information communication and technology for the service delivery, application development and infrastructure improvement of the health sector to improve the health delivery system is also very critical for developing countries [76].

ICTs can be included into healthcare systems to help identify and/or prevent unfavorable public health incidents. The new COVID-19 pandemic, a serious public health emergency, highlights the pressing need for safe, efficient, and evidence-based digital health implementations. The

COVID-19 pandemic has highlighted the potential that information and communication technologies (ICTs) offer, including the uptake of online consultations by health professionals and other creative approaches to delivering healthcare in spite of travel restrictions, public health laws, and anxiety associated with in-person appointments.

To maintain resilience in the event of any of these future unfavorable events, it is necessary to rethink how ICTs could be implemented in healthcare after the COVID-19 pandemic. Using ICTs to build resilient healthcare systems illustrates the range of ways that ICTs may help healthcare systems become more robust. PHI contributes to the analysis, design, implementation, and evaluation of information systems that improve clinical and public health outcomes and processes, improve interactions between clients and healthcare providers and the health system, and increase community and individual capacity to manage health during pandemics and crises in environments with limited resources [76].

The increasing demands, constantly evolving processes, and other influences that potentially shape how health care will be provided in the future are the things the health sector needs to consider. Given the vast constraints for the health sector, the opportunities for implementation of digital health solutions are extensive where the appropriateness of the solution and involving emerging technologies shall be prioritized [56].

References

1. Winslow C. The untilled fields of public health. Science. 1920;51:23–33.
2. O'Carroll PW, Ripp LH, Yasnoff WA, Ward ME, Martin EL. Public health informatics and information systems. New York: Springer; 2003.
3. Imhoff M, Webb A, Goldschmidt A. Health informatics. Intensive Care Med. 2001;27(1):179–86.
4. Magnuson JA, Fu PC Jr. Public health informatics and information systems. Oregon Health and Science University. London: Springer; 2014.
5. Friede A, Blum HL, McDonald M. Public health informatics: how information-age technology can strengthen public health. Annu Rev Public Health. 1995;16:239–52.
6. Yasnoff WA, Carroll PW, Koo D, Linkins RW, Killourne EM. Public health informatics: improving and trasforming public health in the information age. J Public Heal Manag Pract. 2000;6:67–75.
7. Dixon BE. Applied public health informatics: an ehealth discipline focused on populations. J Int Soc Telemed eHealth. 2020;8:e14.
8. European Union. Assessing the impact of digital transformation of health services. European Union; 2019.
9. Aziz HA. A review of the role of public health informatics in healthcare. J Taibah Univ Med Sci. 2017;12(1):78–81.
10. World Health Organization. Global strategy on digital health 2020–2025. Geneva: World Health Organization; 2021.
11. Athavale AV, Zodpey SP. Public health informatics in India: the potential and the challenges. Indian J Public Health. 2010;54(3):131–6.
12. Dani N, Sood SP, Prakash N, Mbarika V, Agrawal R. GIS and telemedicine: tools for public healthcare. e Health. 2006;1:11.
13. McNabb SJN, Ryland P, Sylvester J, Shaikh A. Informatics enables public health surveillance. J Health Spec. 2017;5:55–9.
14. Massoudi BL, Sobolevskaia D. Keep moving forward: health informatics and information management beyond the COVID-19 pandemic. IMIA Yearb Med Informatics. 2021;30(1):75–83.
15. Hoyt RE, Sutton M, Yoshihashi A. Medical informatics: practical guide for the healthcare professional. 3rd ed. Pensacola: University of West Florida; 2009.
16. Getachew E, Adebeta T, Muzazu SGY, Charlie L, Said B, Tesfahunei HA, Wanjiru CL, Acam J, Kajogoo VD, Solomon S, Atim MG, Manyazewal T. Digital health in the era of COVID-19: reshaping the next generation of healthcare. Front Public Health. 2023;11:942703.
17. Mustafa UK, Kreppel KS, Brinkel J, Sauli E. Digital technologies to enhance infectious disease surveillance in Tanzania: a scoping review. Healthcare (Basel). 2023;11(4):470.
18. Perrin PB, Pierce BS, Elliott TR. COVID-19 and telemedicine: a revolution in healthcare delivery is at hand. Health Sci Rep. 2020;3(2):e166.
19. World Health Organization. mHealth New horizons for health through mobile technologies. Based on the findings of the second global survey on eHealth, Global Observatory for eHealth series, vol. 3. World Health Organization; 2011.
20. Alwashmi MF. The use of digital health in the detection and management of COVID-19. Int J Environ Res Public Health. 2020;17(8):2906.
21. Health Information Technology Directorate. Federal Ministry of Health. National Digital Health Strategy, 2020–2029. HITD; 2021.
22. Gabarron E, Rivera-Romero O, Miron-Shatz T, Grainger R, Denecke K. Role of participatory health informatics in detecting and managing pandemics: literature review. Yearb Med Inform. 2021;30(1):200–9.

23. CDC. CDC's vision for public health surveillance in the 21st century. CDC; 2012.

24. Ali G, Deshpande A, Francombe J, et al. Digital technologies for the surveillance, prevention and control of infectious diseases—a scoping review of the research literature—2015–2019. European Centre for Disease Prevention and Control; 2021.

25. Leong KC, Chen WS, Leong KW, Mastura I, Mimi O, Sheikh MA, et al. The use of text messaging to improve attendance in primary care: a randomized controlled trial. Fam Pract. 2006;23(6):699–705.

26. Déglise C, Suggs LS, Odermatt P. SMS for disease control in developing countries: a systematic review of mobile health applications. J Telemed Telecare. 2012;18(5):273–81.

27. Vital Wave Consulting. mHealth in Ethiopia: strategies for a new framework. Vital Wave Consulting; 2011.

28. World Health Organization. Global diffusion of eHealth: making universal health coverage achievable. Report of the third global survey on eHealth. Geneva: WHO; 2016.

29. Fernandez-Luque L, Kushniruk AW, Georgiou A, et al. Evidence-based health informatics as the foundation for the COVID-19 response: a joint call for action. Methods Inf Med. 2020;59(6):183–92.

30. Harding K, Biks GA, Adefris M, Loehr J, Gashaye KT, Tilahun B, Volynski M, Garg S, Abebaw Z, Dessie K, Mersha TB. A mobile health model supporting Ethiopia's eHealth strategy. Digit Med. 2018;4(2):54–65.

31. Shahil Feroz A, Afzal N, Seto E. Exploring digital health interventions for pregnant women at high risk for pre-eclampsia and eclampsia in low-income and middle-income countries: a scoping review. BMJ Open. 2022;12(2):e056130.

32. Manyazewal T, Woldeamanuel Y, Blumberg HM, Fekadu A, Marconi VC. The potential use of digital health technologies in the African context: a systematic review of evidence from Ethiopia. NPJ Digit Med. 2021;4(1):125.

33. Xiong S, Lu H, Peoples N, Duman EK, Najarro A, Ni Z, Gong E, Yin R, Ostbye T, Palileo-Villanueva LM, Doma R, Kafle S, Tian M, Yan LL. Digital health interventions for non-communicable disease management in primary health care in low- and middle-income countries. NPJ Digit Med. 2023;6(1):12.

34. Gashu KD, Gelaye KA, Mekonnen ZA, Lester R, Tilahun B. Does phone messaging improves tuberculosis treatment success? A systematic review and meta-analysis. BMC Infect Dis. 2020;20(1):42.

35. Willis VC, Thomas Craig KJ, Jabbarpour Y, Scheufele EL, Arriaga YE, Ajinkya M, Rhee KB, Bazemore A. Digital health interventions to enhance prevention in primary care: scoping review. JMIR Med Inform. 2022;10(1):e33518.

36. Tambo E, Xia S, Xin-Yu F, Xiao-Nong Z. Digital surveillance and communication strategies to infectious diseases of poverty control and elimination in Africa. J Infect Dis Epidemiol. 2018;4:56.

37. Sittig DF, Singh H. COVID-19 and the need for a National Health Information Technology Infrastructure. JAMA. 2020;323(23):2373–4.

38. Baliga BS, Baliga S, Jain A, Kulal N, Kumar M, Koduvattat N, Kumar BGP, Kumar A, Ghosh SK. Digitized smart surveillance and micromanagement using information technology for malaria elimination in Mangaluru, India: an analysis of five-year post-digitization data. Malar J. 2021;20(1):139.

39. Nema S, Verma AK, Tiwari A, Bharti PK. Digital health care services to control and eliminate malaria in India. Trends Parasitol. 2021;37(2):96–9.

40. Mellor S, Cox J, Roth S, Parry J. Digital health infrastructure: the backbone of surveillance for malaria elimination strong health information systems hold the key to ending malaria in the Greater Mekong Subregion. Asian Development Bank; 2016.

41. Gashu KD, Gelaye KA, Lester R, Tilahun B. Effect of a phone reminder system on patient-centered tuberculosis treatment adherence among adults in Northwest Ethiopia: a randomised controlled trial. BMJ Health Care Inform. 2021;28(1):e100268.

42. Tilahun B, Gashu KD, Mekonnen ZA, Endehabtu BF, Angaw DA. Mapping the role of digital health technologies in the case detection, management, and treatment outcomes of neglected tropical diseases: a scoping review. Trop Med Health. 2021;49(1):17.

43. Assaye BT, Shimie AW. Telemedicine use during COVID-19 pandemics and associated factors among health professionals working in health facilities at resource-limited setting 2021. Inform Med Unlocked. 2022;33:101085.

44. Smith AC, Thomas E, Snoswell CL, Haydon H, Mehrotra A, Clemensen J, Caffery LJ. Telehealth for global emergencies: implications for coronavirus disease 2019 (COVID-19). J Telemed Telecare. 2020;26(5):309–13.

45. Willis K, Tuell C, Marzilli C. Exploring digital health promotion and education in East Texas: pathways to improving access. J Heal Educ Teach. 2020;11(1):43–55.

46. Ahrens C, Negash E, Coder M, Costilla-Reyes O, Trentini YA. The intersection of digital health and equity. Economist Impact; 2022.

47. Campbell JI, Aturinda I, Mwesigwa E, Burns B, Santorino D, Haberer JE, Bangsberg DR, Holden RJ, Ware NC, Siedner MJ. The Technology Acceptance Model for Resource-Limited Settings (TAM-RLS): a novel framework for mobile health interventions targeted to low-literacy end-users in resource-limited settings. AIDS Behav. 2017;21(11):3129–40.

48. Watterson JL, Walsh J, Madeka I. Using mHealth to improve usage of antenatal care, postnatal care, and immunization: a systematic review of the literature. Biomed Res Int. 2015;2015:153402.

49. McCool J, Dobson R, Whittaker R. Moving beyond the individual: mHealth tools for social change in low-resource settings. BMJ Glob Health. 2018;3(6):e001098.

50. Higgs ES, Goldberg AB, Labrique AB, Cook SH, Schmid C, Cole CF, Obregón RA. Understanding the role of mHealth and other media interventions for behavior change to enhance child survival and development in low- and middle-income countries: an evidence review. J Health Commun. 2014;19 Suppl 1(Suppl 1):164–89.

51. Mahmud N, Rodriguez J, Nesbit J. A text message-based intervention to bridge the healthcare communication gap in the rural developing world. Technol Health Care. 2010;18(2):137–44.

52. Hirsch-Moverman Y, Daftary A, Yuengling KA, et al. Using mHealth for HIV/TB treatment support in lesotho: enhancing patient-provider communication in the START study. J Acquir Immune Defic Syndr. 2017;74 Suppl 1(Suppl 1):S37–43.

53. Nhavoto JA, Grönlund Å, Klein GO. Mobile health treatment support intervention for HIV and tuberculosis in Mozambique: perspectives of patients and healthcare workers. PLoS One. 2017;12(4):e0176051.

54. Labrique AB, Vasudevan L, Kochi E, Fabricant R, Mehl G. mHealth innovations as health system strengthening tools: 12 common applications and a visual framework. Glob Health Sci Pract. 2013;1(2):160–71.

55. Manakongtreecheep K. SMS-reminder for vaccination in Africa: research from published, unpublished and grey literature. Pan Afr Med J. 2017;27(Suppl 3):23.

56. World Health Organization. WHO guideline: recommendations on digital interventions for health system strengthening. Geneva: WHO; 2019.

57. Siddiquee NKA, Poudyal A, Pandey A, Shrestha N, Karki S, Subedi R, Sah AK, Dirghayu KC. Telemedicine in resource-limited setting: narrative synthesis of evidence in nepalese context. Smart Homecare Technol TeleHealth. 2019;6:1–14.

58. Stark AL, Geukes C, Dockweiler C. Digital health promotion and prevention in settings: scoping review. J Med Internet Res. 2022;24(1):e21063.

59. Koh A, Swanepoel W, Ling A, Ho BL, Tan SY, Lim J. Digital health promotion: promise and peril. Health Promot Int. 2021;36(Suppl_1):i70–80.

60. Dutta B, Hwang HG. The adoption of electronic medical record by physicians: a PRISMA-compliant systematic review. Medicine (Baltimore). 2020;99(8):e19290.

61. Hamade N, Terry A, Malvankar-Mehta M. Interventions to improve the use of EMRs in primary health care: a systematic review and meta-analysis. BMJ Health Care Inform. 2019;26(1) https://doi.org/10.1136/bmjhci-2019-000023.

62. Ajadi S, Drury P. Health systems, digital health and COVID-19: insights from Bangladesh, Myanmar, Pakistan, Benin, Nigeria and Rwanda. GSMA; 2021.

63. Aranda-Jan CB, Mohutsiwa-Dibe N, Loukanova S. Systematic review on what works, what does not work and why of implementation of mobile health (mHealth) projects in Africa. BMC Public Health. 2014;14:188.

64. AlKnawy B, Kozlakidis Z, Tarkoma S, Bates D, Honkela A, Crooks G, Rhee K, McKillop M. Digital public health leadership in the global fight for health security. BMJ Glob Health. 2023;8(2):e011454.

65. Keesara S, Jonas A, Schulman K. Covid-19 and health care's digital revolution. N Engl J Med. 2020;382(23):e82.

66. Tilahun B, Fritz F. Comprehensive evaluation of electronic medical record system use and user satisfaction at five low-resource setting hospitals in ethiopia. JMIR Med Inform. 2015;3(2):e22.

67. Carney TJ, Kong AY. Leveraging health informatics to foster a smart systems response to health disparities and health equity challenges. J Biomed Inform. 2017;68:184–9.

68. Koehle H, Kronk C, Lee YJ. Digital health equity: addressing power, usability, and trust to strengthen health systems. Yearb Med Inform. 2022;31(1):20–32.

69. Veinot TC, Ancker JS, Bakken S. Health informatics and health equity: improving our reach and impact. J Am Med Inform Assoc. 2019;26(8-9):689–95.

70. Brewer LC, Fortuna KL, Jones C, Walker R, Hayes SN, Patten CA, Cooper LA. Back to the future: achieving health equity through health informatics and digital health. JMIR Mhealth Uhealth. 2020;8(1):e14512.

71. Ethiopian Federal Ministry of Health. Information revolution roadmap. Ethiopian Federal Ministry of Health; 2016.

72. Linde DS, Korsholm M, Katanga J, Rasch V, Lundh A, Andersen MS. One-way SMS and healthcare outcomes in Africa: systematic review of randomised trials with meta-analysis. PLoS One. 2019;14(6):e0217485.

73. Ibeneme S, Karamagi H, Muneene D, Goswami K, Chisaka N, Okeibunor J. Strengthening health systems using innovative digital health technologies in Africa. Front Digit Health. 2022;4:854339.

74. United Nation. Adopted in United Nations General Assembly resolution 70/1. United Nation; 2015.

75. World Health Organization. Atlas of eHealth country profiles. The use of eHealth in support of universal health coverage. Based on the findings of the third global survey on eHealth 2015. Global observatory for eHealth. Geneva: WHO; 2016.

76. Karamagi HC, Ben Charif A, Ngusbrhan Kidane S, Yohanes T, Kariuki D, Titus M, Batungwanayo C, Seydi AB, Berhane A, Nzinga J, Njuguna D, Kipruto HK, Andrews Annan E, Droti B. Investments for effective functionality of health systems towards Universal Health Coverage in Africa: a scoping review. PLOS Glob Public Health. 2022;2(9):e0001076.

77. Atnafu A, Otto K, Herbst CH. The role of mHealth intervention on maternal and child health service delivery: findings from a randomized controlled field trial in rural Ethiopia. mHealth. 2017;3:39.

78. Mekonnen ZA, Gelaye KA, Were MC, Gashu KD, Tilahun BC. Effect of mobile text message reminders on routine childhood vaccination: a systematic review and meta-analysis. Syst Rev. 2019;8(1):154.

79. Gibson DG, Ochieng B, Kagucia EW, Were J, Hayford K, Moulton LH, Levine OS, Odhiambo F, O'Brien KL, Feikin DR. Mobile phone-delivered reminders and incentives to improve childhood immunisation coverage and timeliness in Kenya (M-SIMU): a cluster randomised controlled trial. Lancet Glob Health. 2017;5(4):e428–38.
80. Mekonnen ZA, Gelaye KA, Were M, Tilahun B. Effect of mobile phone text message reminders on the completion and timely receipt of routine childhood vaccinations: superiority randomized controlled trial in Northwest Ethiopia. JMIR Mhealth Uhealth. 2021;9(6):e27603.
81. Shiferaw F, Zolfo M. The role of information communication technology (ICT) towards universal health coverage: the first steps of a telemedicine project in Ethiopia. Glob Health Action. 2012;5:1–8.
82. Tozzi AE, Gesualdo F, D'Ambrosio A, Pandolfi E, Agricola E, Lopalco P. Can digital tools be used for improving immunization programs? Front Public Health. 2016;4:36.
83. Alotaibi YK, Federico F. The impact of health information technology on patient safety. Saudi Med J. 2017;38(12):1173–80.
84. Luna D, Almerares A, Mayan JC 3rd, González Bernaldo de Quirós F, Otero C. Health informatics in developing countries: going beyond pilot practices to sustainable implementations: a review of the current challenges. Healthc Inform Res. 2014;20(1):3–10.

Data Analytics and Public Health

Habtamu Alganeh Guadie

Abstract

Gathering significant amounts of information from different sources and formats is a major real-world challenge. Small amounts of data can only be stored using traditional databases. The old database management systems struggle to extract knowledge from unorganized data. It becomes essential to manage both organized and unorganized data while creating an effective system. Big data technology, which can derive insights from both structured and unstructured data, solves this problem. The goal of big data is to compile information from multiple places and store it in a central location. There are many opportunities to provide high quality patient care at reasonable costs when big data analytics is used in the healthcare industry. Additionally, the proliferation of mobile and internet connected devices has sparked an information explosion. Large amounts of data cannot be handled by current frameworks; new creative approaches must be utilized. This chapter outlines data analytics for public health and its role in health systems overall.

H. A. Guadie (✉)
Department of Health System Management and Health Economics, School of Public Health, College of Medicine and Health Sciences, Bahir Dar University, Bahir Dar, Ethiopia

SMART Health, Research and Publication Department, Bahir Dar, Ethiopia
e-mail: Habtamu.Alganeh@bdu.edu.et

Keywords

Artificial intelligence · Big data · Machine learning · Prediction

3.1 Health Data Analytics

3.1.1 Overview

Information from the healthcare industry is incredibly rich and comes from many different sources, like text from clinical notes, sensors, images, and traditional electronic records. The processing and analysis of the underlying data is significantly hindered by the diversity in how the data is collected and represented [1, 2]. The approaches required to examine these many forms of data are hugely varied. Additionally, the diversity of data unavoidably produces several issues with data combination and examination. Different data types frequently permit the discovery of understandings that would otherwise not be feasible from a single source of information. The immense prospective of such incorporated data analysis strategies has only recently been brought to light [3, 4].

Health information can take many different forms, like clinical and lab results, medical notes, data created by machines from medical equipment or at-home tracking sensors, financial details about health services, hospital invoices, literature data from medical journals, social media posts covering health topics, and more [5].

3.1.2 Why Data Analytics in Public Health?

Analyzing large amounts of data has tremendous potential to reshape healthcare as it evolves into technology's next major trend [6]. The results of the growing capability to examine intricate datasets promise not just process optimization but numerous paths to lift the level of patient care and subsequently patient satisfaction. Applying big data analytics in healthcare also enables swift decision making and as a consequence plays a critical role in saving lives in circumstances where every moment matters [7].

Any organization can enhance the protection of its essential information by adopting big data analytics. Consequently, the data can be utilized later to identify new opportunities. By doing so, you can develop an improved business and make informed decisions that will raise profits and satisfy customers. Predicting, optimization, modeling, and other strategies that help decision-making and provide insight for managers and policymakers are what is referred to as big data analytics approaches [8, 9].

3.2   Data Acquisition

3.2.1 Overview of Data Acquisition

One of the industries that is most reliant on information is healthcare. Medical facilities were able to produce huge volumes of data due to the swift shift to digital technologies [10]. The vast volume of data holds potential to offer some meaningful understandings. It can aid with automated health observation and discovering therapies. Health information requires transferring, handling and retaining in a protected manner since it contains exceptionally sensitive specifics [11, 12].

A health management information system collects, stores, analyses, and evaluates health-related data from health facility to district, regional and national administrative levels. It provides analytical reports and visualizations that facilitate decision making at all these levels. HMIS are also referred to as routine health information systems [13, 14].

Information regarding health is collected, stored, studied, and assessed by a healthcare administration information system at administrative levels varying from district (health post in some countries) to national [15]. Decision making is supported at each of these levels by the analytical reports and visual presentations supplied. Many of the details in an HMIS originate from interactions between patients and healthcare professionals in medical facilities. Healthcare is delivered through preventative, promotional, medical and surgical, rehabilitative, and palliative care initiatives in hospitals, health centers, and community outreach programs [16].

HMISs are complex, demonstrating the varied and different characteristics of overseeing and delivering healthcare. They reference individual patient files, family record cards, admissions and discharge forms, ward registers and count sheets, community level files, infrastructure and resource files, records of community health projects, and routine evaluations of the infrastructure and resources of medical facilities [17].

3.2.2   Types of Health System Data Acquisition

Health system records can be classified as individual patient record systems, facility-based registry systems, community level record systems, and health facility assessments.

3.2.2.1 Individual Patient Record Systems

Most of the data collected by an HMIS at healthcare centers comes from individual documentation of patient-provider interactions, which may contain patient identification, medical diagnoses, results of lab and diagnostic tests, prescriptions, preventative, promotional, curative, and rehabilitative services given, and payments made [18, 19].

The next level of the health system receives summary reports from managers based on a subset of the data, and then aggregates them to create indicators for all facilities. The majority of low- and middle-income nations still maintain individual records using paper-based methods. However, the use of electronic medical records in hospitals is rising. Remote institutions with limited resources may lack the sophisticated management systems, networking expertise, and technology needed to maintain electronic records [20, 21].

3.2.2.2 Facility-Based Registry Systems

Records of patient admissions, discharges, and which ward they were in are all examples of registers based around a specific facility. Some registers focus on tracking individuals who require long-term care over an extended period, like those for prenatal appointments, vaccinations, or chronic illnesses such as cancer. Each type of register only stores the minimum necessary data needed to be able to locate and follow up with the patients in the future [21].

The health team can identify patients who need to be actively pursued to ensure compliance with treatment interventions, such as immunization completion, full tuberculosis treatment, compliance with anti-retroviral regimens, or regular monitoring and control of blood pressure, through regular review of registers [22].

Registries that track patient information can be useful for documenting details of treatments provided and evaluating the quality of healthcare services. These types of registries contain data such as diagnoses at the beginning and end of care, results of laboratory tests, and details of therapies received, in addition to personal identifiers. The registry also notes the cause of death if a patient sadly passes while hospitalized, as classified using the standards of the International Classification of Diseases (ICD). All of this collected information allows for following trends in patient cases and outcomes over time [23].

3.2.2.3 Community Level Record Systems

Data from community-based workers who conduct health promotion and disease preventive initiatives is integrated by HMISs. These community workers may work for the healthcare system, such as Community Health Workers in Kenya or Health Extension Workers in Ethiopia [24].

The data these service providers gather at the moment of delivery is crucial for managing community programs and for making decisions regarding the budget, policy, and human resources. Data are used by community health workers to monitor their patients and manage their care, particularly for initiatives that call for long-term monitoring and connections to community facilities [25, 26].

In order to avoid counting the same health events multiple times, it is essential to combine data from community sources with the data collected by individual healthcare facilities. The tools used for gathering this information require literacy and numerical skills. To guarantee patients are assigned appropriate clinical care, facility staff need to aid and supervise community health workers. For example, employees could help community members locate clients who were receiving services but are no longer engaged in their continued care. This collaboration between different levels of the health system helps provide comprehensive and accurate information [27].

3.2.2.4 Health Facility Assessments

A Health Management Information System (HMIS) combines routine data gathered through regular patient care and running of healthcare centers with additional information collected periodically from facilities beyond what is provided in standard reports. This allows a more complete picture of activities and services by including planned supplementary collection of information alongside the ongoing data generated as a natural part of service delivery and management.

Health Facility Assessments produce data on:

- Service utilization,
- Personnel resources,

- Readiness to deliver specific interventions (such tuberculosis control), and
- Facility infrastructure, equipment, and consumables.

HFAs are a productive technique to gather data on facility distribution and availability. They can pinpoint the areas where the healthcare system needs to improve.

Each level of the health system's HMIS units manages data to support operations at that level and below and to report a necessary subset of data to the level above. A hospital, for instance, manages its patients as well as the supplies and goods required to run the institution using its own information system [28].

Healthcare centers are required by their higher-level managers to regularly submit certain reports through the Health Management Information System (HMIS). These include notifications of communicable diseases, numbers of vaccines administered, prenatal care visits, facility births, and the reasons patients were seen. The reports from all facilities and programs are gathered and collated at the district level.

The HMIS uses routine facility data to evaluate results and impacts. Facilities are also the sole source of details like tuberculosis treatment outcomes, interventions for preventing mother-to-child transmission (PMTCT) coverage rates, and consistent usage of antiretroviral medication. Long-term monitoring of treatment adherence and health outcomes are crucial for managing conditions like diabetes, hypertension, and cancers. The system tracks the administration of therapies for these disorders. This collected information is critical for program planning and assessment as well as individual patient management from various medical perspectives [29].

3.2.3 Challenges of Data Acquisition

Health information collected in lower-income and middle-income countries often has issues related to quality, making the data difficult for end users to rely on or determine if it is suitable for its intended purpose. Limitations to data quality can include missing or absent values, inaccuracies in measurement techniques, and mistakes entered during data collection or subsequent processing. The impression that regular reports from healthcare centers and districts are usually late, contain errors, and have gaps undermine their credibility and make the information harder to utilize. Problems with missing or faulty details introduce doubts about the usability and trustworthiness of such routinely gathered health statistics [30, 31].

The data collected serves as the underlying basis for identifying possible health issues or locating specific subsets within the overall patient group. It also helps healthcare providers determine what additional details may be needed and next steps that should be taken to improve understanding of a patient's concern or to deal with a concern that has been recognized. Having appropriately gathered and organized health information aids clinicians in assessing patients, deciding on follow up questions or exams required, and determining the best course of action for diagnosis or treatment [32].

Seeing health data solely as digital outputs like monitored waveforms or statistical charts fails to capture its full complexities. While laboratory results and quantifiable metrics can be extremely valuable, there are various more nuanced forms of information that may prove equally important for quality care delivery. These include subtle nonverbal cues like an evasive look from a patient avoiding a question during an exam. Details surrounding the nature of a person's health concern, or specifics about family dynamics or financial situation are also key. Additionally, an experienced physician will often gain a subjective sense of severity simply from briefly interacting with the individual. Viewing data too narrowly as just numbers overlooks the richness present in other types of qualitative insights that inform a comprehensive understanding and treatment approach for each unique patient [33, 34].

Medical professionals universally acknowledge the value of observations such as interpersonal cues and qualitative details in forming conclusions about patient evaluation and treatment approaches. However, recording this kind of nuanced information in a manner that fully conveys its actual meaning poses a challenge, given how poorly defined the specific role and applicable metrics are, even among colleagues. While capturing the full richness and subtleties may be difficult, providers still require means of descriptively sharing relevant context that circumvents direct quantification or standardization across caregivers, in order to optimize coordination of care for those in their charge. Structured templates alone cannot suffice without supplemental explanatory insights from experienced peers [35, 36].

Health professionals acquire health information about individuals and populations. Although typical conceptions of the healthcare team conjure up pictures of coworkers attending to sick patients, the team's job entails much more than just patient care; data gathering and recording play a key role [37].

In the process of gathering and interpreting data, health professionals play a significant role. In order to acquire narrative descriptive information on the main complaint, prior illnesses, family and social history, and a system review, they speak with the patient. They assess the patient while gathering important information and documenting it during or after the appointment. They typically arrange laboratory or radiologic testing and assess the patient's reaction to therapeutic interventions to determine what more data to gather [38].

There are several reasons why medical information is recorded. They might be required to support the correct care of the patient from whom they were taken, but they might also benefit society by collecting and analyzing data about populations of people.

Ensuring care teams can deliver connected, continuous care over extended time periods is a core objective of implementing organized health data collection and documentation methods within clinical environments. Most patients facing significant medical conditions will need recurring appointments for issues needing monitoring or management spanning months or years. Records now act as an important conduit allowing varied specialists—such as additional physicians, physiotherapists, nurses, imaging technicians, social workers or discharge coordinators—to exchange relevant insights. This infrastructure likewise preserves the clinical notes and findings initially captured to inform future patient interactions. Only through coordinated, comprehensive care supported by detailed yet accessible records can people receive optimal long-term medical support for their often complex situations [39, 40] (Table 3.1).

It's important to note that the availability and level of detail of these data elements may vary in different healthcare settings and countries, particularly in global south. However, efforts are being made to improve medical record systems in developing countries to ensure better patient care, continuity, and data management.

Table 3.1 Medical record data elements and their explanation included in developing countries

Medical records are meant to offer a thorough compilation of data about specific patients:	
Data elements	Descriptions
Patient identification	This includes basic information about the patient, such as name, age, gender, address, contact details, and unique identifiers like national identification numbers or health insurance numbers.
Medical history	This includes information about the patient's past medical conditions, surgeries, allergies, immunization history, and family medical history.
Vital signs and diagnosis	Measurements like blood pressure, heart rate, respiratory rate, temperature, and oxygen saturation are recorded to assess the patient's overall health status. The medical condition or disease identified by the healthcare provider based on the patient's signs, symptoms, and diagnostic tests.
Treatment plan	Details of the treatment prescribed by the healthcare provider, including medications, procedures, surgeries, or referrals to other specialists.
Follow-up appointments	Information about scheduled appointments for future follow-up or referrals to other healthcare providers.

Ensuring care teams can work together seamlessly over prolonged periods is a primary objective of organized health data gathering and documentation methods within clinical environments. Most patients facing complex medical conditions will need recurring contact with providers for issues requiring sustained follow-up and management. Only through integrated, collaborative efforts sustained by detailed-yet-accessible records can individuals receive optimized long-term support that addresses their multifaceted needs as circumstances change over time. Structured recording plays a pivotal role in enabling different specialists to align their efforts toward maintaining or improving one's health status at all points of interaction along their treatment journey [41].

More than just addressing a patient's immediate or long-term health concerns is required in order to provide high-quality medical treatment. Additionally, it necessitates teaching patients about how their lifestyle choices and environment might either lower their chance of developing disease later on or contribute to it. Similar to this, data collected frequently during a patient's continuous care may indicate that even though the patient may feel healthy and be free of symptoms right now, they are at a high risk of getting a certain condition [42].

Medical data plays a vital role by allowing teams to pinpoint influential factors, monitor how patient risk ebbs and flows over an extended period, and guide tailored education or preemptive steps concerning nutrition, medications or physical activity. Some of the most widespread examples of ongoing risk evaluation at present involve periodic checks for excessive weight, high blood pressure and abnormal cholesterol levels. In these situations, irregular results could foreshadow future issues; therefore, the ideal care involves intervening beforehand, when there is still time to curtail developing problems before they become entirely evident or worse. Structured collection and documentation of pertinent health details is key to this strategic, proactive approach aimed at earlier identification and better management of growing concerns [43].

3.3 Big Data

3.3.1 Basic Concepts

The term "big data"refers to extraordinarily large and intricate datasets that challenge conventional data processing approaches. It is a vast volume of data that is processed swiftly from a variety of various sources to aid in decision-making. Big data is characterized by their volume, variety and velocity—also known as the 3Vs—these information troves are defined by their immense scale, wide-ranging and diverse formats (structured, semi-structured and unstructured) as well as the breakneck pace at which fresh inputs are generated and must be handled. Key obstacles in big data analysis involve the capturing, storage, manipulation and visualization of such voluminous stores, while also preserving privacy, accuracy and consistency. Industries have utilized big data's promising potential through predictive analytics, user behavior profiling and other progressive techniques for extracting meaningful insights. These tools can uncover purpose amidst oceans of information previously too overwhelming to comprehend. Big data is the term used to describe an enormous volume of information that can be in any raw format and is retrieved in its raw form from numerous sources without any modifications. It is widely known with the volume, velocity and variety [44].

Data serves as the foundation for all we do in healthcare system. Patient data refers to medical records that are kept on a specific patient. In the medical field, "big data"describes gathering, reviewing, and using huge amounts of personal details like how people use services and their health histories. It shows a huge amount of info from patients, doctors, tests, and treatments that regular ways can't easily understand and use well. Studying huge and complex sets of numbers requires advanced digital methods to find knowledge that can help diagnose, treat, and prevent disease better across groups of people. If we use advanced strategies well to make sense of info on a scale too big for normal processes, it offers chances to provide care that targets people's needs better, is more proactive, and personal through figuring out patterns in the data.

Big data comes from many different sources, things that happen on their own in nature and things people make. Advancing tech and modern items we use every day have caused huge amounts of organized, partly organized, and unorganized info to flow in from numerous varied makers all over the world. Whether from social media or sensors, satellites or surveillance, applications generate ambient data exhausts telling tales as they accumulate from distributed entities into centralized silos. Opportunities await those developing the strategies for gleaning insights from the exabytes exhaled by an exponentially connected cosmos. Whether through digital interactions, scientific observations or daily human activities—data generation now proliferates endlessly from every sphere. Making sense of these powerful informational currents created both directly and indirectly by humankind, and indirectly by planetary processes as well, presents immense opportunities and complex challenges that will influence global progress far into the future [3, 45].

Big data is defined by the 3Vs—volume, variety, and velocity. Volume means how huge the info is. Variety includes the different types like organized, partly organized, or unorganized data. Velocity refers to how fast new data is made and has to be analyzed. Big data can have structure, no structure, or some structure and comes from many places. Veracity is about the quality and how true the info is. Value refers to what useful insights can be found in the data. Variability is another feature—it's always changing. Big data needs special methods and techs to find patterns in datasets too big and complex for regular analyzing approaches [46, 47].

3.3.2 Characteristics of Big Data

Big data can be defined by five key aspects—volume, velocity, variety, veracity, and value. The volume refers to the large amount of data. The velocity looks at the speed at which data is generated and processed. The variety covers the differ-

ent types and formats of data. The veracity considers the reliability and accuracy of the data. And the value evaluates the usefulness and insights that can be extracted from the data. Together, these 5Vs provide a comprehensive way to characterize big data and understand its unique challenges and opportunities. As indicated in Fig. 3.1.

3.3.2.1 Volume

Volume is the primary data property and the basis for all subsequent attributes. In the context of big data, volume refers to the massive size of the data. The name "big data" itself is related to a size which is enormous. To determine the value of data, the size of data plays a very crucial role. If the volume of data is very large, then it is actually considered as a "big data." The amount of information in big data can truly be huge—measured in terabytes (thousands of gigabytes) and petabytes (thousands of terabytes)! The sheer size of these datasets means traditional storage and processing just can't handle it alone. Laptops and regular desktops usually don't have enough memory, computing power, or storage space to break down super large big data properly. Specialized distributed computing systems are often better suited for the job. They can share the massive workload across many connected machines and servers working together. This helps make analysis of truly huge datasets more feasible compared to trying on a single ordinary computer. The other qualities of the data will be more clearly defined the more data that is supplied [46, 47]. To summarize volume is about quantity, depth, and the dependability of inferences

3.3.2.2 Velocity

When talking about processing and analyzing information, velocity is one of the key factors of big data, along with volume and variety. Velocity refers to how quickly new data is created, received, and studied. It shows that data is now developing and moving faster than ever before. The term "velocity" really emphasizes how important it is to handle data in real-time or almost real-time. When data is understood and acted on as soon as possible. Advances in tech-

Fig. 3.1 Framework of
Big data elements

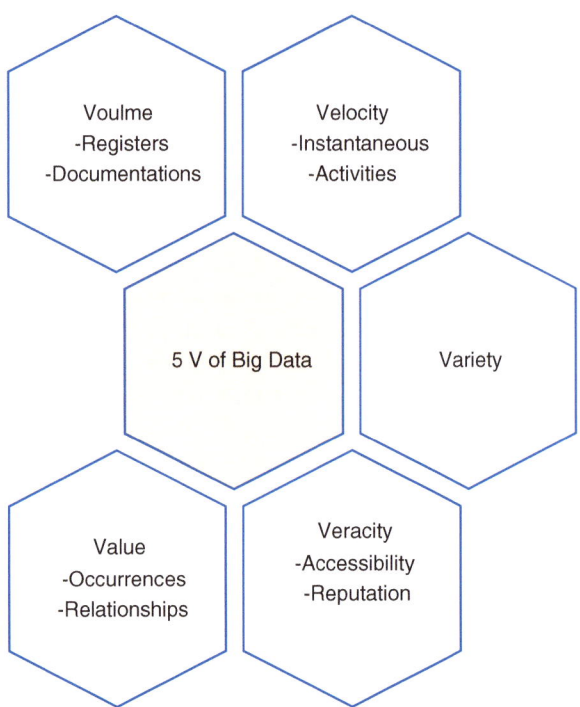

nology and all the different systems connecting
to each other mean huge amounts of info are
being made and sent around in many forms like
sensor readings, social media, computer logs and
more. By managing velocity well, organizations
can gain understanding and make smart choices
on time. It involves dealing with super-fast
streams of data, making sure intake, processing,
and analysis can keep up with how quickly the
info flows, and using methods like stream processing and real-time analysis. Working
effectively with velocity is key to realizing the
value of big data [46, 47].

3.3.2.3 Variety

Variety describes the different kinds of information that can be looked at. It also explains how
widely things are covered. Big data isn't always
neatly organized, and combining it with regular
databases isn't necessarily straightforward. So
data analysts need to understand the category big
data falls in when they work with structured and
unstructured—which makes storing and studying huge amounts of data much more complicated. It points to the diversity of types of data.

Big data has the ability to originate from several
places, both internally and externally of an organization. It also has the capability to be organized, somewhat organized, or non-organized.
Data that is organized has a conventional structure and is arranged in a formatted collection.
Non-organized data does not have a structure
and comes in many documents or formats.
Somewhat organized data has affiliated details,
like metadata, making it less complicated to process than non-organized data. The diversity in
types of data generally necessitates unique handling abilities and specialized algorithms. For
instance, data sets with many types could join
organized data from databases, somewhat organized data such as XML or JSON documents,
and non-organized data like text files, graphics,
or videos [46, 47].

3.3.2.4 Veracity

Veracity in big data talks about how good quality,
consistent, right, and trustful the information is.
It's extremely important to be sure the data can be
relied on and is worthwhile for making smart
choices based on evidence. Veracity includes

checking the data for unfair biases, interference, strange parts, and mistakes that could affect how useful it is [46, 47].

3.3.2.5 Value

Value in big data talks about how useful and important the gathered info is for companies. While the data itself may not automatically have value on its own, its real worth comes from what can be learned from it after processing and carefully studying it. By changing basic data into ideas that can be put into action, businesses can improve how they make choices, spot possibilities, enhance how things run, and ultimately sell more and better please customers. The value of big data appears when companies make the most of it in the right way to gain an advantage over others and do better in their work [46, 47].

The major aspects of healthcare data values are listed in the following table (Table 3.2).

3.3.3   The Role of Big Data in the Health System

Data analytics serves healthcare domains in diverse capacities. It bolsters practitioner development, enhances diagnostic precision through pattern discernment in scans, and empowers early outbreak identification. Cost reductions and strategic planning are augmented through business intelligence gleaned from retrospective exploration. Personalized care quality also increases as evidence-guided decision making emerges from analytics. Population health management gains from predictive AI models customized for targeted groups constructed from analytics insights. Preventative strategies too are strengthened by uncovering obscure risk factors. Overall, comprehensive data integration empowers institutions to prioritize excellent patient-centered outcomes and longevity through optimized resource deployment. The prominence of analytics was made clear amidst COVID-19 challenges, and prospects similarly brighten other spheres such as disease investigation, therapeutic evaluation and genome comprehension moving ahead.

The improvement of healthcare quality is a result of several factors, and big data analytics are very beneficial to the healthcare sector. Some of these benefits are discussed below.

3.3.3.1 Patient-Centered Services Delivery

Big data analytics plays an expanding role empowering customized care through enlightened choices. Analyzing vast records, care pro-

Table 3.2 The major aspects of healthcare data values

Major aspects	Definition
Adequate expertise	All medical professionals need robust training to help patients with suitable abilities for achieving excellent outcomes. All medical experts guiding care require ample preparation so their expertise aligns with each patient's distinctive requirements for achieving optimal results.
Worthwhile quality	The standard of care delivered to every individual seeks quality assurance through assessment emphasizing worth realization.
Innovation advances	Novel innovations promise furthering therapeutic and systemic enhancements to benefit communities. New discoveries will lead to novel therapies and methods of healthcare delivery.
Appropriate treatment	Every person deserves well-timed, rehabilitation suited to their circumstances. Collaborative efforts empowered by centralized information sharing optimize assistance. Streamlined coordination prioritizes individual needs. It is certainly right that every patient receives suitable, timely care. Coordinated efforts from all health service providers with access to centralized data to deliver top services to patients is preferable rather than excessive procedures.
Self-care responsibilities	Education encourages personal responsibility through health-sustaining decisions over diet, exercise, screening and lifestyle influences. Patients must be educated to take responsibility for their own health by choosing a proper diet, exercise, preventative care, and other lifestyle factors.

viders comprehend individuals holistically, optimizing results while reducing expenses. Discerning clusters and correlations, practitioners cater interventions responding to each situation's subtleties. Identifying elevated risk profiles through algorithms, practitioners preempt complications through preventive remedies tailored for wellness sustainability. Rather than solitary snapshots, big data illuminates patients' contexts across time—genetics, behaviors, milieus affecting health. This elucidation supports relationship-centered care addressing medical as well as socioeconomic determinants through consistent care coordination. Beyond transactions, the focus shifts to preservation through comprehensive life course sustainment within communities' constraints.

Big data can also help healthcare providers to optimize staffing, forecast operating room demands, streamline patient care, and improve the pharmaceutical supply chain. All of these factors can lead to a reduction in healthcare costs and an improvement in patient outcomes. In summary, big data analytics is essential for healthcare providers who want to deliver patient-centered services that are personalized, efficient, and effective.

Doctors can help patients more rapidly by giving indication-related medication, recognizing symptoms and viruses early on using the medical data available, lowering painkiller dosages to lower side effects, and giving effective medication based on heritable features. Because of these benefits, readmission rates are reduced, which benefits the patients [48].

3.3.3.2 Identifying Illness Outbreaks Sooner

Big data analytics holds potential importance for public health through recognizing disease emergence more rapidly via surveillance of diverse digital indicators. Mining information from online searches, social platforms and electronic records permits discernment of population-level symptom patterns that could foreshadow outbreaks. By aggregating such distributed population health clues, analytics may pinpoint

abnormal presenting issues earlier through location-tagging or abnormalities in frequency/ character. Early detection supports strategic, data-driven allocation of screening and prevention resources toward slowing spread. With emerging conditions, each hour of head start matters—accelerated recognition through big data mining signposts affords aiding communities before crises peak. If leveraged judiciously, these novel multidimensional insights into symptom trends offer hope to safeguard populations through agile, targeted interventions informed by real-time digital epidemiology.

Looking the trends of viral infections prior to the live investigations dispersing. Examining the local logs of individuals experiencing illness-related suffering in a particular location can help identify this. By having important defense techniques, it helps the medical professionals to guide the patients.

3.3.3.3 Evaluating the Hospital's Standards

Big data plays a significant role in evaluating hospital standards and improving healthcare services. By analyzing large volumes of data from various sources such as hospital records, medical examinations, and patient medical records, healthcare organizations can extract deeper insights to enhance the functionality and services of the healthcare system. Big data analytics can help in better management, care, and low-cost treatments, leading to improved patient outcomes and reduced healthcare costs. It enables the creation of a holistic view of consumers, patients, and physicians, improves care personalization and efficiency, and identifies geographic markets with growth potential. Additionally, it optimizes hospital growth by improving care efficiency, effectiveness, and personalization. Furthermore, big data analytics can be used to evaluate and improve the quality of healthcare services, assess diagnoses and treatment methods, and identify more cost-effective ways to diagnose and treat patients. It also helps in reducing the cost of healthcare delivery and improving the overall quality of life. Therefore, the systematic management and analysis of big data are essential for healthcare organizations to harness the potential of big data and convert it into better services and financial advantages. To determine whether the health facilities are set up in accordance with national minimum medical standards. In contrast to forbidding health facilities, it helps administration to monitor crucial actions.

3.3.3.4 Changing the Methods of Treatment

Big data is transforming therapeutic approaches by enabling customized, evidence-driven treatment roadmaps. Through insight mining from voluminous health records, clinicians gain enhanced foresight enabling superior care guidance. Analytic insights reveal risk tendencies and disease progressions, assisting clinicians to preemptively optimize protocols. By recognizing patient clusters and outcome correlations, big data equips practitioners to differentiate care catered to each individual's profile. Anticipating those facing elevated burdens through predictive algorithms, professionals can proactively reduce complications or delay illness manifestation through targeted preventative measures. Personalized therapy design leverages big data to consider a patient holistically—not simply their current condition, but hereditary predispositions and socioeconomic contexts. This level of customization shows much promise for long-term well-being through programs tailored for sustainability within each patient's unique circumstances. Overall, big data places the focus on prevention to preserve health—representing a step forward for patient-centered, compassionate and cost-efficient services.

It can also help in optimizing treatment plans by analyzing the effectiveness of different treatments and identifying the most effective ones for specific patients. Big data can also help in developing new drugs and medical devices by analyzing patient data and identifying new targets for drug development. Additionally, big data analytics can help in predicting the outcomes of different treatments and identifying the most cost-effective treatment options. In summary, big data analytics is essential for healthcare provid-

ers who want to deliver personalized and effective treatment plans that improve patient outcomes and reduce healthcare costs.

The examination of a modified patient continuously reports the effects of medications, and by means of this study, dosages of medications can be changed for rapid outcomes. An expert can help other victims by delivering actual tablets by examining a patient's energetic symptoms to offer active precaution to patients and by conducting research on the records created by patients who have previously experienced the same signs.

3.3.3.5 Improving Efficiency and Effectiveness in Public Health Interventions

Big data plays a key role in the area of public health. Some of the major advantages of big data in the health system include:

1. **Cost Reduction**: Big data analytics can help in identifying areas for improved efficiency and cost reduction, potentially saving billions in healthcare costs.
2. **Minimizing Medical Errors**: By analyzing large volumes of data, healthcare providers can identify patterns and trends that can help in reducing medical errors and improving patient safety.
3. **Improving Diagnostics and Predictions**: Big data analytics can lead to more accurate and timely diagnostics, as well as better predictions for patient outcomes and disease progression.
4. **Increasing Health Indicators**: By leveraging big data, healthcare organizations can gain a better understanding of patient health indicators, leading to more personalized and effective care.
5. **Enhancing Patient-Centered Services**: Big data analytics can help in providing more personalized and efficient patient care, leading to improved patient outcomes and satisfaction.

In summary, big data presents extensive possibilities to advance health and healthcare when responsibly applied. By revealing hidden connec-

Table 3.3 Summary of advantages of big data in healthcare industry

The roles of big data	Ways and means
Reduces the cost incurred	Cost savings are made possible by utilizing big data technologies and different data manipulation techniques.
Enables the safe storage of a significant amount of acquired data in order to protect user privacy	A lot of data can be safely saved, and it can be used to find business practices that are more effective.
Rids in making decisions more quickly and with higher quality	Various resources and data can be merged with the use of quick analytical tools to assess fresh sources of data.

tions within comprehensive patient information resources, organizations can reduce expenses, strengthen error prevention, enhance diagnostic precision and tailor treatment to individual characteristics—contributing to improved wellness results and a more streamlined system (Table 3.3).

In low- and middle-income nations, the spread of new technology typically involves a combination of appropriation, diffusion, and, frequently, skipping some of the intermediary development phases seen in high-income countries. In low-resource environments over the past 20 years, mobile phones have become increasingly common before a widespread landline phone system was developed. This is an example of leapfrogging.

There is a lot of interest in "mobile health" or "m-health" programs because of the opportunities that the prevalence of mobile phones in these contexts presents for improving the delivery of healthcare. There have been several small-scale m-health projects that have shown proof of concept, but not many of the confirmed strategies have been used widely.

3.4　The Nature of Data

3.4.1　Structured Data

With big data analytics, "structured data" refers to information that conforms to a predefined framework or blueprint, making it straightforward to evaluate systematically. It follows a consistent tabular format with discernible associations between rows and columns. Familiar examples include spreadsheets and relational databases—both adhere to an unambiguous organization where specific cell positions correlate to designated features or cases.

This consistent structure is highly advantageous because tools can readily search through, query meaning from, and subject the data to diverse analytical methods. The organized layout assigns defined slots for each element and distinguishes separate records through rows, lending itself to powerful interrogation and elucidation of patterns. Its schematic precision renders such structured information a uniquely valuable big data asset with significant potential to derive insights from large and complex stores of numeric documentation. Organizing information into predefined formats with specific fields and attributes is known as structured data. This conventional method allows for swiftly combining related pieces across a database during queries. The rigid design facilitates speedy aggregation of pertinent details from across the entire storage system.

It is also easier to keep secure and is ideal for data-driven applications such as business intelligence and analytics, as well as for machine learning and artificial intelligence applications. 'Structured' data refers to any data that can be accessed, processed, and stored in a fixed way. Over time, computer science talent has had more success creating methods for handling this type of data and also extracting value from it [49].

Structured data has a predefined format where all parts have clear definitions, making it user-friendly. Individual data characteristics and their interrelationships through established positions are known due to following templates that guide the role and position of each variable. This organized nature stems from templates that clarify what can be found and where, eliminating uncertainty and streamlining retrieval and analysis tasks. These schemas describe the location and significance of each item. Because it needs little to no preprocessing, structured data is the simplest type of data to analyze. Data may need to be cleaned up and reduced to simply the pertinent information, but it won't require much interpretation or conversion before a real enquiry can be carried out. The simple procedure of combining relational and enterprise data is one of the main benefits of adopting structured data. Little preparation is required to make all sources compatible because relevant data dimensions are typically defined and specific elements are in a uniform format. Information arranged in a consistent template with particulars in an ordered table provides clear access. Structured data establishes predictable layout of related facts and figures within tables. The uniform organization readily conveys significance and associations between stored specifics.

3.4.2 Unstructured Data

The term "unstructured data" when used regarding large and diverse data sets known as "big data"indicates any accumulation of information that lacks a fixed design or schema. It has an organic structure that emerges from its creation and application rather than a prescribed format. While hard to categorize, examples include text documents, emails, photos, videos, audio files and more. Without designated classifications, analyzing and extracting insights from unstructured data presents more challenges compared to coded and standardized structured data.

"In the realm of huge data sets, unstructured data is a compilation of records which has" no organized or clearly defined. It is chaotic and challenging to handle, comprehend, and evaluate. Unstructured data does not have a set structure and can change at different times. It includes social media comments, tweets, shares, posts, YouTube videos users view, emails, text documents, images, videos, and sensor data. Unstructured data is the most abundant type of data in big data, accounting for up to 90% of it.

Not all varieties of recorded information are as methodically compiled and supplied with codes for utilization identical to data that has been organized into a predefined format. Most experts agree that only 20% or less of all data is organized. What are the remaining four fifths of the information that is currently available? We naturally refer to this data as unstructured as it isn't. Your entire unorganized data is unstructured data [2, 50].

You might be able to determine why it takes up so much space in the current data library. Unstructured data is produced by almost all computer-related activities. No one is recording their phone calls or giving each tweet a semantic tag. Organizing information into standardized templates facilitates analysis through structured queries and calculations. However, obtaining the same functionality for irregular records requires extensive effort. Not only character and numeric data sequences but also audiovisual content like photographs and videos diverge from rigid field descriptions and roles within an overall schema design.

3.4.3 Semi-Structured Data

Data that is semi-structured is between structured and unstructured data. This typically corresponds to unstructured data that has metadata attached. Data with some order but not completely rigid design is considered semi-structured. This shares trait of both structured and unstructured data. Unlike strictly structured data requiring exact conformity, semi-structured data can adapt and change to a degree while maintaining a framework for simpler interpretation than random unorganized data. There is a predictability to how elements associate allowing easier analysis than fully unstructured information, even if not fully standardized.

Data that is described as semi-structured often employs supplemental indicators beyond just the raw information itself, such as metadata tags or annotations, to provide context around what is contained. These extra details serve to illuminate the type of data and give additional understanding of its nature compared to just looking at it alone without explanatory labels. The inclusion of metadata aids in interpreting the real meaning and significance of the data elements. This information may already be collected, such as the time, place, and email address, or it may be added later as a semantic tag [50]. It has a fused content of both structured and unstructured data.

3.5   Predictive Modeling

3.5.1   What Is Predictive Modeling?

Predictive modeling refers to statistical techniques that analyze past and present data to recognize patterns informing forecasts of likely future states. This predictive analytics methodology represents a core means of generating projections. Essentially, relevant information is compiled to build a statistical algorithm. As new situations emerge, the model then makes principled guesses as to probable outcomes based on past trends recognized during development. Predictive modeling cycles through continuous data accrual, hypothesis formation, testing predictions, and refining the model calibration. Over iterative enhancements, a mature solution emerges for utilizing healthcare data evidence to guide strategic planning and clinical decision-making with disciplined expectations setting given present understandings. Though probabilistic rather than definitive, the approach supports optimized resource management and risk estimation—assisting both population and precision health goals—when properly tailored and judiciously blended with clinical insight to respect medicine's empirical foundations. This technique can be used to predict a wide range of outcomes, from customer behavior and credit risks to corporate earnings and market trends. Predictive modeling is often used in various industries, including healthcare, finance, and marketing, to make informed decisions and manage risks. It is a valuable tool for businesses seeking to forecast future events and make data-driven plans and strategies. Some common types of predictive modeling techniques include regression, neural networks, decision trees, and time series data mining. The method of examining data through analytical processes to develop forecasts or estimations concerning potential outcomes and future trends, and this approach is referred to as predictive analytics.

In contrast to descriptive and diagnostic models, predictive models are used to forecast future events, assist in expediting the decision-making process, and generate fresh insights that result in better judgments [51].

In order to describe, query, and understand complicated data, predictive analytics uses sophisticated mathematical formulations, potent statistical computer algorithms, effective software tools, and services. Predictive analytics seeks to identify patterns and trends in the data [52].

Predictive analytics' main objective is to find patterns in the dataset—relationships, correlations, arrangements, or motifs—in terms of place, time, and features (variables) that could be used to minimize the complexity of the data and prune its dimensionality. Predictive analytics may make predictions of unknown events, estimations of likelihoods or parameters, categorization labels, or other general or specific projections using these process features [51, 53].

Predictive analysis aims to discern upcoming likelihoods through numeric profiling or progressive machine learning. In health, balancing costs with outcomes proves perennially pivotal. Considering symptoms primarily, staff historically prescribe personalized regimens for presenting patients. Yet fresh modalities might expand such options. Aggregating population patterns across diversities using anonymized inputs captures subtle influences predictive alone would miss. Outcomes could improve through teaming quantification with clinicians' intuitions born of eons honing observation skills beyond dataset's present capacities. Staying open to symbiotic human-digital pairings respects medicine's art while technology empowers its science [48].

Based on the information at hand, more informed decisions concerning the patient's care are required. The ideal treatment plan for a patient could be rapidly and precisely determined using predictive modeling in the healthcare industry using the patient's demographic information and other medical histories [51].

Predictive analytics can be utilized effectively for screening purposes, treatment selection, and treatment tailoring because to the massive amounts of health data that healthcare systems and treatment facilities collect in digital form [8].

Under supervised learning, when the training data is labeled, predictive modeling falls. This indicates that all of the training data set's records have known input variables and outcomes. The outcome is an output variable having a continuous (regression) or categorical (classification) output space [54].

In order to form forecasts potent in illuminating overlooked correlations, predictive investigation utilizes ancestral particulars, arithmetical schemas or automated perceptive refining. Examination of these crafted modes facilitates projections of forthcoming probabilities. Illuminating the puzzle meriting solving, or pinpointing the ideal result, initiates model-building efforts. Only with lucidity regarding objectives can variables yield purpose, patterns clarify, and derivatives emerge robust in translation yet delicate to life's richness escaping terms. Wisdom starts in clarity; prediction finds footing there as well [4, 54].

Predictive analytics within medical settings addresses diverse topics, including but not limited to anticipating readmission hazard (the probability of a patient returning within 1 month), estimating novel therapies, trials and remedies, and boosting results by empowering patients with optimized care tailored to their circumstances. Additional applications involve forecasting demand for services to appropriately allot resources, identifying patients needing particular interventions to most favorably impact care trajectories, and signaling potential complications requiring proactive prevention. As with any domain, the goal centers on progressing from reaction to action through insight—illuminating avenues to elevated wellness, reduced suffering and health care empowering humanity at both individual and collective scales [51].

The general steps of predictive analytics are as following;

1. Defining the objective:—the first thing to understand is the problem to be solved.

2. Second thing is to gather various types of data for the problem or objective
3. Choose an algorithm to build the model
4. Build a predictive model using the sample training data

3.5.2   Techniques of Predictive Analytics

Different machine learning methodologies can be used to create predictive models. A prediction model is developed using prediction approaches like k-nearest neighbors (kNN), artificial neural networks (ANNs), and support vector machines (SVMs) [54, 55].

3.5.2.1 k-Nearest Neighbors | kNN
A supervised machine learning algorithm for classification problems is called kNN. Case-based reasoning of disease in healthcare are best suited for kNN algorithms. In the classified data set, the kNN classifier finds the k cases of the problem that are the most similar, and it selects one of those cases as the majority class for the k selected data. The nearest neighbor class is used by the kNN classifier to categorize the unlabeled observation. Both the training set and the test set keep track of the observational characteristics [54, 56].

3.5.2.2 Naïve Bayes Classification Modeling
Nave Bayes can be used to build effective illness prediction models. Because the outcome variable's class label is ambiguous, classification problems are fundamentally probabilistic in nature. The classification to which a record is comparatively more likely to belong will be estimated by a predictive model created using a training data set and a data mining approach. As a result of variables like noisy data, imbalanced data, or the exclusion of significant factors from the data set during model development, the predictions are not always accurate [57].

A misdiagnosis of an illness can have major consequences in the medical field. A clinician must consider a range of symptoms and reach a conclusion about a number of potential outcomes. Additionally, incorrect estimation of the relationship between symptoms and results may result in a misdiagnosis. The costs of making incorrect predictions and the advantages of being accurate are frequently unknown. As a result, it is necessary to use classification models that explain the probabilistic link between attributes and class outcomes [58].

3.5.2.3 Artificial Neural Networks

ANNs are mathematical models made up of a number of concurrent, interconnected processing components. As information flows, all connected components change or adapt at once, negating the need for centralized control. For difficult classification issues like disease diagnosis in healthcare, ANN can be used. Once the target disease has been identified, a patient's medical history will be used to determine whether the patient has the disease or not [59].

The first step in making the right diagnosis is choosing the signs (symptoms, lab results, and instrument readings) that can correctly identify the illness. After carefully selecting the signs, a collection of past cases is made, checked to confirm it is valid, and looked over for unusual entries. Then the system is trained. The final results given by the AI system can help expect the chances of risks and survival for people with sicknesses like cancer and heart problems by assigning importance to each symptom during the system's preparation. Similar to that, it can help pick the best treatment by finding the right medicine containing the drug needed for a particular condition [60, 61].

3.5.2.4 Decision Trees

Data mining tasks like classification, diagnosis, and inductive learning all make use of decision trees. It is a trustworthy classification tool that is constructed by repeatedly splitting the training data set into smaller subsets until each subset contains records with outcome variables belonging to the same class. It also features nodes and branches [62].

Decision trees are used in healthcare for illness diagnosis. Models are trained on a variety of input variables, such as age, weight, and body mass index (BMI), to a specific result (for example, diabetes risk), and then used to predict the outcome of an unviewed patient record [63, 64].

3.5.2.5 Linear Regression

A continuous dependent variable's value can be estimated using the statistical approach of linear regression based on one or more independent variables [65].

3.5.2.6 Logistic Regression

A statistical method for categorization problems is called logistic regression. It is employed to calculate the discrete values of a dependent variable (Yes/No, True/False, Risk/No Risk) from a set of independent variables, which may be continuous, discrete, dichotomous, or a combination of these [66].

3.5.3   Key Application Areas of Predictive Modeling in Health Care

Some major spheres where predictive analytics hold promise for enhancing health and healthcare delivery are:

1. **Medical Decision Making:** determining illnesses and deciding the appropriate treatments

   By focusing on preventative care, which includes immunization, screening, and precise disease diagnosis, primary health care can be improved. Health care workers may now precisely diagnose illnesses and offer efficient medical assistance thanks to technology. It's possible that a predictive model that was trained in the past won't forecast current trends with the same level of accuracy. The choice of the model and the frequency of retraining the model with appropriate data affect prediction accuracy [8, 67].

2. **Health Care Management**

   Management in healthcare companies is primarily concerned with demand forecasting, which is a difficult task due to the daily census's high degree of variability (the number of admissions and discharges). In addition to personnel (ambulatory staffing, nurses, doctors, and surgeons), ancillary services, and support services like housekeeping, food services, and linen, it has an impact on hospital-wide decisions. Forecasting the daily census and overall demand can aid in capacity utilization and efficient resource planning, both of which can greatly enhance service quality [8].

For the purpose of prescribing personalized medication and population health management, the future course of a disease must be predicted. To understand the severity of the condition, it is not always possible to find a single biomarker because the symptoms of many chronic diseases are heterogeneous. Prognostic risk prediction algorithms are quite helpful in these situations [68].

3. **Reducing Health Care Costs**

State and federal budgets are consistently under pressure from rising health care expenses. Policymakers who oversee medical aid work hard to reduce spending [69]. The technique of using sophisticated mathematical formulations, robust statistical computer algorithms, effective software tools and services to represent, query, and understand complicated data is known as predictive modeling [70].

A core goal of predictive analytics is forecasting trends, correlations, and behavior over time based on patterns learned from existing health data sources. These techniques leverage proxy indicators—representing real-world processes that may be indirectly observed—to gain new understandings. Through examining inherent characteristics in collected data, predictive models potentially reveal underlying system dynamics even where direct measurements are limited or look beyond current records into subsequent periods. Healthcare predictive analytics thereby seeks to infer likely future outcomes, resource needs and scenarios based on deep scrutiny of available feature information as a window onto larger healthcare mechanisms and their responses to various inputs. If properly developed and tailored, such forecasting aids strategic planning as well as personalized risk estimation and care optimization.

Predictive analytics' main objective is to find patterns in the dataset—relationships, correlations, arrangements, or motifs—in terms of place, time, and features (variables) that could be used to minimize the complexity of the data and prune its dimensionality. Predictive analytics may make predictions of unknown events, estimations of likelihoods or parameters, categorization labels, or other general or specific projections using these process features. The usability, impact on predicted accuracy, and direction of (human) activities arising from (machine) projections are all determined by the underlying assumptions of a given predictive analytics technique.

Big data analytics has the enormous potential to revolutionize healthcare as it develops into the next big thing in information technology. The outcomes of the increasing ability to analyze complex datasets not only promise process optimization but also offer numerous ways to raise the standard of patient treatment and, consequently, patient happiness.

3.5.4 Key Elements of Big Data Analytics in Healthcare

Big data analytics has four major elements in health system including inputs, processes, security, and human expertise, knowledge and governance as shown in the Fig. 3.2.

3.5.4.1 Data Input

The data enables the use of analytics to produce insights that can be put to use. Healthcare information, which is incredibly rich, can be used to increase both operational effectiveness and the quality of care. All the information needed to address specific issues must be sourced in order to make the most of such data. Additional infrastructure may be needed for locating and gathering the sources of pertinent data [1, 9, 51].

Fig. 3.2 The key
elements of big data
analytics in healthcare

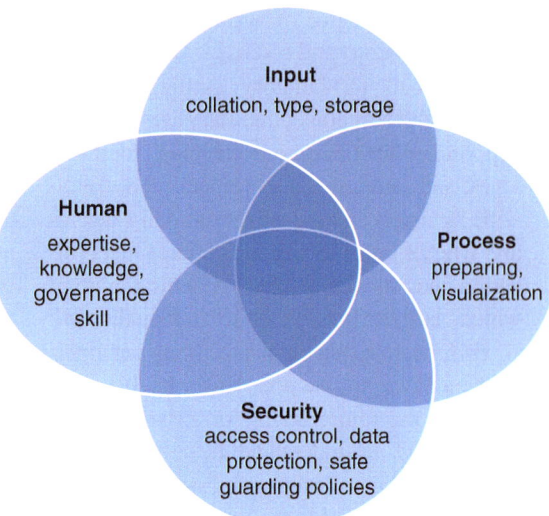

Healthcare data is very diverse in nature, taking into account the complexity of diseases and therapeutic approaches. It is difficult to handle because to the variety of health-related data and differences in how it is structured. Data might be unstructured (health care professional notes), semi-structured or weakly structured (diagnostic data), or highly structured (demographic data) [51].

3.5.4.2 Process
Data Processing and Preparation:

- Organizing and structuring the information to guarantee results are high quality: through formatting consistency and cleaning to remove errors and irregularities.
- Transforming raw clinical information from its original organized/semi-organized state into a structured table format suitable for evaluation.

Visualization:

- Effectively translating results into clear, visual forms through techniques like graphs, charts, diagrams or summarized highlights/take-aways.
- Displaying output on user-friendly dashboards for straightforward access and comprehension.

- Tools such as Tableau, Google Charts and Jupiter can produce interactive visualizations to help experts interpret and apply findings.

The goal is distilling insights from data in a manner facilitating informed decision-making through presentation styles optimized for the human perception system. This translates knowledge into actionable guidance benefitting both individuals and the larger healthcare community.

3.5.4.3 Human
Better data analysis and event prediction depend on the human factor. Big data analytics needs the proper individuals who can comprehend the output of analytical models and determine which information is crucial. Extraction of significant inferences from processed data and the logic underlying that data is made possible by human intuition and skills. Clinical data specialists are essential for treating critically ill patients and saving lives in the healthcare industry because these services include saving human lives. These experts must be able to explain the results of analytical tools [51].

3.5.4.4 Security
Access Control: In the healthcare industry, the standard access control guideline of "denying access when in doubt" is changed to "allowing

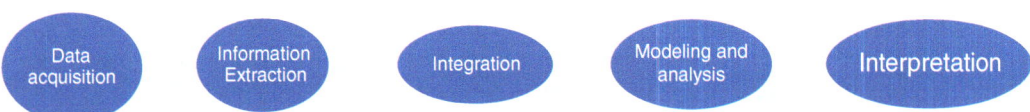

Fig. 3.3 Illustrating the overall process of big data analytics

access when in doubt" so that health-related data is easily accessible in emergency situations. Although patient privacy may be at jeopardy, methods for retroactive auditing must be taken to establish a balance between privacy and accessibility [35]. Data protection is about safeguarding healthcare data in all the aspects of data protection through:

Securing sensitive healthcare information involves guarding it from risks and upholding best practices at every stage through:

- Establishing an explicit rationale for why details are being gathered in the first place;
- Thoughtful selection of applicable information directly germane to the indicated purpose;
- Confirming the truthfulness and precision of the information being retained. Overall, carefully planning and managing information access and use helps maximize the benefits of data utilization while minimizing any attendant privacy/security issues—reassuring both providers and patients that patient welfare is the top priority.

The workflow in the whole process of valuable information extraction from large datasets can be used to describe big data analytics, a technique employed in vast datasets. Big data analytics' fundamental steps can be distilled into a list of five. Data management refers to the first three steps, whereas analytics refers to the final two (Fig. 3.3):

Big data analytics in healthcare involves analyzing enormous datasets, identifying clusters, and correlating them, as well as using data mining and artificial intelligence to enhance predictive models [6, 9, 70].

The analysis of extensive healthcare data (known as big data analytics) draws upon understandings from a range of scientific domains that contribute their respective expertise and knowledge to the field. These influences include health informatics applying information technology to medicine, bioinformatics decoding biological information, medical imaging science around technologies like x-rays and scans, medical informatics promoting digital health tools, as well as computational biomedicine advancing medicine through computational techniques. By drawing together multidisciplinary perspectives and capabilities, big data analytics in health systems can develop a more sophisticated and nuanced view of issues, leading to better solutions and ultimately improving patient care. The field exemplifies the benefits of an integrated approach across research communities.

Big data analytics techniques can improve patient-centered care, generate fresh insights into the causes of disease, detect infectious diseases before they spread, keep track of how effectively medical and healthcare facilities are performing, and ensure better treatment options. Big data analytics can boost revenue while cutting costs. Additionally, it aids in the treatment of illnesses, increases life expectancy, and lowers the number of avoidable fatalities [1].

3.6   Machine Learning

Predictive analytics is a field of data analysis that uses statistical techniques to analyze historical and current data to make predictions about future events. It involves the use of various techniques, including machine learning, to identify patterns and trends in data and make predictions based on those patterns.

Machine learning is a subfield of artificial intelligence that involves the use of algorithms to enable machines to learn and improve from data analysis without explicit programming. Machine learning algorithms can be trained in many ways, with each method having its pros and cons. Within the overarching area of machine learning, there are several core approaches based on how the computational models obtain information to learn. The main categories include: supervised learning where data is labeled for the algorithms; unsupervised learning using unlabeled information; semi-supervised learning applying both labeled and unlabeled inputs; and reinforcement learning where models are rewarded or penalized for responses. Some frequently utilized techniques under these branches include decision trees for solving decision-making problems, neural networks modeled after the human brain, and regression analysis determining relationships between variables. The methodologies employed depend on the nature and objectives of each specific application being developed. Overall, these techniques represent the different paradigms under machine learning for automating analytical tasks across industries including healthcare.

Predictive analytics and machine learning are widely used in various industries, including healthcare, finance, and marketing, to make informed decisions and manage risks. Machine learning, a branch of computer science that tries to create systems and algorithms that learn from data, is a fundamental paradigm in data analytics [71]. Data mining, which is defined as the processing and modeling of huge volumes of data to find previously undiscovered patterns or relationships, is one of the main methods used in machine learning [72]. Text mining is a branch of data mining that uses data mining methods primarily on unstructured text data. Machine learning is a group of algorithms that extract knowledge from data. Humans or other machines may utilize the information to guide their decision-making [73, 74]. The learning process for ML is self-learning and is carried out in accordance with the installed algorithms [75].

3.6.1 Machine Learning Techniques

Big data analytics utilizes machine learning (ML) approaches because of their capacity to mix heterogeneous, varied, and enormous data [76]. ML techniques can be classified into the following:

3.6.1.1 Supervised Methods
Supervised methods that use labeled training data as input include regression and classification. Using a technique that provides the highest level of performance accuracy on the training set, a model is created. Then, to map fresh samples, this model can make use of the current labels. Patient data separated into control and case groups, for instance, could make up an input. A model that may provide the greatest difference between the control and cases is created. After then, the fresh data will be classified using this model. Using labeled data for training, supervised learning creates a framework and uses that framework to classify new observations. Logistic regression, kernel-based techniques, and support vector machines are a few examples of widely used supervised approaches [56].

3.6.1.2 Unsupervised Approaches
Unlabeled training data are the starting point for unsupervised approaches like dimensionality reduction and clustering. Finding the concealed patterns and dividing the data into pertinent subsets allows for the development of a model. Unsupervised learning techniques are typically used for molecular subtyping of cancer patients and pattern recognition in gene expression data. K-means and hierarchical clustering strategies are two frequently used unsupervised learning techniques. The determination of hidden constitutions in untagged data occurs through unsupervised learning [77].

3.6.1.3 Semi-Supervised Approaches
The input for semi-supervised approaches consists of both labeled and unlabeled samples. A model is created that explains the data structure and can forecast new samples [77]. The following are a few of the most popular machine learning algorithms includes k-Nearest Neighbors (KNN), support Vector Machine (SVM), artificial Neural Network (ANN).

K-Nearest Neighbors (KNN)

KNN is an algorithm for supervised machine learning. This approach can be applied to regression issues that also involve forecasting actual values as well as classification challenges that divide problems into K classes. However, classification problems are where this algorithm is most frequently applied. It is a non-parametric sort of model, meaning that there are no preset parameters that define the items. To obtain predictions, it is employed Procedures for the KNN machine learning algorithm, as indicated in Fig. 3.4 [48, 78].

Support Vector Machine (SVM)

It is most frequently used for problem classification. Support vectors (SV) are employed in this approach to separate the classes. The SVM algorithm is ideally suited for classification since it uses two SVs to represent the worst case of each class. This algorithm aids in the discovery of a line or hyper-plane that divides two classes. The data points closest to the dividing hyper-plane are known as SVs in SVMs [79].

Pros:

- Provides higher accuracy
- Gives better result on clean data set and
- Provides better efficiency because it uses subset of training points.

Artificial Neural Network (ANN)

One of the popular forms of machine learning algorithms that mimics the human brain is the ANN [74].

3.6.2   Common Applications of Machine Learning in Healthcare

Machine learning is a subfield of artificial intelligence that enables computers to learn and improve from data without explicit programming. In healthcare, machine learning is used to analyze vast amounts of data, identify patterns, and make predictions with remarkable accuracy. Some common applications of machine learning in healthcare include:

- Improving diagnostic accuracy
- Personalizing patient treatment plans
- Predicting patient outcomes
- Assisting in the early detection of diseases
- Developing new drugs and medical devices
- Automating medical billing and clinical decision support
- Organizing medical records
- Enhancing data security
- Streamlining medical administrative systems

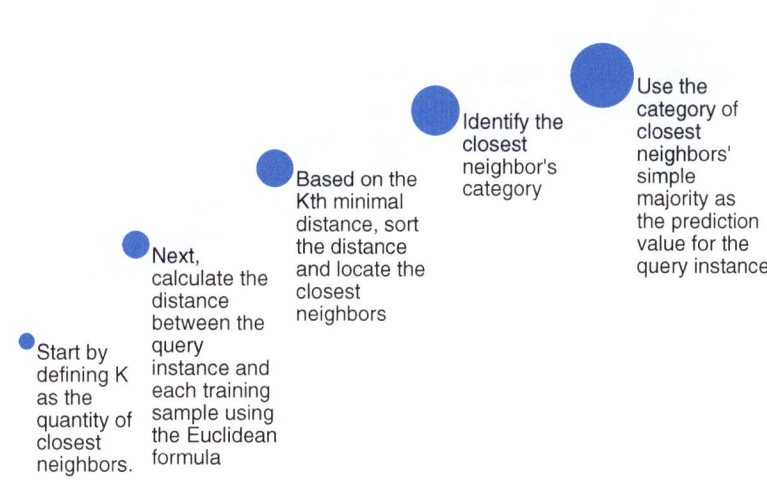

Fig. 3.4 Phases involved in KNN machine learning algorithm

- Improving the quality of care and patient health outcomes

Computerized models utilizing machine learning techniques have the ability to examine retinal scans to identify signs of diabetic retinopathy, gauge potential cardiovascular issues based on data within digital health files, or help specialists identify cancerous growths sooner through diagnostic images. As these types of data-driven solutions continue advancing, they offer hope to overhaul significant parts of how care is provided to patients, from earlier detection and diagnosis of illnesses to monitoring disease progress. Additionally, artificial intelligence applications hold promise to streamline many backend operations at medical facilities through tasks like automatic information retrieval and reporting, freeing up valuable staff time that can then be reallocated to direct patient care activities. Overall, developing AI-assisted tools grounded in machine learning principles shows exciting prospects to improve diverse segments of healthcare delivery and management for both those seeking treatment and provider organizations.

Two main tasks include the use of machine learning. Predicting future results is the first task. For instance, it may be desirable to improve the traffic light sequences at a congested crossing. To forecast the traffic flow 5 min in advance, a machine learning system might be created [80]. The second stage is categorizing things into distinct classes. Coffee beans, for instance, are often categorized into one of four grades: specialty, premium, exchange, and standard. A large-scale bean buyer may create a machine learning algorithm to rate bean quality automatically [74].

After gathering the sample data and identifying its features, a machine learning algorithm is chosen. The chosen model is subsequently trained using the training set or train sample, which is a carefully chosen subset of the data. A separate test set is used to further validate the model whether the classification or prediction performance is satisfactory. This is a portion of the original sample's data that the model had not previously seen. Iterations make up the entire procedure. Before a final model is chosen, usually several iterations are necessary. Then, this model (or models) is/are applied to fresh, real-world data that was not previously observed. While the main goal of machine learning is precise prediction or classification, other empirical sciences, like econometrics, place a greater emphasis on understanding model parameters, frequently in the context of earlier economic theory.

Often, outcomes from machine learning models are incomparable to those from more established empirical methods. Unfortunately, it is frequently impossible to understand model parameters in a useful way. In most cases, there is a definite trade-off between predictability and interpretability.

To learn from, analyze, and estimate from data, machine learning uses a number of methods. Deep learning has become a subset of machine learning as a result of advancements and advancements in the field.

Machine learning (ML) offers users some notable advantages: It can compile, combine and make sense of huge amounts of complex medical information, ML systems are capable of processing and studying vast datasets in ways that would be extremely challenging or impossible for humans alone, and it allows for the analysis, evaluation and assessment of complex and detailed data in healthcare in order to better understand patterns and trends.

Overall, ML provides abilities surrounding the assimilation, investigation and judgment of extensive complicated data in the medical field that can benefit users.

With the use of machine learning techniques, we may evaluate already-collected data and determine the links that exist within the data set as well as the essential traits of significant data. Precision medicine, or anticipating which treatment procedures will be most effective, is the most popular application of machine learning in the medical field. Applications of machine learning and precision medicine that have a high probability of success on a patient typically require a training dataset with a known outcome variable. These methods may identify patterns and relationships in sophisticated datasets and use those patterns and associations to make precise predictions about probable cancer outcomes [81].

All types of data can be used to train the machine to predict future outcomes using ML-based methodologies. For instance, if 1000 patient records are used to train the computer with features that contain disease, depending on attributes, the computer may be able to predict the presence of disease when a fresh dataset is provided. A significant advancement in the combined fields of computers and health care is the era of disease prediction.

3.7   Application of Artificial Intelligence (AI)

Artificial intelligence (AI) is the product of the fusion of numerous technologies, algorithms, and methodologies. Artificial intelligence (AI) is the ability of computers and systems to learn and apply knowledge in order to carry out a variety of cognitive tasks, such as sensing, processing oral language, reasoning, learning, and making decisions, essentially imitating human behavior [82]. This would help us understand how things work better if it were combined with data collection and analytics.

The delivery of medical care is undergoing dramatic improvements and enhancements thanks to the development of technologies like artificial intelligence. These tools have abilities to understand information, continue learning over time, and take appropriate actions. Whether assisting researchers explore new links between genetic profiles or aiding surgeons through robotic instruments, AI is demonstrating unmatched skills to detect hard-to-see connections within data that people would likely overlook. Overall, artificial intelligence has great potential to revolutionize healthcare and significantly boost patient care through its sophisticated cognitive capabilities.

In today's world, artificial intelligence is a major player in every industry. The traditional methods for storing patient information are no longer adequate due to the sharp rise in patient numbers in healthcare. Artificial intelligence (AI) has numerous applications in healthcare, including:

1. **Medical diagnosis**: AI can help in diagnosing diseases and identifying patterns in medical images, X-rays, and scans.
2. **Drug discovery**: AI can help in identifying new drug targets and predicting the efficacy of new drugs.
3. **Patient engagement and adherence**: AI can help in engaging patients and improving adherence to treatment plans.
4. **Administrative activities**: AI can automate administrative tasks, such as medical billing and clinical documentation.
5. **Precision medicine**: AI can help in tailoring healthcare interventions to individuals or groups of patients based on diagnostic or prognostic information.

AI has the potential to transform many aspects of patient care, as well as administrative processes within healthcare organizations. It can help in faster and more accurate diagnoses, predicting the development of diseases, supporting doctors with treatment decisions, and managing the demand for hospital beds. However, there are also concerns about how AI might be used, including risks to privacy and distortions to decision making. Research is essential to realize AI's potential, and regulators and public bodies have set safety standards that innovations must meet. Some of the areas AI developments in health sector are as following:

- Uncovering conditions early
- Support evidence-based decision making
- Support treatment process
- Support personal health care through wearable devices

3.7.1   Common Techniques of Artificial Intelligence

Most common techniques of AI in healthcare setting are machine learning, natural language processing, and deep learning (Fig. 3.5).

By foreseeing the outcomes of a molecule and determining its safety, artificial intelligence can support the development of structure-based drug discovery [83]. It is crucial in cutting healthcare

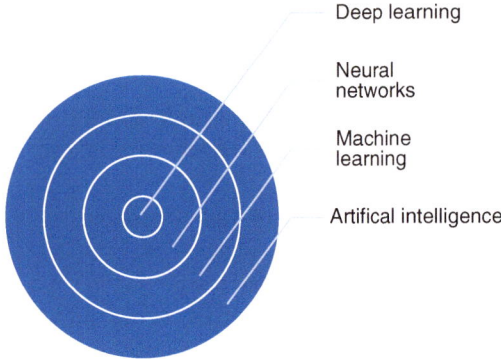

Deep learning

Neural
networks

Machine
learning

Artifical intelligence

Fig. 3.5 Artificial intelligence framework

costs and accelerating the process. Artificial intelligence methods, including:

- Deep learning- used for drug discovery,
- Natural language processing—to reinvent medicine.

3.7.1.1 Deep Learning

Deep learning is a subfield of machine learning that focuses on artificial neural networks and their algorithms. It is inspired by the structure and function of the human brain, where information is processed through interconnected neurons. Deep learning algorithms are designed to automatically learn and extract representations or features from large amounts of data. These algorithms typically consist of multiple layers of interconnected nodes, known as artificial neurons or units. Each neuron takes a set of inputs, performs a weighted sum, applies an activation function, and produces an output. The outputs from one layer of neurons serve as inputs to the next layer, forming a hierarchical representation of the data.

Deep learning methods can be supervised, semi-supervised, or unsupervised, and they are capable of learning features automatically without the need for manual feature engineering, and falls under the umbrella of artificial intelligence, is deep learning. Deep learning employs algorithms that are modeled after the composition and operation of the human brain. The important difference between deep learning and machine learning is that deep learning requires more train-

ing time and less testing time. In comparison to machine learning, deep learning can handle a big amount of input data to carry out an analysis more effectively [84].

Deep learning diverges from traditional approaches to AI by taking a brain-inspired perspective on how systems can analyze information. Unlike other techniques that demand data formatting like a spreadsheet before processing, deep learning networks can learn directly from raw information without prearranging the material. Through a multitiered design of interconnected processing units akin to neurons in the brain's structure, deep learning develops an intuitive grasp instead of relying on step-by-step procedures. By emulating biology's strategy, deep learning achieves a flexibility lacking in approaches limited to set formulas or particular use cases. Overall, it brings a unique vantage to how to solve challenges through a thinking style more natural and expansive than what came before. Deep learning can be applied to increasingly challenging tasks and can evaluate photos, sounds, and other high-dimensional data [85].

3.7.1.2 Natural Language Processing in Health System

Some common ways natural language processing is used in healthcare involve helping to organize and examine clinical notes and medical articles. Tasks like sorting documents, extracting useful information from written reports, and combining published studies can all benefit from NLP methods. Analyzing both structured and unstructured data sources lets doctors and researchers more easily notice important links and angles that expand knowledge of medicine. Whether dealing with transcribed voice recordings, translated documents or online health questions, the overall goals revolve around aiding enhanced healthcare, more precise diagnoses and better patient results through sophisticated language-focused computer techniques [86]. NLP systems can have AI conversations, document patient interactions, assess unformatted clinical notes on patients, and generate reports. NLP is needed to deal with clinical details as more and more kinds of medical information and evidence are collected in an unorganized or partly organized form. Handling clinical information in its various states requires advanced language processing abilities to glean meaningful insights from diverse data sources for improved decision making and care coordination [75].

One of NLP's objectives is to extract knowledge from natural language writings that are found in many contexts, such as medical records, reports, or social media [87, 88]. AI is having a significant impact on the healthcare industry, changing healthcare and its core functions. Five areas where artificial intelligence can be used:

(a) Digital consultation
(b) Smart diagnosis
(c) Drug discovery
(d) Robot assistance
(e) Virtual follow-up system

3.7.1.3 Digital Consultation

Live interaction between patients and physicians can now occur thanks to artificial intelligence being applied in healthcare. Remote advising is not a novel idea, but past advising programs had numerous limitations. Advancements in AI have enabled more efficient, flexible and scalable virtual consultation solutions to expand access to care. By leveraging technologies like natural language processing, conversational platforms can facilitate patient-clinician communication to discuss symptoms, treatment options and answer health questions in real-time regardless of physical location. This represents significant progress for telehealth and demonstrates how AI is enhancing connectivity within the patient experience [89–91].

Due to recent, highly-developed improvements in artificial intelligence, several problems have been addressed. First, breakthroughs in deep learning have enabled users to make better-informed choices. Through studying numerous real patient scenarios, these AI-guided platforms have learned to ask relevant questions regarding a person's medical details instead of reacting hastily to queries. Second, responding to patients' inquiries has become simpler thanks to enhanced natural language learning. It has substantially changed how computers answer by comprehending and analyzing complex terms and phrases more adeptly.

Overall, these sophisticated technological upgrades demonstrate artificial intelligence's growing potential to enhance healthcare through more nuanced dialog and informed discussion [92].

3.7.1.4 Smart Diagnosis

AI tools have helped doctors diagnose patients more quickly and precisely. Artificial intelligence resources have enabled physicians to diagnose patients more rapidly and accurately. New technologies assisted by AI can help uncover and tackle patient concerns while minimizing mistakes. Moreover, the preemptive finding of significant medical problems has been achievable through AI's use in radiology and cardiology areas. By augmenting clinical expertise with data-driven insights, doctors can make faster, supported decisions leading to improved outcomes. The implementation of advanced computing continues to strengthen core areas of healthcare through more informed diagnostic abilities and proactive patient monitoring [69, 93].

3.7.1.5 Drug Discovery

AI is being applied to drug discovery and development to improve efficiency, reduce costs, and enhance the quality of new drug candidates. However, the field also faces challenges related to bias and discrimination, which can lead to unintended consequences in drug development and clinical applications.

Now, artificial intelligence (AI) technologies are helping in pharmaceutical production. Massive datasets and essential knowledge are being used to find fresh medicinal targets. The application of AI in the pharmaceutical industry may help researchers find drugs that are more effective in treating fatal diseases.

AI for drug discovery and development is a promising field, but it must address the challenges of bias and discrimination to ensure that new drugs are safe, effective, and equitable for all patients. Regulatory frameworks and policy changes are being developed to address these challenges and ensure that AI-based drug discovery and development are conducted in a responsible and ethical manner.

It can detect minor medical patterns, allowing researchers and experts to more precisely track the development of new drugs [69].

3.7.1.6 Robots Assistance in Health System

AI in healthcare merely requires fusing the robustness of robotics with the convergent skills of surgeons, without necessarily implying that robotics will eventually replace all medical professionals. In settings like factories and warehouses, robots carry out preset activities like lifting, moving, or assembling goods, as well as delivering medical supplies in hospitals. Robots and androids with more complex operating systems and advanced degrees of AI have lately developed into more collaborative with humans and are capable of being trained through specific tasks [94].

The ability of surgeons to diagnose, see, and perform precise operations within microscopic distances in challenging tasks like gynecologic surgery, prostate surgery, and head and neck surgery has significantly increased thanks to embedded knowledge systems and surgical robots, though the majority of crucial decisions are still made by surgeons. These embedded knowledge systems should give physicians advice instead of directives because relying too heavily on electronic knowledge can often result in errors. The integration of physician knowledge and expertise with those of embedded knowledge systems and surgical robots ought to be the primary goal [95].

3.7.1.7 Virtual Follow-Up System

Patients who require routine care and examinations have significant difficulties due to the constant high demand for doctors. Applications of AI then start to work [93]. Chatbots powered by AI help to solve this issue by providing constant support to patients who require continuing care [96, 97]. Patients with problems must first join instantly, and the chatbots can respond appropriately in a matter of seconds.

AI-powered virtual follow-up systems are being used in various industries, including healthcare, sales, and marketing, to improve efficiency and personalize interactions with customers or patients. These systems use AI-powered tools to analyze customer or patient responses and provide appropriate contextual messages in real-time. They can also automate routine tasks, such as lead qualification, nurturing campaigns, and appointment scheduling, freeing up human resources to focus on building meaningful relationships with customers or patients. AI-powered virtual assistants can work round-the-clock, ensuring that customers or patients receive responses and engagement even outside regular business hours. These systems can also handle multiple leads or patients simultaneously and ensure consistent and systematic follow-up, preventing leads or patients from falling through the cracks. Additionally, thanks to recent advancements, patients no longer need to type out their symptoms because chatbots can easily decipher handwritten notes and images [78].

3.7.2 Goals of Artificial Intelligence in Healthcare

AI has the power to enhance diagnosis, expand therapeutic alternatives, increase patient adherence and engagement, and promote operational and administrative efficiency. Artificial intelligence has incredible potential in the medical industry to do tasks that require little human involvement. Artificial intelligence appears to be most suited to support clinical judgment, analysis, and training. It has been demonstrated that when this technology is used properly, an accurate and quick diagnosis may be made. The major objective of artificial intelligence (AI) is to eliminate the risk of potential human error in medical care and surgery. The medical staff could look into the extensive diagnostic procedures and the gathered information. It is used to establish a patient's genetic profile. Case studies, medical issues, and patient histories are all maintained in this system [98, 99].

3.7.2.1 Improve Diagnostics

By examining symptoms, recommending individualized treatments, and assessing risk, artificial intelligence (AI) technology can assist medical practitioners in diagnosing patients. It can also spot unexpected results. Intelligent symptom checkers are already being used by many healthcare organizations and healthcare providers. By asking people a series of questions about their symptoms, this machine learning technology can determine the best course of action for getting medical attention [100].

By synthesizing data and making conclusions, AI technology can also advance precision medicine—healthcare that is catered to the individual—by enabling more knowledgeable and individualized therapy. Deep learning algorithms are able to examine enormous volumes of data, including details about a patient's genetic makeup, further molecular/cellular analyses, and lifestyle factors—and discover pertinent studies that might assist physicians in making treatment decisions [67, 101].

3.7.2.2 Detecting Disease

For healthcare providers, imaging technologies can accelerate the diagnostic process. By recognizing any possible dangers linked to an individual, AI can provide several benefits for preemptive identification. For the aim of establishing a care roadmap and ensuring patients' welfare, precise illness identification is fundamental. Advanced visualization assets empowered by machine learning analytics help practitioners more quickly pinpoint medical problems and abnormalities. This supports swifter determination of the most effective therapy approach. Overall, AI-assisted diagnostic modalities enhance clinicians' ability to deliver timely, informed care centered on patients' needs [102, 103]. Particularly in general medical practice settings and remote areas, human mistakes can constrain diagnostic exactness and productivity because interpreting clinical information is a complex mental job. Convolutional neural networks, knowledge maps, and transformers are a few illustrations of man-made brainpower strategies that have been appeared to be viable and promising in helping with and enhancing sickness analysis and actually treatment also. The utilization of AI in the analytic cycle assists specialists with expanding the accuracy and viability of their judgments, bringing about the arrangement of

recently accessible computerized wellbeing administrations. By limiting human blunder and giving continuous scientific asset admittance, AI upgrades basic leadership regardless of area or asset restrictions [83, 104].

3.7.2.3 Advancing Treatment

Medical AI is becoming into a useful tool for patient care. Patients who have lost their capacity to talk and move could benefit from brain-computer interfaces. Additionally, this technology may enhance the quality of life for ALS, stroke, and spinal cord injury patients. The development of new technologies may open up new possibilities for tailoring medicines to each patient's particular genetic profile [105].

AI is advancing treatment in various ways, including drug discovery, personalized medicine, and improving patient care. Some examples of AI's impact on treatment include:

1. **Precision medicine and drug discovery:** AI examines vast genetic and health datasets linked to illnesses to recognize potential medical targets and forecast drug effectiveness as well as adverse reactions.
2. **Personalized clinical trials:** AI enables smaller trial sizes with fewer patients randomly assigned to standard care. This enhances cost-efficiency of medication development through virtual comparison groups.
3. **Early cancer identification:** AI tools can accurately spot cancer in its early stages, speeding diagnosis and improved prognoses through earlier treatment start times.
4. **Medical imaging analysis:** AI algorithms inspect intricate scans from CT, MRI and X-rays to assist surgeons enhance skills and refine techniques.
5. **Accelerating research:** AI hastens the research process through optimized study planning, enrollment figures and revealing deeper links between diseases and therapies.
6. **Reusing current medications:** AI examines present medications to fight specific illnesses, advancing new drugs through cost-effective development leveraging existing knowledge.

7. **Generative design:** AI can model molecular structures de novo, aiding discovery and progress of novel pharmaceutical candidates from the start."
8. **Patient engagement and adherence:** AI can be used to personalize and contextualize care, improving patient outcomes
9. **Virtual follow-up systems:** AI can automate routine tasks, such as lead qualification and appointment scheduling, freeing up human resources to focus on building meaningful relationships with patients

Additionally, by examining historical, current, and future patient data, clinical decision support systems (CDSSs) can support healthcare professionals in making better medical decisions. Lastly, AI has the potential to speed up medication development by cutting down on the time and expense associated with discovery. AI tools assist in data-driven decision making, assisting researchers in determining which chemicals merit further investigation [106].

3.7.2.4 Boosting Patient Engagement

With wearable innovation and customized restorative gadgets like action trackers and keen watches, both patients and experts can screen wellbeing. By obtaining and breaking down measurements about people, these innovations can in addition advance the investigation of public wellbeing elements on a more extensive scale. As day by day use of such advanced wellbeing apparatuses becomes more common, huge informational collections are created that offer valuable bits of knowledge when dissected utilizing man-made brainpower. This permits recognized examples and conceivable wellbeing hazards to be recognized all the more rapidly, encouraging anticipatory medicinal services and counteractive action [107]. In order to foster lasting client relationships, this degree of involvement makes use of AI's potential in the healthcare industry. It enables medical professionals and healthcare facilities to use technology to improve patient pleasure and experience [108, 109].

Additionally, these tools can be helpful in encouraging patients to follow medical advice. Patient adherence to treatment regimens may influ-

ence the outcome. The care plan may not succeed if individuals are not obedient and do not alter their behavior or take prescription medications as instructed [110]. AI's ability to individualize therapy may empower patients to take an increasingly dynamic part in their care. Machines with man-made brainpower can convey customized updates or substance intended to inspire input from patients. By sending tailor-made wellbeing data and proposals, counteracting dangers or self-administration tips, AI has potential to enhance patient responsibility for wellbeing administration. This progressive correspondence could expand consistency with treatment designs. Additionally, AI-curated substance considers singular preferences, ways of life and wellbeing objectives. Personalized intercessions and minding may fortify the quiet-doctor relationship, prompting improved personal satisfaction and results over the long haul [79].

3.7.2.5 Supporting Administration and Overall Flow

By taking a portion of the functions off of staff, AI can upgrade the authoritative and operational work process in the human services framework. Takers invest some place in the scope of 34–55% of their opportunity on clinical records documentation and audit, making it one of the key reasons for brought down profitability. Note taking and record keeping utilizes critical clinical assets that could be redirected to people. AI arrangements involving mechanical language handling can help streamline this documentation errand, freeing doctors to spend more energy focusing on thoughtful care conveyance. Reducing the documentation workload through astute frameworks could upgrade efficiencies and enable providers to expand accessibility of high-worth administrations for patients [111].

3.7.3 Major Challenges of Artificial Intelligence

The implementation of AI in public health faces several challenges that need to be addressed for successful integration. Some of the major challenges of AI in public health include:

3.7.3.1 Data Scarcity

An AI system needs trained data to function. The majority of individuals might not be aware that labeling training data requires a significant amount of human labor in order to obtain high-quality data sets. Additionally, the data set must be sufficiently extensive and sizeable to be used for training. The capacity to acquire these high-quality data is important for classifying AI systems as "good" or "bad" in general. These would frequently be the difficulties for new applications or startup businesses [112, 113].

3.7.3.2 Data Privacy and Security

The use of AI in healthcare requires large amounts of patient data, raising concerns about data privacy and security. It is essential to ensure that patient data is protected from unauthorized access and that patients have control over how their data is used [79, 114].

3.7.3.3 Transparency of Algorithms

Some forms of AI remain difficult for people like doctors and nurses to fully comprehend and trust since the inner workings leading to a given output or diagnosis may not be apparent. Without transparency into what drove the machine to its conclusion, professionals have less insight into assessing the reasoning and making use of an AI tool's analysis. If a system functions more as an opaque "black box", accepting its result without perceiving how it was derived presents a challenge for acceptance and incorporation into clinical practice. Greater explainability of AI decision-making may be important to establish reliance in the care environment.

Algorithms are used by AI systems, in particular machine learning, to make decisions and predictions. These machine learning algorithms frequently get more complicated as they work to get the necessary accuracy. Consequently, they become increasingly challenging for human observers to understand. A "black box" with little transparency, some machine learning algorithms, like deep learning, may involve multiple layers of features and thousands of variables. Anyone finds it difficult to articulate the reasoning behind a decision or prediction [114].

3.7.3.4 Knowledge Gap

Many within the medical field including those providing care and receiving it may not truly understand how artificial intelligence works and what it can and cannot do compared to human abilities. This could lead to thinking the technology is able to do more than it really can or being too doubtful of it. Without the right context, people interacting with AI may develop wrong ideas. Spending more time teaching about what AI is currently good at and what still needs human thinking, watching, or choice would help develop a more factual view of what AI brings to healthcare now and later. This could foster improved confidence in AI tools used for suitable medical needs.

3.7.3.5 Data Quality and Interoperability

Healthcare data is frequently incomplete, inconsistent, and inaccurate, which can introduce biases and errors in AI models. In addition, the inconsistency of data formats and protocols hampers the ability to compare and exchange data across different healthcare systems, limiting the potential for insights derived from large-scale data analysis.

3.7.3.6 Data Access, Control and Use

Compared to conventional health technology, AI has a number of distinctive qualities. Notably, they sometimes make mistakes and have biases that make it difficult or impossible for human medical professionals to supervise them. The latter is due to the "black box" problem, in which the methods and "reasoning" employed by learning algorithms to arrive at their conclusions may be partially or completely opaque to human observers. If the proper controls are not in place, this opacity might also apply to how health and personal information is used and exploited [113, 114].

3.7.3.7 Legal and Policy Framework

At present, there are no definite rules or standards for how AI should and should not be applied within medical settings in global south. Without such direction, healthcare providers face an unclear path forward regarding responsible utilization. It can also present difficulties in confirming these systems serve all patient groups fairly and respect ethical practices. Establishing regulatory guidance backed by thoughtful discourse could ultimately smooth adoption of AI by creating a shared understanding around accountability, patient rights and equal access to advances across communities.

References

1. José Sousa M, Jamil G, Eduardo Walter C, Au-Yong-Oliveira M, Moreira F. Big data analytics on patents for innovation public policies. Wiley Online Libr. 2021;40(1):e12673. https://doi.org/10.1111/exsy.12673.
2. Belle A, Thiagarajan R, Soroushmehr SMR, Navidi F, Beard DA, Najarian K. Big data analytics in healthcare. Biomed Res Int. 2015;2015:370194.
3. Raghupathi W, Raghupathi V. Big data analytics in healthcare: promise and potential. Health Inf Sci Syst. 2014;2(1):1–10. https://doi.org/10.1186/2047-2501-2-3.
4. Alharthi H. Healthcare predictive analytics: an overview with a focus on Saudi Arabia. J Infect Public Health. 2018;11(6):749–56.
5. Galetsi P, Katsaliaki K. A review of the literature on big data analytics in healthcare. J Oper Res Soc. 2019;71(10):1511–29. https://doi.org/10.1080/01605682.2019.1630328.
6. Putchala B, Kanala LS, Donepudi DP, Kondaveeti HK. Applications of big data analytics in healthcare informatics. In: Health informatics and patient safety in times of crisis; 2023. https://www.igi-global.com/chapter/applications-of-big-data-analytics-in-healthcare-informatics/314115.
7. Marichamy VS, Natarajan V. Blockchain based securing medical records in big data analytics. Data Knowl Eng. 2023;144:102122.
8. Sarker IH. Data science and analytics: an overview from data-driven smart computing, decision-making and applications perspective. SN Comput Sci. 2021;2(5):1–22. https://doi.org/10.1007/s42979-021-00765-8.
9. Do Nascimento IJB, Marcolino MS, Abdulazeem HM, Weerasekara I, Azzopardi-Muscat N, Goncalves MA, et al. Impact of big data analytics on people's health: overview of systematic reviews and recommendations for future studies. J Med Internet Res. 2021;23(4):e27275.
10. Nutley T, Gnassou L, Traore M, Bosso AE, Mullen S. Moving data off the shelf and into action: an intervention to improve data-informed decision making in Cote d'Ivoire. Glob Health Action. 2014;7:25035.
11. Wagenaar BH, Sherr K, Fernandes Q, Wagenaar AC. Using routine health information systems for well-designed health evaluations in low-and middle-income countries. Health Policy Plan. 2016;31(1):129–35.
12. Siegler EL. The evolving medical record. Ann Intern Med. 2010;153(10):671–7.
13. Feyzabadi VY, Emami M, Mehrolhassani MH. Health information system in primary health care: the challenges and barriers from local providers' perspective of an area in Iran. Int J Prev Med. 2015;6:57.
14. Hotchkiss DR, Diana ML, Foreit KGF. How can routine health information systems improve health systems functioning in lowand middle-income countries? Assessing the evidence base. Adv Health Care Manage. 2012;12:25–58.
15. Wude H, Woldie M, Melese D, Lolaso T, Balcha B. Utilization of routine health information and associated factors among health workers in Hadiya Zone, Southern Ethiopia. PLoS One. 2020;15(5):e0233092.
16. Munda Mucee E, Odhiambo-Otieno G, Wambui Kaburi L, Kainyu KR. Routine health management information use in the public health sector in Tharaka Nithi County, Kenya. Imp J Interdiscip Res. 2016;2(3):660–72.
17. Hagel C, Paton C, Mbevi G, English M. Data for tracking SDGs: challenges in capturing neonatal data from hospitals in Kenya. BMJ Glob Health. 2020;5(3):e002108.
18. Kassie SY, Demsash AW, Chereka AA, Damtie Y. Medical documentation practice and its association with knowledge, attitude, training, and availability of documentation guidelines in Ethiopia, 2022. A systematic review and meta-analysis. Inform Med Unlocked. 2023;38:101237.
19. Korst LM, Eusebio-Angeja AC, Chamorro T, Aydin CE, Gregory KD. Nursing documentation time during implementation of an electronic medical record. J Nurs Adm. 2003;33(1):24–30.
20. Tamir T, Geda B, Mengistie B. Documentation practice and associated factors among nurses in harari regional state and dire dawa administration governmental hospitals, Eastern Ethiopia. Adv Med Educ Pract. 2021;12:453–62.
21. Demsash AW, Kassie SY, Dubale AT, Chereka AA, Ngusie HS, Hunde MK, et al. Health professionals' routine practice documentation and its associated factors in a resource-limited setting: a cross-sectional study. BMJ Heal Care Inform. 2023;30(1):e100699.
22. Kebede M, Endris Y, Zegeye DT. Nursing care documentation practice: the unfinished task of nursing care in the University of Gondar Hospital. Inform Health Soc Care. 2016;42(3):290–302. https://doi.org/10.1080/17538157.2016.1252766.
23. Bhattacharya AA, Umar N, Audu A, Allen E, Schellenberg JRM, Marchant T. Quality of routine facility data for monitoring priority maternal and newborn indicators in DHIS2: a case

study from Gombe State, Nigeria. PLoS One. 2019;14(1):e0211265.

24. Hermann K, Van Damme W, Pariyo GW, Schouten E, Assefa Y, Cirera A, et al. Community health workers for ART in sub-Saharan Africa: learning from experience—capitalizing on new opportunities. Hum Resour Health. 2009;7(1):1–11. https://doi.org/10.1186/1478-4491-7-31.

25. Maes K, Kalofonos I. Becoming and remaining community health workers: perspectives from Ethiopia and Mozambique. Soc Sci Med. 2013;87:52–9.

26. Silva R, Amouzou A, Munos M, Marsh A, Hazel E, Victora C, et al. Can community health workers report accurately on births and deaths? Results of field assessments in Ethiopia, Malawi and Mali. PLoS One. 2016;11(1):e0144662.

27. Nguefack-Tsague G, Tamfon BB, Ngnie-Teta I, Ngoufack MN, Keugoung B, Bataliack SM, et al. Factors associated with the performance of routine health information system in Yaoundé-Cameroon: a cross-sectional survey. BMC Med Inform Decis Mak. 2020;20(1):339.

28. Dessie G, Jara D, Alem G, Mulugeta H, Zewdu T, Wagnew F, et al. Evidence-based practice and associated factors among health care providers working in public hospitals in Northwest Ethiopia during 2017. Curr Ther Res. 2020;93:100613.

29. Shayan SJ, Kiwanuka F, Nakaye Z. Barriers associated with evidence-based practice among nurses in low- and middle-income countries: a systematic review. Worldviews Evid Based Nurs. 2019;16(1):12–20. https://doi.org/10.1111/wvn.12337.

30. Adane A, Adege TM, Ahmed MM, Anteneh HA, Ayalew ES, Berhanu D, et al. Exploring data quality and use of the routine health information system in Ethiopia: a mixed-methods study. BMJ Open. 2021;11(12):e050356.

31. Guadie HA, Shiferaw AM, Gashu KD. Health workers' perceptions on data-informed decision-making practices in primary health care units at Awi Zone, Northwest Ethiopia. Ethiop J Heal Dev. 2022;36(2) https://doi.org/10.20372/ejhd.v36i2.

32. Lander J, Curbach J, von Sommoggy J, Bitzer EM, Dierks M-L. Awareness, information-seeking behavior, and information preferences about early childhood allergy prevention among different parent groups: protocol for a mixed methods study. JMIR Res Protoc. 2021;10(1):e25474.

33. Greenhalgh T, Hinder S, Stramer K, Bratan T, Russell J. Adoption, non-adoption, and abandonment of a personal electronic health record: case study of HealthSpace. BMJ. 2010;341:c5814.

34. Flanagan ME, Saleem JJ, Millitello LG, Russ AL, Doebbeling BN. Paper- and computer-based workarounds to electronic health record use at three benchmark institutions. J Am Med Informatics Assoc. 2013;20(e1):e59–66.

35. Wassie MA, Zeleke AA, Dachew BA, Kebede M. Evidence-based practice and its associated fac-

tors among medical laboratory professionals in West Amhara hospitals, Northwest Ethiopia. Int J Evid Based Healthc. 2018;16(1):66–72.

36. Nicol E, Bradshaw D, Uwimana-Nicol J, Dudley L. Perceptions about data-informed decisions: an assessment of information-use in high HIV-prevalence settings in South Africa. BMC Health Serv Res. 2017;17(Suppl 2):765.

37. Kreps GL, Neuhauser L. New directions in eHealth communication: opportunities and challenges. Patient Educ Couns. 2010;78(3):329–36.

38. Cooper CJ, Cooper SP, Del Junco DJ, Shipp EM, Whitworth R, Cooper SR. Web-based data collection: detailed methods of a questionnaire and data gathering tool. Epidemiol Perspect Innov. 2006;3:1.

39. Nguyen L, Bellucci E, Nguyen LT. Electronic health records implementation: an evaluation of information system impact and contingency factors. Int J Med Inform. 2014;83(11):779–96.

40. Leon N, Balakrishna Y, Hohlfeld A, Odendaal WA, Schmidt BM, Zweigenthal V, et al. Routine Health Information System (RHIS) improvements for strengthened health system management. Cochrane Database Syst Rev. 2020;2020(8):CD012012.

41. Worku T, Yeshitila M, Feto T, Leta S, Mesfin F, Mezmur H. Evidence-based medicine among physicians working in selected public hospitals in eastern Ethiopia: a cross-sectional study. BMC Med Inform Decis Mak. 2019;19(1):1–8. https://doi.org/10.1186/s12911-019-0826-8.

42. Mheidly N, Fares J. Leveraging media and health communication strategies to overcome the COVID-19 infodemic. J Public Health Policy. 2020;41(4):410–20.

43. Yehualashet DE, Melese Yilma T, Takele A, Nebiyu J, Gedlu M, Jemere AT, et al. Factors associated with practicing evidence-based medicine among medical interns in amhara regional state teaching hospitals, northwest Ethiopia: a cross-sectional study. Adv Med Educ Pract. 2021;12:843–52.

44. Vishnoi SK, Virmani N, Pant D, Virmani N, Garg A. Big data in healthcare. In: Designing intelligent healthcare systems, products, and services using disruptive technologies and health informatics. CRC Press; 2022. p. 211–27.

45. Mota AL, Ferraciolli SF, Ayres AS, Polsin LLM, da Costa LC, Kitamura F. AI and big data for intelligent health: promise and potential. In: Trends of artificial intelligence and big data for E-health. Cham: Springer; 2022. p. 1–14.

46. Ishwarappa AJ. A brief introduction on big data 5Vs characteristics and hadoop technology. Procedia Comput Sci. 2015;48(C):319–24.

47. Millham R, Agbehadji IE, Frimpong SO. The paradigm of fog computing with bio-inspired search methods and the "5Vs" of big data. In: Fong S, Millham R, editors. Bio-inspired algorithms for data streaming and visualization, big data management, and fog computing, Springer tracts in nature-inspired

computing. Singapore: Springer; 2021. p. 145–67. https://doi.org/10.1007/978-981-15-6695-0_8.

48. Srivastava D, Pandey H, Agarwal AK. Complex predictive analysis for health care: a comprehensive review. Bull Electr Eng Inform. 2023;12(1):521–31.

49. Galetsi P, Katsaliaki K, Kumar S. Big data analytics in health sector: theoretical framework, techniques and prospects. Int J Inf Manag. 2020;50:206–16.

50. Adnan K, Akbar R, Khor SW, Ali ABA. Role and challenges of unstructured big data in healthcare. Adv Intell Syst Comput. 2020;1042:301–23. https://doi.org/10.1007/978-981-32-9949-8_22.

51. Venkatesh R, Balasubramanian C, Kaliappan M. Development of big data predictive analytics model for disease prediction using machine learning technique. J Med Syst. 2019;43(8):272.

52. Luo J, Wu M, Gopukumar D, Zhao Y. Big data application in biomedical research and health care: a literature review. Biomed Inform Insights. 2016;8:1–10.

53. Hulsen T, Friedecký D, Renz H, Melis E, Vermeersch P, Fernandez-Calle P. From big data to better patient outcomes. Clin Chem Lab Med. 2022;61(4):580–6.

54. Benramdane MK, Kornyshova E, Bouzefrane S, Maupas H. Supervised machine learning for matchmaking in digital business ecosystems and platforms. Inf Syst Front. 2023; https://doi.org/10.1007/s10796-022-10357-3.

55. Roberts L, Dhanoa H, et al. Machine learning for enhanced healthcare: an overview for operational and clinical leads. Br J Healthc Manage. 2023;29(1):12–9. https://doi.org/10.12968/bjhc.2022.0096.

56. Murugesan M, Yu J-H, Singh Bhandari K, Chung W, Jung K-S, Cho S-M, et al. Supervised machine learning approach for modeling hot deformation behavior of medium carbon steel. Wiley Online Libr. 2022;94(2):2200188. https://doi.org/10.1002/srin.202200188.

57. Chen S, Webb GI, Liu L, Ma X. A novel selective naïve Bayes algorithm. Knowl-Based Syst. 2020;192:105361.

58. Jackins V, Vimal S, Kaliappan M, Lee MY. AI-based smart prediction of clinical disease using random forest classifier and Naive Bayes. J Supercomput. 2021;77(5):5198–219. https://doi.org/10.1007/s11227-020-03481-x.

59. Reddy S, Fox J, Purohit MP. Artificial intelligence-enabled healthcare delivery. J R Soc Med. 2019;112(1):22–8. https://doi.org/10.1177/0141076818815510.

60. Suwarno I, Cakan A, Raharja NM, Baballe MA, Mahmoud MS. Unexpected alliance of cardiovascular diseases and artificial intelligence in health care. In: Machine learning, image processing, network security and data sciences, Lecture notes in electrical engineering, vol. 946. Singapore: Springer. p. 481–92. https://doi.org/10.1007/978-981-19-5868-7_35.

61. Yuan G, Lv B, Hao C. Application of artificial neural networks in reproductive medicine. Hum Fertil (Camb). 2023;26(5):1195–201.

62. Tulasi Bhavani T, Rao MK, Reddy AM. Network intrusion detection system using random forest and decision tree machine learning techniques. Adv Intell Syst Comput. 2020;1045:637–43.

63. Kaparthi S, Bumblauskas D. Designing predictive maintenance systems using decision tree-based machine learning techniques. Int J Qual Reliab Manage. 2020;37(4):659–86.

64. Jijo BT, Abdulazeez AM. Classification based on decision tree algorithm for machine learning. JASTT. 2021;2(1):20–8.

65. Ye T, Liu B. Uncertain hypothesis test with application to uncertain regression analysis. Fuzzy Optim Decis Mak. 2022;21(2):157–74.

66. De Menezes D, Prata D, Secchi AR, Pinto JC. A review on robust M-estimators for regression analysis. Comput Chem Eng. 2021;147(8):107254.

67. Secinaro S, Calandra D, Secinaro A, Muthurangu V, Biancone P. The role of artificial intelligence in healthcare: a structured literature review. BMC Med Inform Decis Mak. 2021;21:125.

68. Nutley T, Reynolds HW. Improving the use of health data for health system strengthening. Glob Health Action. 2013;6:20001.

69. Kumar M, Nguyen TPN, Kaur J, Singh TG, Soni D, Singh R, et al. Opportunities and challenges in application of artificial intelligence in pharmacology. Pharm Rep. 2023;75(1):3–18.

70. Benzidia S, Bentahar O, Husson J, Makaoui N. Big data analytics capability in healthcare operations and supply chain management: the role of green process innovation. Ann Oper Res. 2023;333:1077–101. https://doi.org/10.1007/s10479-022-05157-6.

71. Atkinson JG, Atkinson EG. Machine learning and health care: potential benefits and issues. J Ambul Care Manage. 2023;46(2):114–20.

72. Rajendran S, et al. Health informatics system using machine learning techniques. 2023. https://books.google.com/books?hl=en&lr=&id=Kg-mEAAAQBAJ&oi=fnd&pg=PA179&dq=healthcare+informatics+big+data+analytics&ots=lZLz40rfDV&sig=dFUeh1D9KZ35p4wWvCicDdiAWho.

73. Patil R, Shah K. Machine learning in healthcare: applications, current status, and future prospects. Handb Res Mach Learn. 2022;23:163–86.

74. Langenberger B, Schulte T, Groene O. The application of machine learning to predict high-cost patients: a performance-comparison of different models using healthcare claims data. PLoS One. 2023;18(1):e0279540. https://doi.org/10.1371/journal.pone.0279540.

75. Silvestri S, Islam S, Papastergiou S, Tzagkarakis C, Ciampi M. A machine learning approach for the NLP-based analysis of cyber threats and vulnerabilities of the healthcare ecosystem. Sensors. 2023;23:651.

76. Strang KD. How could machine learning help healthcare informatics predict coronavirus? In: Health informatics and patient safety in times of crisis. IGI Global; 2023. https://www.igi-global.com/chapter/how-could-machine-learning-help-healthcare-informatics-predict-coronavirus/314107.

77. Roberts L, Dhanoa H, Lanes S, Holdship J. Machine learning for enhanced healthcare: an overview for operational and clinical leads. Br J Healthc Manag. 2023;29(1):12–9.

78. Solanki R, Rajawat A, Gadekar AR, Patil ME. Building a conversational chatbot using machine learning: towards a more intelligent healthcare application. In: Handbook of research on instructional technologies in health education and allied disciplines. IGI Gloabal; 2023. https://www.igi-global.com/chapter/building-a-conversational-chatbot-using-machine-learning/320385.

79. Jiang F, Jiang Y, Zhi H, Dong Y, Li H, Ma S, et al. Artificial intelligence in healthcare: past, present and future. Stroke Vasc Neurol. 2017;2(4):230–43.

80. Jentzer J, Kashou A, Murphree DH. Clinical applications of artificial intelligence and machine learning in the modern cardiac intensive care unit. Intell Based Med. 2023;7:100089.

81. Kumar K, Kumar P, Deb D, Unguresan ML, Muresan V. Artificial intelligence and machine learning based intervention in medical infrastructure: a review and future trends. Healthcare. 2023;11:207.

82. Sinha A, Kumar G. Artificial intelligence in healthcare and its application in brain stroke diagnosis. In: Bioinformatics tools and big data analytics for patient care. Chapman and Hall/CRC; 2023. https://www.taylorfrancis.com/chapters/edit/10.1201/9781003226949-6/artificial-intelligence-healthcare-application-brain-stroke-diagnosis-ambarish-kumar-sinha-gaurav-kumar.

83. Mahdi S, Battineni G, Khawaja M, et al. How does artificial intelligence impact digital healthcare initiatives? A review of AI applications in dental healthcare. Int J Inform Manage Data Insights. 2023;3:100144.

84. Xiao C, Choi E, Sun J. Opportunities and challenges in developing deep learning models using electronic health records data: a systematic review. J Am Med Informatics Assoc. 2018;25(10):1419–28.

85. He T, Liu H, Zhang Z, Li C, Zhou Y. Research on the application of artificial intelligence in public health management: leveraging artificial intelligence to improve COVID-19 CT image diagnosis. Int J Environ Res Public Health. 2023;20:1158.

86. Khurana D, Koli A, Khatter K, Singh S. Natural language processing: state of the art, current trends and challenges. Multimed Tools Appl. 2023;82(3):3713–44.

87. Khurana D, Koli A, Khatter K, Singh S. Natural language processing: state of the art, current trends and challenges. Multimed Tools Appl.

2023;82(3):3713–44. https://doi.org/10.1007/s11042-022-13428-4.

88. Tinmouth J, Swain D, Chorneyko K, et al. Validation of a natural language processing algorithm to identify adenomas and measure adenoma detection rates across a health system: a population-level study. Gastrointest Endosc. 2023;97(1):121–129.e1.

89. Stoves J, Connolly J, Cheung CK, Grange A, Rhodes P, O'Donoghue D, et al. Electronic consultation as an alternative to hospital referral for patients with chronic kidney disease: a novel application for networked electronic health records to improve the accessibility and efficiency of healthcare. Qual Saf Health Care. 2010;19:e54.

90. Skeith L, Mohamed M, Karovitch A, Liddy C, Afkham A, Archibald D, et al. The use of eConsults to improve access to specialty care in thrombosis medicine. Thromb Res. 2017;160:105–8.

91. Banks J, Farr M, Edwards H, Horwood J, Salisbury C, Northstone K, et al. Use of an electronic consultation system in primary care: a qualitative interview study. Br J Gen Pract. 2018;68(666):e1–8.

92. Marziniak M, Brichetto G, Feys P, Meyding-Lamadé U, Vernon K, Meuth SG. The use of digital and remote communication technologies as a tool for multiple sclerosis management: narrative review. JMIR Rehabil Assist Technol. 2018;5(1):e5.

93. Anthony B Jr. Use of telemedicine and virtual care for remote treatment in response to COVID-19 pandemic. J Med Syst. 2020;44(7):132.

94. Kyrarini M, Lygerakis F, Rajavenkatanarayanan A, Sevastopoulos C, Nambiappan HR, Chaitanya KK, et al. A survey of robots in healthcare. Technology. 2021;9(1):8.

95. Tavakoli M, Carriere J, Torabi A. Robotics, smart wearable technologies, and autonomous intelligent systems for healthcare during the COVID-19 pandemic: an analysis of the State of the Art and Future Vision. Adv Intell Syst. 2020;2(7):2000071. https://doi.org/10.1002/aisy.202000071.

96. Broussard BS, Broussard AB. Using electronic communication safely in health care settings. Nurs Womens Health. 2013;17(1):59–62.

97. Eysenbach G. The role of chatgpt, generative language models, and artificial intelligence in medical education: a conversation with chatgpt and a call for papers. JMIR Med Educ. 2023;9:e46885.

98. Davenport T, Kalakota R. The potential for artificial intelligence in healthcare. Futur Healthc J. 2019;6(2):94.

99. Sun L, Gupta RK, Sharma A. Review and potential for artificial intelligence in healthcare. Int J Syst Assur Eng Manag. 2022;13(1):54–62. https://doi.org/10.1007/s13198-021-01221-9.

100. Amann J, Blasimme A, Vayena E, Frey D, Madai VI. Explainability for artificial intelligence in healthcare: a multidisciplinary perspective. BMC Med Inform Decis Mak. 2020;20(1):1–9. https://doi.org/10.1186/s12911-020-01332-6.

101. Panch T, Szolovits P, Atun R. Artificial intelligence, machine learning and health systems. J Glob Health. 2018;8(2):020303.

102. Kumar Y, Koul A, Singla R, Ijaz MF. Artificial intelligence in disease diagnosis: a systematic literature review, synthesizing framework and future research agenda. J Ambient Intell Humaniz Comput. 2023;14(7):8459–86.

103. Mirbabaie M, Stieglitz S, Frick NRJ. Artificial intelligence in disease diagnostics: a critical review and classification on the current state of research guiding future direction. Health Technol (Berl). 2021;11(4):693–731.

104. Szolovits P, Patil RS, Schwartz WB. Artificial intelligence in medical diagnosis. Ann Intern Med. 1988;108(1):80–7.

105. Bohr A, Memarzadeh K. The rise of artificial intelligence in healthcare applications. In: Artificial intelligence in healthcare. Academic Press; 2020. p. 25–60.

106. Manne R, Kantheti SC. Application of artificial intelligence in healthcare: chances and challenges. Curr J Appl Sci Technol. 2021;40(6):78–89.

107. Bates DW, Levine D, Syrowatka A, Kuznetsova M, Craig KJT, Rui A, et al. The potential of artificial intelligence to improve patient safety: a scoping review. NPJ Digit Med. 2021;4(1):54.

108. Holtz B, Nelson V, Poropatich RK. Artificial intelligence in health: enhancing a return to patient-centered communication. Telemed J E Health. 2023;29(6):795–7.

109. Antel R, et al. The use of artificial intelligence and virtual reality in doctor-patient risk communication: a scoping review. Patient Educ Couns. 2022;105:3038–50.

110. Butow P, Hoque E. Using artificial intelligence to analyse and teach communication in healthcare. Breast. 2020;50:49–55.

111. Shaheen MY. Applications of artificial intelligence (AI) in healthcare: a review. Sci Prepr. 2021; https://doi.org/10.14293/S2199-1006.1.SOR-.PPVRY8K.v1.

112. Kumar P, Sharma S, Dutot V. Artificial intelligence (AI)-enabled CRM capability in healthcare: the impact on service innovation. Int J Inform Manage. 2023;69:102598.

113. Petersson L, Larsson I, Nygren JM, Nilsen P, Neher M, Reed JE, et al. Challenges to implementing artificial intelligence in healthcare: a qualitative interview study with healthcare leaders in Sweden. BMC Health Serv Res. 2022;22(1):1–16. https://doi.org/10.1186/s12913-022-08215-8.

114. Kumar P, Chauhan S, Awasthi LK. Artificial intelligence in healthcare: review, ethics, trust challenges & future research directions. Eng Appl Artif Intell. 2023;120:105894.

The Digital Ecosystem and Major Public Health Informatics Initiatives in Resource-Limited Settings

4

Kassahun Dessie Gashu

Abstract

The advent of digital technologies holds great promise for enhancing primary healthcare and transforming the way governments address emerging and re-emerging public health threats in settings with limited resources. The potential of digital health solutions to revolutionize healthcare accessibility and delivery cannot be overstated. Particularly in low- and middle-income countries with unmet healthcare needs, innovation is rapidly advancing. Policymakers are actively exploring avenues to harness this potential and ensure the long-term sustainability of digital health solutions, given the positive outcomes observed thus far.

However, establishing a solid foundation for digital health in resource-limited settings remains a complex endeavor. The achievement of such progress is often a challenging task. The successful implementation of digital health hinges on a multitude of internal and external factors. This chapter will be discussing how the digital ecosystem is fundamentally affecting the sustainable adoption of digital health in resource-limited settings. In addition, the chapter discussed the lessons learnt from some major public health informatics initiatives in the area.

Keywords

Digital health · Info-structure · Leadership · Readiness · Digital literacy · Maturity

4.1 Introduction

Digital health adoption and sustainability are intricate processes. In resource-limited settings, the achievement of successful implementation and scale-up largely hinges on a variety of factors and obstacles. Public health informatics, both as a research field and as a public service, is a relatively recent development that necessitates a comprehensive foundation for its realization. The field heavily relies on information technology and encompasses various disciplines, imposing numerous prerequisites for the adoption and expansion of public health informatics. Furthermore, the contextual factors play a crucial role in effectively adopting information technology for public health purposes.

In resource-limited settings, access to and quality of infrastructure are lacking, along with various complex contextual factors that impact the adoption of digital health. Despite the growth of infra-

K. D. Gashu (✉)
Department of Health Informatics, Institute of Public Health, College of Medicine and Health Sciences, University of Gondar, Gondar, Ethiopia

SMART Health, Research and Publications Department, Bahir Dar, Ethiopia
e-mail: kassahun.dessie@uog.edu.et

structure and information and communication technology (ICT) penetration, challenges such as digital exclusion, poor quality, unaffordability, and unsustainability persist in these settings. To effectively implement digital health in resource-limited settings, it is necessary to overcome challenges related to infrastructure, shortage of skilled manpower, competing priorities, public digital literacy, financing, and other factors.

In this chapter, we discussed the fundamental groundwork and initiatives related to public health informatics within resource-limited settings. It particularly emphasizes groundworks such as, the role of leadership, digital health infrastructure (referred to as "info-structure"), manpower development, digital literacy, and readiness for digital health implementation. Additionally, it explores major initiatives and the level of digital health maturity in resource-limited settings.

4.2   Digital Health Leadership

As per the eHealth strategy outlined by the World Health Organization (WHO), there exist seven essential components or building blocks that contribute to the long-term viability of a nation's digital health system [1]. These components are as follows:

1. Leadership, Governance, and Multi-Sector Engagement: This component emphasizes the importance of effective leadership, governance structures, and collaboration across multiple sectors involved in digital health implementation.
2. Strategy and Investment: Developing a comprehensive strategy and allocating adequate resources and investments are crucial to successfully and sustainably implement digital health initiatives.
3. Legislation, Policy, and Compliance: Establishing appropriate legislation, policies, and ensuring compliance with regulatory frameworks are essential to protect privacy, security, and ethical considerations in digital health.

4. Workforce: Building a skilled and diverse workforce capable of effectively utilizing and maintaining digital health systems is vital for sustained success.
5. Standards and Interoperability: Implementing standardized protocols and ensuring interoperability enable seamless data exchange and integration between different digital health systems and stakeholders.
6. Infrastructure: Establishing robust and reliable digital infrastructure, including hardware, software, and network capabilities, is fundamental for supporting digital health services and applications.
7. Services and Applications: Providing a range of high-quality digital health solutions to achieve meaningful impact related to access, quality and cost of healthcare.

4.2.1   Why Leadership and Governance Are the Success Factors?

Governmental entities often take the lion's share for the successful digital health revolution. Top decision-makers and political figures have the power to bring change in organizational norms relating to digital health. Leadership and governance is not simply a component but also a sub-component across all other elements in the building blocks of a national digital health. For instance: It is impossible to develop and deploy strategies, investments, legislations policies and workforce development, etc. without the full engagement of leadership and governance.

The methods for creating strategies significantly vary not only on the context of the nation but also the role of the government plays significant role. While some strategies are meticulously thought out, others emerge in a more collaborative way. It indicates that the role of leadership is beyond making a decision to develop a strategy, it also includes how the leadership played a role in the strategy development process in a way to bring change.

When it comes to the successful application of innovative technology, two key components of leadership stand out: governance and the commitment of political leaders. These elements are key to ensure the innovative digital health initiatives can successfully overcome barriers in the healthcare delivery particularly in resource-limited settings.

4.2.1.1 Political Commitment

Realizing digital health transformation largely depends on higher level of investment and commitment than does technological innovation. Political leaders ought to make a commitment to articulating a vision for digital health, creating a strategy for it, and seeing to its implementation. According to the World Health Organization's guiding principles [2], the choices and dedication of a country play a crucial role in a worldwide plan that prioritizes the responsible and enduring implementation of digital healthcare technology in the context of country's healthcare policies. The governments have to make decisions to incorporate eHealth into their national healthcare systems and demonstrate a commitment to following through with this decision.

Within the global strategy, it is acknowledged that each nation, in its distinct national context, bears the responsibility of developing appropriate strategies specific to the national contexts. In order to achieve the SDGs major health domains, nations are required to embrace a viable adoption of health information systems putting the key unique national identities into consideration including, the unique cultural values, existing policies, and visions.

For a particular health information system to be scaled up in resource-limited settings, financial viability must be achieved, which is a major hurdle. Pilot financing is crucial for demonstrating a digital health solution's cost-effectiveness. In fact, a number of digital health pilot programs in LMICs lack long-term viability planning and are unable to complete their implementation due to financial constraints. Historically, an early stage research and development and pilot programs have received 85% of financing for digital health in Africa [3]. Therefore, it is also essential for policymakers to maintain their commitment in order to secure the funds required to implement the nation's long-term health strategy.

4.2.1.2 Governance

Governance pertains to the structural organization of entities involved in advising, coordinating, supporting, regulating, overseeing, and implementing a digital health strategy. According to literatures, governance tends to encompass matters such as rights, regulations, responsibilities, and risks within the realm of digital health [4]. Governance, plays bigger role in any developmental agenda including digital health system development. Currently, digital health governance has come to the government's attention as a key strategy to realize the digital health transformation. As recommended by studies, the national governments should undertake the following measures in their governance to transform into health system digitalization in resource-limited countries [5]:

1. Prioritize digital health as a key agenda item for the country.
2. Extend explicit, transparent, and widespread support to the digital health strategy.
3. Allocate long-term funding platforms to sustain the initiatives
4. Harmonizing the digital agenda and healthcare plans to mutually reinforcing one another.
5. Promote the training of IT engineers to enhance their skills in healthcare technology.
6. Encourage IT professionals and medical staff to undergo training in digital health practices.
7. Establish robust connectivity and provide the necessary infrastructure to hospitals, clinics, and other healthcare facilities.
8. Support the enactment of legislation that offers legal clarity to all stakeholders involved in digital health.

It has been suggested three models of digital health governance that can be adopted to effectively and sustainably implement the digitalization processes. The selection of the models depends up on the contexts of the particular settings in which the system is implemented. The digital health governance models include:

(a) Centralized Model: The government takes a leading role in formulating and implementing digital health policies and strategies. The Ministries of Health promote digital health and recruits the technical expertise of other ministries, and agencies to implement digital health systems.

(b) Collaborative Model: The government collaborates with various stakeholders, such as healthcare providers, technology companies, and research institutions, to jointly develop and implement digital health initiatives. The Ministries of Health act as the driving force behind digital health initiatives.

(c) Decentralized Model: The government delegates decision-making authority to regional or local authorities, allowing them to design and execute digital health programs tailored to their specific needs and resources. The Ministry of Health directs health strategy, while a designated outside agency or directorate, using its own technical resources and ability, directs strategy and solution implementation for digital health.

Hence, effective leadership is vital at each levels of the national governmental structures to ensure sustainability of health system digitalization. In order to fully leverage the complete capabilities of health information technologies and synchronize it with the goals of societal health and the progress of universal healthcare, it is crucial to establish a comprehensive strategy, demonstrate strong leadership, and foster collaborative endeavors across various sectors.

Policymakers need to take the lead in crafting a strong health information strategy that includes persuasive idea and offers strong direction to end-users including other actors within the healthcare system. While the strategic frameworks are crucial starting point, the effective execution of a national health information strategy demands more than just strong leadership. It necessitates collaborative efforts between IT and healthcare professionals across different sectors, as well as transparent governance. The government's responsibilities include enacting necessary legislation, providing financial support and infrastructure, openly endorsing digital transformation, and ensuring coherence and synergies among various programs.

Conversely, it is important to recognize that digital transformation can directly impact fundamental rights such as privacy, bodily integrity, health, liberty, private life, and confidentiality. Therefore, any advancements in digital health should adhere to professional ethical standards. The establishment of human rights in this context necessitates the application of appropriate laws. Consequently, laws governing digital health should, at the very least, encompass the following areas [4]:

1. The legitimacy of telemedicine, electronic prescriptions, and the storage of health records in electronic format.

2. The obligation to accurately document medical information and ensure its safety and security, encompassing all aspects of data protection within the realm of information security.

3. The specifications regarding the content of health records, including the types of medical records to be maintained, their organization, and other pertinent details.

4. The prescribed governance procedures to ensure interoperability, as well as the protocols and standards to be implemented.

5. The specific rights bestowed upon patients with regard to their data.

6. The various purposes for which health records may be utilized, including research, legal proceedings, and healthcare-related matters.

4.2.2 Practical Leadership Experience in Resource-Limited Settings

Since the WHO's Resolution WHA58.28 in 2005 [6], which urged member states to incorporate eHealth into their health systems and services, there has been a notable increase in strong governmental commitments to digital health. This has led to the exploration of various digital health initiatives aimed at addressing specific healthcare challenges in resource-limited settings. Alongside the establishment of advanced data exchange platforms, the utilization of widespread ICT has been harnessed.

Initially, the emphasis of digital health initiatives was on testing various strategies through pilot programs. However, there has been a transition concerning prioritizing scalable, multifunctional, and long-term viability to overcome barriers such as inefficiency, inequity, low access and quality of healthcare in the existing health system particularly in resource-limited settings. Despite the efforts, there has been limited progress over time in addressing the issues of quality, integration, and sustainability of digital health systems in resource-limited settings. Consequently, there is a need for increased funding and political assistance to overcome these challenges.

Fortunately, there is evidence supporting the potential of digital health, particularly mHealth to enhance the delivery of health services in low- and middle-income countries. Collaborations between governments, technologists, non-governmental organizations, academia, and industry are forming to harness the benefits of digital health and drive progress in this field. By working together, these stakeholders can contribute to the advancement of digital health and its positive impact on healthcare delivery [7].

The successful implementation of digital health is often attributed to effective leadership, but it is important to recognize that the opposite can also hold true. Weak leadership can be responsible for the failure of digital health initiatives. Research conducted in resource-limited settings has consistently shown a correlation between poor implementation of digital health and weak leadership. This highlights the critical role that leadership plays in determining the success or failure of digital health projects.

Strong and capable leadership is essential to navigate the complexities, overcome challenges, and ensure the smooth adoption and integration of digital health solutions [8]. The gaps may be due to perceived values related to digital health, misconception, competing priorities, etc. Scalability of digital health advances are undoubtedly be hampered by insufficient policies, standards, or an unstable infrastructure in developing countries.

4.2.3   Effective Leadership Approaches

Researchers recommended some important leadership approaches for successful digital health adoption in resource-limited settings.

4.2.3.1 Start with Evidence-Based Digital Health Initiatives

The foundation of effective leadership in digital health begins with the careful selection of technology. With a plethora of digital health applications available in the global market, it is crucial to establish a rigorous selection criteria. The mere existence of numerous applications does not guarantee their usability in all contexts. Therefore, to ensure successful adoption and long-term sustainability of digital health technologies, it is essential to choose tools based on robust scientific evidence and take into account contextual factors [9, 10].

By employing a thoughtful and evidence-based approach to selection, leaders can identify the most suitable digital health tools for their specific needs and circumstances. This involves considering factors such as the target population, healthcare infrastructure, technological capabilities, and regulatory requirements. Rigorous selection criteria help to mitigate risks and maximize the potential benefits of digital health interventions.

Ultimately, effective leadership in digital health involves making informed decisions about which technologies to implement, guided by scientific evidence and a deep understanding of the contextual factors at play. By prioritizing careful selection, leaders can set the stage for successful adoption and long-term sustainability of digital health solutions.

4.2.3.2 Aligning National Priorities with Local Needs

The concept of aligning national priorities with local needs is crucial for facilitating the adoption of digital health. To foster collaboration with investors and donors and align their interests with regional and local health priorities, it is important for the government to invest in robust governance systems. By sharing knowledge about potential sources of financing support or incentives, investments can be optimized [8].

This process should involve the establishment of a solid corporate architecture and effective interoperability, both of which rely on digital standards—both technical and managerial—that contributors and investors agree to follow or gradually converge towards. Additionally, investments in interoperability testing facilities and support for innovation centers that nurture regional digital health entrepreneurs should be evaluated based on their socioeconomic impact.

Public-private partnerships present both new opportunities and challenges for investments in digital health. By leveraging these partnerships, governments can tap into additional resources and expertise. However, it is essential to carefully navigate the complexities associated with such collaborations to ensure that investments in digital health are effectively utilized.

By aligning national priorities with local needs, investing in governance systems, and fostering collaboration with investors and donors, governments can create an enabling environment for successful digital health initiatives. This approach encourages innovation, maximizes the socioeconomic impact, and promotes sustainable development in the field of digital.

4.2.3.3 Engaging Stakeholders

The recommendation from many researchers is to establish close partnerships and engage all stakeholders throughout the entire process, from the inception to the scale-up of innovative digital health solutions, particularly in resource-limited settings. To facilitate sustainable implementation, digital health innovators must actively involve and collaborate with all stakeholders, advocating for investments in external elements that support scaling up. It is crucial for the scaling process to be dynamic and flexible, with the private sector playing a significant role in initiating and expanding digital health initiatives. Achieving clarity regarding the nature and duration of partnerships is critical to ensure the scalability and sustainability of digital health initiatives [11].

The stakeholders involved in digital health implementation are diverse and encompass various sectors. These stakeholders include, but are not limited to, governmental sectors, international organizations, non-governmental organizations (NGOs), civil society organizations, donor agencies, foundations, universities and research institutions, development banks, faith-based organizations, the private sector including technology developers, health providers, community leaders, patients, and public representatives. Engaging and involving these stakeholders in a collaborative manner is essential for the successful implementation and long-term sustainability of digital health initiatives.

4.2.3.4 Global Collaborations

Global collaborative efforts aimed at achieving a more cohesive approach to scaling and integrating digital health have the potential to provide the leadership necessary to make new solutions accessible to healthcare practitioners and patients in low- and middle-income countries [11]. Collaborative endeavors that encompass global organizations, governmental officials, charitable organizations and partner, and the academia can play a pivotal role in expediting evolvement and supporting the widespread and effective adoption of health information technologies.

Monitoring hidden expenses and adopting a shared finance strategy are integral parts of partnerships that help keep costs low for investors and minimize the financial burden on users throughout the program's duration. By addressing these financial aspects, partnerships can ensure affordability and accessibility of digital health solutions.

With increasing consensus and understanding about the responsibilities of local administrative actors, system implementers and donors, the pursuit of sustainability becomes more attainable. Defining clear roles and responsibilities among stakeholders lays the foundation for coordinated endeavors and the enduring success of digital health initiatives.

By fostering collaboration, shared financing strategies, and clear delineation of roles, the global community can work together to overcome fragmentation and achieve sustainable scaling and integration of digital health solutions. This will ultimately lead to improved healthcare outcomes for individuals in LMICs [12].

By fostering collaboration, shared financing strategies, and clear delineation of roles, the global community can work together to overcome fragmentation and achieve sustainable scaling and integration of digital health solutions. This will ultimately lead to improved healthcare outcomes for individuals in LMICs.

4.2.3.5 Embedding to the Routine Program

The process of embedding a program into routine operations involves integrating its goals, activities, and resources into existing structures and practices. This integration ensures that the program becomes an integral part of the organization or system rather than an isolated initiative. Despite efforts made to promote ownership and local engagement from the very beginning, there is a notable absence of locally driven investment. Locally driven investment refers to the commitment of resources, both financial and non-financial, from local stakeholders such as government entities, organizations, or communities. This investment is crucial for the program's sustainability and long-term success.

The absence of locally driven investment in the program has substantial implications for its budget. Insufficient investment makes it difficult to allocate the necessary resources and secure funding to support the program's objectives and activities. As a result, there may be limitations in implementing essential components of the program and achieving the desired outcomes. Moreover, the lack of local investment can indicate a lack of responsibility and ownership among local stakeholders. When stakeholders have a financial or resource investment in a program, they are more likely to take ownership of its implementation and outcomes. This sense of ownership is crucial for driving the program's success and ensuring its seamless integration into routine operations.

To address this challenge, it is essential to engage and involve local stakeholders in the decision-making process. Creating opportunities for them to contribute through financial or in-kind investments is key. This can be accomplished through collaborative partnerships, advocacy efforts, and capacity building initiatives that empower local stakeholders to take ownership and contribute to the program's long-term sustainability. By actively addressing the issue of locally driven investment and promoting ownership among local stakeholders, the program can be embedded more effectively into routine operations. When local stakeholders, such as community members, organizations, or institutions, have a sense of ownership and investment in the program, they are more likely to actively participate and contribute to its success. This involvement helps to embed the program into routine operations, making it a sustainable and integral part of the community or organization. This approach maximizes the program's effectiveness and its ability to bring about positive outcomes for the intended beneficiaries.

4.2.3.6 Knowledge Management Approach

There is a pressing need to implement a knowledge management approach that identifies, archives, and shares best practices to benefit the global community and future generations. This approach should capture the knowledge of how new digital solutions are implemented, including evidence and lessons learned regarding the methods and techniques for adopting and sustaining digital health initiatives in countries and international communities. By effectively managing this knowledge, resources can be conserved, and the need to reinvent the wheel can be minimized. The establishment of a robust knowledge management system ensures that valuable insights and experiences are preserved and accessible, facilitating the advancement and widespread adoption of digital health solutions [2].

Based on the above leadership approaches, there are various scenarios; for instance the lessons learned from the successful "SMS-based smoking cessation programmes" in Samoa [13], and India [14], is summarized in Box 4.1.

Box 4.1 Lessons Learned on the Impact of Leadership for Successful Digital Health in Public Health

Lesson 1: The significant success factor in Samoa's smoking cessation efforts was the alignment of the intervention with the country's Non-Communicable Disease (NCD) strategy and regional priorities. Through close collaboration with the government, civil society, and the World Health Organization, trust in the tool has been established. As a result, the government has assumed ownership of the program, recognizing its importance and taking responsibility for its implementation. This alignment, collaboration, and ownership have played a crucial role in the success of Samoa's smoking cessation initiative.

Lesson 2: The mCessation (SMS-based smoking cessation) program implemented in India in 2015 was found to be both feasible and effective. Engaging various stakeholders and tailoring the program to the local context, it was able to effectively reach and engage the population, contributing to positive outcomes in smoking cessation efforts. Several success factors contributed to its positive outcomes, including:

• *Multi-sector support: The program received support from various sectors, including governmental sectors, the World Health Organization, the International Telecommunication Union, and others. This collaboration and endorsement from multiple stakeholders played a significant role in the program's success.*

• *Cultural and linguistic adaptation: The program was tailored to be culturally and linguistically appropriate for the diverse population in India. It included*

regional languages and a voice-based response system to ensure that it effectively addressed the specific needs and preferences of the population. This adaptation helped overcome barriers related to language and cultural differences, increasing the program's accessibility and relevance.

4.3 Digital Health Infrastructure

According to WHO [15], A digital health platform can be defined as a shared digital health information infrastructure, known as an "Info-structure," which serves as the foundation for building and delivering consistent and integrated digital health services to support healthcare delivery. The following are some of the key infrastructures that support digital health systems.

4.3.1 Power Infrastructure

Electricity is essential for deployment and operation of a digital health service. All computing devices need consistent electric power. Globally, access to electricity is growing every day. However, reliability and affordability of electricity remains an issue in LMICs [16]. For example, studies in rural areas of India [17], Pakistan [18], Malaysia [19], and many other resource-limited settings indicated that, electric power outages is a major challenge. Moreover, flooding, bureaucratic delays, shortage of local skilled manpower for maintenance, lack of incentives, etc. worsening the shortage and inconsistency of power [19].

Practical experience has revealed that the main extrinsic limiting constraints affecting the scalability of digital health projects in LMICs are the dependability and bandwidth of networks, as well as the accessibility of electricity to charge devices [11].

4.3.2 Mobile Network Infrastructure

Globally, mobile signal coverage is growing more than ever. Despite the mobile networking is growing fast, it is still lower in resource-limited settings as compared with developed world. The percentage of the population in Africa that can access a mobile cellular signal, or mobile cellular coverage, is estimated by the ITU to be 88.4%. A 3G signal is now accessible to over 77% of people, and a long-term evolution (LTE) mobile broadband signal is now available to 44.3% [20].

The growth network coverage on the other hand is not evenly distributed. In 2019, the number of active mobile broadband subscriptions in Africa per 100 people reached 33.1, much behind the global average of 75 per 100 people [21]. The mobile network coverage also showed much disparities which is a greater in urban than rural areas [22].

4.3.3 Internet Infrastructure

Following the fast growth of mobile cellular coverage, the access and use of internet is growing in resource-limited settings. For instance: According to the ITU in 2019, 14.3% of homes in the African region had access to the Internet, compared to 57.4% globally. In Africa, the proportion of people utilizing the Internet in 2019 was 28.6% (20.2% females, 37.1% men), compared to an average of 51.4 (48.3% females, 55.2% males) globally [20].

Internet usage is generally low in resource-limited settings. The low internet usage is not solely due to poor internet network coverage [23]. One of the major reasons include digital-divide such as lack of affordability of smart mobile phones and poor digital literacy among rural and less literate communities.

4.3.4 5G Infrastructure

Among other factors, the COVID-19 pandemic, created network congestion people due to the shift towards virtual networks for entertainment and education, as face-to-face contacts were risks for transmission of the disease. These situation has raised the demand of using more online resources and hastened the development of 5G infrastructure. Now a days, the coverage and use of 5G infrastructure is even growing in resource-limited settings.

Lessons from the 3G and 4G eras highlight the need for governments and other stakeholders to address critical policy imperatives for the 5G era, both in the broader context of next-generation connectivity and growth of the digital economy [24].

4.3.5 Data Infrastructure

Evidence showed that data infrastructures such as healthcare databases, warehouses, virtualization systems and cloud resources are demonstrating significant advancements in under developed nations. Regarding cloud computing implementations in health care is still low, but growing interests [25]. Cloud computing is an emerging technology, which has benefits and drawbacks [15]. Some of the benefits include:

- Cost savings: Cloud-based solutions can provide cost savings for healthcare institutions with limited IT staffing, funds, and infrastructure. By leveraging the cloud, organizations can avoid substantial direct cost spent in hardware and software including running budget of the project. Instead, they can pay for cloud services on a subscription basis, which can be more cost-effective and scalable.
- Scalability and flexibility: Cloud-based solutions offer scalability, allowing healthcare institutions to easily scale up or down based on their needs. This flexibility is beneficial for accommodating expansions, seasonal changes, and evolving health situations. Organizations can quickly adjust their resources and infrastructure without the need for significant investments in additional hardware or software.
- Interoperability focus: With cloud-based solutions, IT staff can dedicate their efforts to

improving interoperability between different health systems and applications. By focusing on interoperability, organizations can enhance the efficiency and effectiveness of their health system business processes, streamline data exchange, and improve care coordination.

- Offsite data backup: Cloud-based solutions provide the advantage of offsite backup for data and applications. Storing data and applications in the cloud ensures that critical information is protected from physical damage or loss. In the event of a disaster or system failure, organizations can recover their data and applications from the cloud, minimizing downtime and preserving continuity of care.

Whereas the drawbacks associated with relying on external cloud-based solutions for digital health systems include:

- Limited control: The deployment, management, and customization of the system may be restricted due to external ownership of the hardware and software components. This lack of control can hinder the flexibility and customization options needed to tailor the system to specific healthcare requirements.
- Security and privacy concerns: Entrusting sensitive health data to external cloud providers raises concerns about data security and privacy. It is essential to ensure robust security measures and adherence to privacy regulations to protect patient information from unauthorized access or data breaches.
- Data storage limitations and scalability: The capacity for data storage and scalability may be constrained by data caps imposed by the cloud provider. This limitation can impact the system's ability to handle large volumes of data and scale up as the healthcare organization's needs grow.
- Dependency on internet connectivity: A dependable and consistent internet connection is necessary for accessing and utilizing cloud-based digital health systems. Reliance on internet connectivity introduces a potential point of failure, as system functionality may be compromised in the event of network disruptions or outages.

4.3.6 The Role of Digital Health Infrastructure

The digital health infrastructure (Info-structure) can be defined as a cohesive collection of interconnected and recyclable constituents for supporting a wide range of health information system applications [15]. This integrated infrastructure provides a foundation for the development, deployment, and operation of various digital health solutions, ensuring interoperability and efficiency across the ecosystem. By leveraging common and reusable components, the digital health infrastructure enables seamless integration and collaboration among different applications and systems, ultimately enhancing the delivery of healthcare services and improving patient outcomes. The sustainability of digital health interventions is interdependent with complex factors including availability and functionality of the digital infrastructure [26]. Digital health infrastructure fulfills an essential and irreplaceable role [15]. Among numerous functions, we have outlined below the objectives of digital infrastructures.

4.3.6.1 Connecting All Functions of the Health System

The digital health infrastructure plays a vital role in enabling the efficient delivery of diverse healthcare and public health services by seamlessly connecting all functions within the health system. Through the utilization of the Internet, telecommunication networks and electric power infrastructures, combined with resilient health information systems, the digital health infrastructure establishes linkages between different elements of the healthcare system. The interconnectedness between the different components of the health system and with other essential sectors would facilitates the smooth flow of information, collaboration, and coordination among different healthcare functions. As a result, healthcare providers can leverage the digital health infrastructure to deliver services more effectively, improve healthcare outcomes, and enhance the overall functioning of the health system.

4.3.6.2 Facilitate Public and Patient Engagement

The utilization of digital infrastructure plays a crucial role in enhancing public and patient engagement in healthcare by leveraging various digital communication tools. For instance, the telecom and internet infrastructure serves as a facilitator for seamless communication among stakeholders within the healthcare ecosystem. This enables effective and timely information exchange, empowering individuals to actively participate in their own healthcare journey. By leveraging digital communication tools, such as telemedicine platforms, mobile health applications, and secure messaging systems, healthcare providers can engage with patients and the public more efficiently. These tools enable remote consultations, health monitoring, appointment scheduling, personalized health education, and real-time communication between healthcare professionals and patients. Furthermore, digital infrastructure enables the dissemination of health-related information and resources through online portals, social media platforms, and interactive websites. This empowers individuals to access reliable health information, participate in health promotion activities, and make informed decisions about their well-being.

4.3.6.3 Simplify Data Management and Use

The digital health infrastructure plays a vital role in supporting public health functions, encompassing activities such as research data collection, disease outbreak surveillance, vital statistics monitoring, and health facility data tracking. Digital health infrastructure can also help us to develop a centralized repository for diverse datasets, enabling efficient data management and utilization. For instance, cloud computing and data warehouses are instrumental in facilitating these processes.

4.3.6.4 Support Administrative Functions in the Health System

The digital health infrastructure enhances the overall efficiency, transparency, and effectiveness of healthcare administration. It streamlines finan-cial management, optimizes workforce utilization, improves supply chain operations, facilitates equipment maintenance, and simplifies payment and insurance processes. Ultimately, these advancements contribute to a more streamlined and effective healthcare system [15].

4.3.6.5 Provide/Track Health Information and Support Health Care

In the evolving landscape of healthcare, clinicians are increasingly utilizing apps for telemedicine, enabling remote consultations and virtual healthcare delivery. Patients, on the other hand, receive informative messages on health education and timely reminders for appointments and medication schedules through digital platforms. Additionally, users can actively monitor and track their health indicators, such as blood pressure and exercise statistics, using dedicated health applications. These advancements signify a shift in the point of care, extending beyond the traditional doctor's office and empowering patients to take a more active role in managing their own health.

Telemedicine apps allow clinicians to provide medical consultations, diagnoses, and treatment recommendations remotely, bridging geographical barriers and improving access to healthcare services. This technology enables patients to connect with healthcare professionals from the comfort of their own homes, reducing the need for in-person visits for certain conditions or follow-ups. Through health education messages and reminders delivered via digital platforms, patients receive valuable information on various health topics and are prompted to adhere to their healthcare routines. These reminders ensure that patients attend appointments on time, take their medications as prescribed, and follow recommended self-care practices, ultimately contributing to better health outcomes. Furthermore, health applications empower users to actively engage in monitoring and managing their health. With the ability to track vital signs, exercise activity, and other health indicators, individuals gain insights into their own well-being and can make informed decisions regarding their lifestyle choices. The self-tracking and self-management approach promotes a proactive and personalized approach to healthcare.

4.3.7 Financing the Digital Health Infrastructure

There are six common models of financing the digital health infrastructure. These includes direct government financing, public reimbursement, private reimbursement, licensing, donor grants and out-of-pocket financing platforms. Of these, licensing, donor grants and out-of-pocket financing models are commonly practiced in resource-limited settings [3].

4.3.7.1 Direct Government Financing

To incentivize the development of digital infrastructure, governments implement direct financing incentives that encourage them to cover a significant portion, typically around 30% to 50%, of the associated costs. These financial incentives serve as a means to promote and support the implementation of digital infrastructure projects across various sectors. By providing funding support, governments aim to facilitate the adoption of digital technologies, enhance connectivity, and foster digital inclusion within their jurisdictions. This financial backing helps offset a substantial portion of the financial burden associated with establishing and maintaining robust digital infrastructure, encouraging both public and private entities to invest in these critical initiatives. Ultimately, these financing incentives play a pivotal role in driving the expansion and accessibility of digital infrastructure, enabling societies to harness the benefits of a digitally connected world.

4.3.7.2 Public Reimbursement

Public reimbursement programs are implemented by public health insurers to cover the costs of digital health solutions that are deemed to have a substantial positive impact on the overall health of the population. These programs serve as an alternative to relying solely on donor funds to finance such initiatives. By incorporating digital health solutions into their reimbursement policies, public health insurers aim to promote the adoption and utilization of innovative technologies that can contribute to improving health outcomes.

Under these reimbursement programs, public health insurers evaluate the effectiveness and potential benefits of specific digital health solutions. If a solution is determined to have a significant positive impact on population health, the insurer will provide coverage and bear the associated costs. This approach ensures that individuals, including those who may not have the financial means to access these solutions independently, can benefit from their potential advantages.

By integrating digital health solutions into public reimbursement programs, governments and public health insurers actively support the use of technology to enhance healthcare delivery, preventive care, and health management. This approach encourages healthcare providers and patients to embrace digital innovations, fostering the widespread adoption of solutions that have demonstrated their effectiveness in improving population health outcomes.

4.3.7.3 Private Reimbursement

Solutions for digital health are now receiving financial assistance from private companies. Several of these private insurance-led options take advantage of the growing adoption of mobile payment systems in low-income communities (LMICs) by offering low rates and mobile delivery to satisfy the needs of low-income patients.

4.3.7.4 Licensing

Businesses that provide digital health services can rely on licensing to generate revenue from their platforms or goods. Digital health solutions that instruct healthcare professionals on how to deliver services more efficiently and meaningfully are covered under this license model.

4.3.7.5 Donor Grants

Donor funding may not be the usual means of long-term, sustainable financing for digital health initiatives. However, if funders commit to a long-term partnership in close collaboration with the governments, it is still feasible to scale it up to a national level and ensure its sustainability.

4.3.7.6 Out-of-Pocket

In low resource-limited settings, the out-of-pocket payment poses the greatest risk of financial hardship. It still remains a typical model financing to obtain digital health services. Another possible problem is that because donor financing is typically directed at specific projects, it can result in walled programs that duplicate already-existing national initiatives.

Generally, about 85% of the funding for digital health related infrastructure spent on early stages of research, development and pilot programs in Africa has been [3]. The digital health pilot programs require a long-term viability planning and sufficient funding allocated before being completely adopted.

4.3.8 Drivers and Challenges of Digital Health Infrastructure in Resource-Limited Settings

An effective implementation of digital health technologies require supportive policies, digital infrastructure, and understanding of the socio-economic contexts [27]. Despite the rapid growth of digital infrastructure, still significantly larger group of global communities were still out of the benefits of digital infrastructure. For instance: In 2022, around three billion people were still without connectivity, with the vast majority were living in developing nations. In addition, the utilization gap still poses a problem. Despite residing in places with mobile broadband coverage, about 43% of the world's population did not use mobile internet last year [28]. This indicates that coverage in digital infrastructure alone does not guaranty to ensure the potential benefits of ICT. Therefore, to get the full benefits of digital infrastructure, it needs to work on both the physical coverage as well as digital literacy, creating access to computing devices, and improving public awareness. We identified some drivers and challenges of digital infrastructure in resource-limited settings.

4.3.8.1 Driving Factors

Various known and unknown driving factors have shaped the landscape of digital health infrastructure in resource-limited settings. They have fostered the development of innovative solutions, improved access to healthcare services, and contributed to the overall advancements in healthcare delivery. Recognizing and understanding these driving factors is essential for furthering the progress of digital health initiatives in resource-constrained environments. Some of the known driving factors include:

4.3.8.2 Emerging and Re-emerging Public Health Disasters as a Driving Factor

The emergency related to COVID-19 opened an opportunity for promoting the global expansion of ICT infrastructure in resource-limited settings. Virtual communication and remote healthcare services became paramount as physical distancing and social restrictions were implemented to control the spread of the virus. This surge in demand for digital solutions has been discussed in previous sections of the book [29, 30]. The pandemic highlighted the importance of contingency planning and the scaling of digital health programs during public health emergencies. For instance, during the outbreak of Ebola Virus Disease (EVD) in West Africa, contingency planning played a crucial role in rapidly implementing and expanding digital health programs. These programs enabled effective communication, surveillance, and response strategies to be deployed in a timely manner.

The experience of the COVID-19 pandemic and previous public health emergencies has underscored the value of digital infrastructure in mitigating the impact of crises and ensuring the continuity of essential healthcare services. By leveraging digital technologies, healthcare systems can adapt to sudden disruptions, maintain communication channels, and deliver care remotely when physical access is limited.

4.3.8.3 Development of Digital Strategies

The growth of digital infrastructure in resource-limited settings can be significantly influenced by the development of comprehensive digital strategies at the global, regional, and national levels. These strategies, when coupled with collaborations with international communities, have the potential to make a profound impact on advancing digital infrastructure in resource-constrained environments [31]. Global digital strategies provide a framework for harmonizing efforts and coordinating initiatives across countries and regions. They foster collaboration, knowledge sharing, and resource mobilization on a global scale. By aligning priorities and leveraging expertise from international partners, these strategies can drive the development and implementation of digital infrastructure projects in resource-limited settings.

Regional and national digital strategies play a crucial role in tailoring digital solutions to address specific challenges and needs within their respective contexts. These strategies take into account the local socioeconomic conditions, healthcare systems, and technological landscapes. They facilitate the identification of priority areas, allocation of resources, and establishment of policies and regulations that promote the growth of digital infrastructure.

Collaborations with international communities, including governments, non-governmental organizations, and private sector entities, are vital for supporting the development of digital infrastructure in resource-limited settings. Such collaborations bring together diverse expertise, resources, and experiences, enabling the sharing of best practices, capacity-building initiatives, and joint investment in digital health projects. These partnerships can enhance the sustainability and effectiveness of digital infrastructure initiatives by fostering knowledge exchange and leveraging shared resources.

4.3.8.4 The Digital Economy

The global digital economy exerts a significant influence on the expansion of digital infrastructure worldwide. Governments and policymakers rec-

ognize the necessity of robust digital infrastructure to participate in the digital economy, capitalize on economic opportunities, and drive sustainable development. By investing in digital infrastructure, countries position themselves to harness the transformative power of the digital economy and create a conducive environment for innovation, economic growth, and global connectivity.

The influence of the global digital economy serves as a compelling driving force behind the rapid growth of digital infrastructure worldwide. The interconnectedness and pervasive nature of the digital economy have created a strong incentive for countries and regions to invest in and expand their digital infrastructure. It encompasses a wide range of activities, including e-commerce, digital services, and digital communication platforms. It has revolutionized the way businesses operate, transformed industries, and facilitated global connectivity. As a result, countries recognize the need to develop robust digital infrastructure to participate in and benefit from the opportunities presented by the digital economy.

To effectively engage in the global digital economy, countries must have reliable and high-speed internet connectivity, advanced telecommunications networks, and secure digital platforms. These infrastructure elements are essential for businesses to operate efficiently, access global markets, and leverage digital technologies to enhance productivity and innovation. Moreover, the progress towards digital economy increasingly becoming the cause of invention for new commercial models, job opportunities, and economic growth. Governments and policymakers understand the potential economic benefits associated with a thriving digital-based economy and therefore prioritize the development of digital infrastructure as a means to stimulate economic growth, attract investments, and foster innovation in resource-limited settings and globally at large.

4.3.8.5 Challenges

Generally physical coverage of the digital infrastructure rapidly growing and becoming no more a challenge. However, poor infrastructure quality, digital exclusion, lack of interoperability, unaffordability, unreliable financing were some of the challenges of digital infrastructure in resource-limited settings.

Poor Quality of Infrastructure

Practical experience has demonstrated that the scalability of digital health projects in low- and middle-income countries (LMICs) is significantly hindered by various external constraints. The primary limiting factors affecting scalability include the reliability and bandwidth of networks, as well as limited or unreliable access to electricity. Additionally, the absence of high-quality hardware in the region further constrains the ability to scale up digital health initiatives [11, 32].

Reliable and robust network infrastructure is indispensable for the efficient implementation and expansion of digital health projects. Many low- and middle-income countries face limitations in network connectivity, including issues such as limited coverage, intermittent connectivity, and insufficient bandwidth. These challenges hinder the seamless transmission of data, impeding the scalability of digital health solutions.

Access to reliable electricity is another critical constraint that impacts the scalability of digital health projects in LMICs. Insufficient or unreliable power supply can disrupt the operation of digital health systems, rendering them ineffective, particularly in resource-constrained settings where power infrastructure may be inadequate.

Furthermore, the availability of high-quality hardware, including devices, servers, and diagnostic equipment, plays a crucial role in the successful deployment and scalability of digital health solutions. However, LMICs often face difficulties in accessing and affording such hardware due to limited resources.

To overcome these constraints and promote scalability, partnerships with the private sector can play a pivotal role. Private sector involvement, particularly through funding support, can address the hardware needs of digital health projects in LMICs. Collaborating with private entities facilitates the procurement of high-quality hardware and ensures its availability for the expansion of digital health initiatives.

Digital Exclusion

Despite the global expansion of digital infrastructure, there remains a significant disparity in the distribution of development and investment. This imbalance is particularly evident in resource-limited settings, exacerbating the issue of digital exclusion. For instance, the availability of internet connectivity in rural communities is limited, with only approximately 6% having access to some form of connectivity. This disparity can be attributed, in part, to the lack of adequate incentives to attract private sector investment. As a result, urban areas tend to benefit more from private sector investment, which often surpasses public investment in terms of coverage, quality, and scale [33].

If we see African region, over two-third of the people in the continent was not connected to broadband. Twenty-one of the world's 25 least connected nations are in Africa [28]. According to the ITU, over 300 million people in Africa reside over 50 kilometers away from a fiber or cable broadband connection. Africa's rate of internet adoption, which stands at approximately 36%, is notably lower than the global average of 63%.

Lack of Interoperability

Interoperability refers to the capacity of applications and devices within the healthcare system to communicate and share data in a clear and predictable manner. It enables accurate, effective, and consistent exchange of data, allowing for a comprehensive understanding and utilization of the information exchanged [34]. The design of numerous systems overlooked the importance of an integrated architecture that could unify various components into a cohesive and well-coordinated entity. Consequently, devices and information systems faced challenges in communicating with each other due to the absence of a cohesive architecture.

The absence of standardization and interoperability poses a significant challenge when it comes to adopting and maintaining digital health systems in resource-limited settings [35]. The absence of standardization and interoperability is frequently linked to the wastage of digital resources, inadequate data management, and the burden of managing disconnected applications, which adds unnecessary workload for workers and hinders innovation. Moreover, prioritizing the creation of standalone applications hampers the progress and implementation of national systems and infrastructure [15].

Unaffordability

According to ITU's data [24], the costs of telecommunication and ICT services, such as mobile voice, mobile data, and fixed broadband, have generally decreased and become more accessible on a global scale. Nevertheless, affordability remains a challenge in resource-limited settings. Africa represents the region with the highest pricing, followed closely by the Arab States region. In low- and middle-income countries, the cost of mobile broadband is approximately ten times higher as a percentage of income compared to high-income countries [36].

Unviable Financing

Demonstrating the cost-effectiveness of digital health systems in low- and middle-income countries faces a fundamental obstacle in achieving financial sustainability for the expanding digital health infrastructure.

4.4   Digital Health Workforce

The Health Information System (HIS) leverages the interplay among processes, individuals, and technology to enhance healthcare operations and elevate the quality of healthcare services [37, 38]. Skilled workforce is core element of the health system. Evidence suggests workforce development leads to improved achievement of the targeted results [39, 40]. To fulfill the objectives of a specific service, it is essential to ensure a sufficient quantity and diverse range of trained human resources across all levels of the healthcare system.

4.4.1   Who Are HIT Professionals?

The question of whether "informatics" should be considered as a "profession" was examined and following a subsequent inquiries, it was con-

cluded that informatics is in the early stages of professional development [41, 42]. This determination was based on several key factors, including a strong intellectual foundation and methodology, alignment with core societal values, specialized training, a dedication to the "service ideal" above personal interests, professional autonomy, long-term commitment to the field, a sense of community, and the presence of a well-developed code of ethics.

There is a growing consensus that a proficient healthcare information technology (HIT) worker should possess knowledge across diverse domains, encompassing information technology, healthcare, business, and management. However, there is an ongoing debate regarding the specific skills and competencies that are in high demand and most effective. Further research is recommended to comprehensively assess the HIT workforce, explore capacity-building options, and determine the optimal strategies for deploying the workforce most effectively [43].

4.4.2   Why HIT Workforce Is Demanding?

The integration of information and communication technology (ICT) into the healthcare system has been widely acknowledged for its ability to enhance the efficiency of healthcare delivery and improve health outcomes. It is progressively enhancing the quality and safety of healthcare services, all while reducing healthcare costs [44, 45]. Based on available evidence, having a skilled workforce is crucial for the successful adoption and long-term sustainability of Health Information Technology (HIT) implementation [43].

The recognition of the necessity for a health information technology workforce and its integration with health programmes occurred early in England [46] then followed by other countries [47, 48]. However, very little was known about how the HIT workforces is integrated in the existing healthcare system. Work force development in health informatics domain in general has received recognition worldwide even in developing nations [49]. The American Health Information Management Association (AHIMA) identified HIM professionals as "medical records and health information technicians" and emphasized their importance during the transition from manual patient records to electronic medical record system [50].

A considerable number of higher education institutions in developing nations are involved in the education of professionals in health informatics, ranging from lower-level to advanced-level degrees. However, the training and development process is hindered by various barriers. The field of health informatics is still in its developmental stage, leading to a lack of standardized professional training, non-aligned professional characterization, and incomplete job specifications, which remain unresolved issues.

4.4.3 Skills and Number of Workforce

The importance of skilled manpower in Health Information Technology (HIT) is recognized globally, even in resource-limited settings. However, there is still a lack of sufficient research to inform the national demand for manpower and identify the specific competencies required by the industry [43]. Nevertheless, some countries, such as Ethiopia, have undertaken a national survey of their existing manpower and developed a 10-year national roadmap [51]. The study conducted in Ethiopia highlighted the scarcity of manpower within the current health system, along with a high turnover rate among HIT staff. It estimated that by 2030, there would be a need for over 50,000 professionals in fields related to Health Information Systems (HIS).

Further research is required in resource-limited settings to provide a comprehensive understanding of the manpower requirements, including the ideal educational levels, specific roles, necessary competencies, and unique contextual needs [52]. Furthermore, examining factors such as professional satisfaction, skill gaps, staff turnover, and forecasting future needs can contribute to enhancing the process of human resource development in resource-limited settings.

4.4.4 Continuous Professional Development

Continuing Professional Development (CPD) for the health workforce entails deliberate and ideally continuous education pursued after the completion of basic training. Its purpose is to uphold core competencies, as well as update knowledge, skills, and practices [53]. Health informatics is a relatively new field of study, and the curricula and professional standards are still in the process of maturing in low- and middle-income countries (LMICs). Consequently, establishing a robust system for continuous professional development is essential to enhance the competency of professionals in the field of Health Information Technology (HIT).

In resource-limited settings, human resource development necessitates cost-effective approaches, such as blended approaches that combine training, supervision, and mentoring. These methods should strike a balance between maintaining quality and standards while alleviating the strain on already overwhelmed healthcare systems [54, 55]. As technologists, HIT professionals also leverage the benefits of technology-assisted capacity development.

4.4.5 Collaboration for HIT Workforce Development

There is a widespread recognition of the significance of collaborating with local and international higher education institutions and working groups to foster the development of human resources in Health Information Technology in a sustainable manner [49]. The establishment of collaborations with initiatives such as AMIA's Global Partnership Program and Fogarty Informatics Training for Global Health (ITGH) has played a crucial role in offering various capacity-building programs [49]. It still needs to look for more potential collaborators to come aimed with human resource development including Pre- and in-service capacity building activities in HIT.

One of the challenges in the development of the Health Information Technology workforce has been the absence of standardized curricula and professional characterization. Consequently, there has been a lack of informed curriculum development and implementation. Furthermore, the characterization of job profiles, including roles, competencies, and required training, remains unanswered [49].

Therefore, it requires to find the way outs in standardizing the training tools starting from local context [52], then stepping up to regional and global levels.

Generally, recognizing the significance of human resources for Health Information Technology (HIT) is vital for advancing healthcare systems in resource-limited settings. However, there is a practical shortage of technical personnel with the necessary qualifications in the field of HIT.

Therefore, based on the evidence mentioned above, we listed the essential remedies that may help to improve the human resource development in resource-limited settings:

- Developing a nationally relevant HIT human resource roadmap based on scientifically sound evidence and contextual considerations.
- Implementing continuous professional development programs for HIT professionals.
- Collaborating with national and international working groups and higher education institutions.
- Conducting pre- and in-service capacity building activities for HIT professionals.
- Assessing and standardizing the competencies of HIT professionals, along with ongoing monitoring and evaluation of outcomes.

4.5   eHealth Literacy

eHealth literacy, also known as digital health literacy, pertains to the capacity to actively search for, locate, comprehend, and evaluate health information obtained from electronic sources, and subsequently utilize the acquired knowledge to address or resolve health-related issues [56].

eHealth and health literacy are distinct but interconnected concepts. eHealth literacy can enhance health literacy, both are vital components of the healthcare system. Health literacy involves accessing, comprehending, evaluating, and utilizing information and services to make informed decisions about one's health. Research indicates that low health literacy among patients can heighten the risk of extended hospital stays, mortality rates, adverse health outcomes, increased healthcare costs, and reduced patient engagement in their treatments [57, 58].

Digital literacy emphasizes the importance of information technology within the healthcare system. Individuals who possess eHealth literacy skills have cognitive advantages, allowing them to proficiently self-manage their healthcare needs, adopt healthy behaviors, maximize the benefits of health insurance, and experience interpersonal advantages. All the advantages emanated from the proficiency of actors involved in the healthcare in searching for information from digital sources such as from the Internet [59].

4.5.1   How eHealth Literacy Works?

The primary goal of eHealth literacy is to effectively address the health issues of individuals. This applies to both end users of digital health solutions, who can be either health service providers or recipients of services.

4.5.1.1 Health Service Providers

Health service providers, including healthcare workers, leaders, and administrative staff, who possess strong information technology skills, can efficiently and effectively address the health issues of patients or clients. This may involve the ability to actively listen to patient complaints, assess their medical significance, consider appropriate interventions, and simultaneously document relevant notes. Such tasks require a high level of concentration, accurate typing, and familiarity with the user interface of the software or application being used, skills that may not be commonly found even among experienced computer users [60].

To gain a deeper comprehension of the importance of eHealth literacy among health service providers, it is crucial to acknowledge the fact that Electronic Medical Record (EMR) developers often underestimate the level of computer skills required by physicians to effectively utilize EMR systems. In reality, doctors face significant challenges in utilizing these systems. Additionally, some physicians may lack the necessary typing skills to efficiently enter patient medical data, notes, and prescriptions into electronic medical records [61].

4.5.1.2 Health Service Takers

These individuals encompass patients, clients, guardians, at-risk groups, communities, and others who directly or indirectly seek health services. In today's era, technology is leading us towards personalized care. People has access to abundant information to make informed decisions regarding their own, their family's or their community's health. Therefore, eHealth literacy plays a crucial role in effectively engaging service recipients in various eHealth solutions. Proficiency in information technology skills also facilitates searching, comprehending, and utilizing health information for decision-making purposes [59].

4.5.2 Measuring eHealth literacy

eHealth literacy is broad concept that requires a composite measure. A review [62] of eHealth literacy instruments has compiled seven widely used measuring tools as follow.

4.5.2.1 eHealth Literacy Scale (eHEALS)

An 8-item measure of eHealth literacy developed by Norman and Skinner [63], commonly employed assessment of eHealth literacy is a measure that evaluates consumers' knowledge, comfort, and perceived skills in utilizing and applying eHealth in various health domains.

Generally, the concepts of the eight-item tool is summarized below. Each of the tools describes about individual's ability to:

- Search useful learning materials in the web.
- Manipulate digital sources for searching valuable information for their health inquiry
- Assess the type of learning material available

- Assess the right portal for searching information
- Utilize the available information
- Appraise credibility of the available learning materials
- Labeling the quality of available learning materials
- Trust the ability to change their health conditions

4.5.2.2 eHealth Literacy Scale–Extended (eHEALS-E)

It is an extended version of the eHEALS with 16 items developed for online health community users [64]. Each items use a 5-point Likert scale ranging from "strongly agree" to "strongly disagree". The notions of the *eHEALS-E* items are summarized in Box 4.2.

> **Box 4.2 The Summarized Descriptions of the eHEALS-E Items for Assessing Digital Health Literacy**
> *The tool illustrates the individual's ability/ understanding of internet to:*
>
> - *The first eight items are similar to eHEALS such as, searching ability, ability to manipulation, type of learning materials, identifying the source of use information, ability to utilize information, ability to appraise credibility of the information, labeling quality of information and self-confidence on its contribution.*
> - *In addition, this tool included eight more items illustrating about:*
>   - *Ability to extract useful meaning*
>   - *Information selection ability*
>   - *Clearing confusion on bulk data*
>   - *Understanding jargons*
>   - *Understanding where to start*
>   - *Perceived usefulness of the information*
>   - *Making the personal decisions based on the information obtained*
>   - *Trusting as a reliable source of health information*

4.5.2.3 Electronic Health Literacy Scale (e-HLS)

It has 19 items developed for online administration considering the general population [65]. Each item rated with 5-point Likert scale (1 = "strongly disagree" to 5 = "strongly agree). The concepts of the 19-item questions have been summarized below. In summary, the items in e-HLS describes about the individual's capabilities to:

- Understand the portal's information disclosing policy
- Assess for credibility of the source
- Assess the address, proprietorship and sponsorship including financial agreements
- Assessing the goals and how sufficiently addressing information
- Clarity and up-to-date and comprehensiveness of the information
- Assess alternative sources of information
- Capability of assessing the credibility of source and quality of information
- Capability of triangulating the information consulting with healthcare providers
- Trusting the source, and non-biasedness of the information

4.5.2.4 Other Tools

Including Digital health literacy instrument (DHLI) with 21 items with a 4-point Likert scale targeting the general population [66]; eHealth literacy assessment toolkit (eHLA) with 42 items [67]; eHealth literacy questionnaire (eHLQ) with 35 items [68]; Transactional eHealth literacy instrument (TeHLI); with 18 items [69]; etc.

4.5.3 The eHealth Literacy Models

According to the Berkman et al. [56], Health literacy, a term coined in the 1970s, can be broadly defined as the extent to which individuals are able to acquire, comprehend, process, and communicate health-related information necessary for making informed decisions about their health. This definition underscores the significance of eHealth literacy in accessing and effectively uti-

lizing the most up-to-date health information, thereby enabling individuals to make informed decisions regarding their own well-being.

In 2006, Norman and Skinner [56], A conceptual model has been introduced, encompassing six distinct categories of literacy: traditional literacy, health literacy, information literacy, scientific literacy, media literacy, and computer literacy. Over time, this concept has evolved to encompass a broad range of competencies and skills. These include knowledge, motivation, and the ability to access, comprehend, evaluate, and apply health information, as well as engage in prevention and promotion activities [70]. This indicates that eHealth literacy shall include more health concepts than sticking with information technology in order to impact the health outcomes.

4.5.4 eHealth Literacy in Resource-Limited Settings

It is evident that the overall state of eHealth literacy is closely tied to a nation's socio-demographic and economic conditions. For example, the educational status of a community plays a significant role in digital literacy, as it determines the ability to use basic information and communication technologies (ICT) such as the internet and mobile phone communications. Communities or individuals with higher educational attainment are more likely to be digitally literate and have a better understanding of innovative technologies. Economic status also influences literacy, as individuals with access to smartphones and other computing devices have a greater chance of experiencing and becoming familiar with technology.

The most critical concern arises from the fact that technology-disadvantaged groups in resource-limited settings face multiple burdens. These challenges affect not only entire regions categorized as resource-limited settings but also more vulnerable subgroups within those regions. Therefore, it is imperative for all relevant stakeholders to promptly collaborate and identify innovative interventions tailored to the specific contexts of this underprivileged segment of the global population.

In general, there is an urgent need to address the growing disparity in eHealth literacy. As information technology continues to play a significant role in transforming the world, it also contributes to widening the gap in access to and quality of healthcare, exacerbating inequalities.

4.6   Intention and Readiness to Use Digital Health

This section highlights the importance of willingness and intention to utilize digital health solutions in resource-limited settings. The knowledge, attitude, willingness, intention, and ability of stakeholders to embrace and effectively employ digital technologies are crucial prerequisites for the successful adoption and sustainability of any digital health initiative.

Efforts should be focused on raising public awareness, promoting attitude change, and engaging all stakeholders at every stage of the digital health adoption process. This inclusive approach ensures a more sustainable implementation of digital health solutions. It becomes particularly relevant in resource-limited settings where the adoption of digital technologies may involve complex challenges that need to be effectively addressed.

4.6.1   Willingness Versus Intention to Use Digital Health

4.6.1.1 Willingness
In general, willingness to utilize or undertake a particular task can be described as the degree to which an individual or group possesses the confidence, commitment, and motivation necessary to successfully accomplish that specific task [71]. On the other hand, Behavioral Willingness (BW) pertains to the inclination to participate in a specific behavior within a given context. It represents an individual's eagerness to engage in a particular conduct when circumstances are conducive to that behavior, or their receptiveness to seizing opportunities.

4.6.1.2 Intention to Use
Intention signifies the underlying motivations that drive behavior or the level of commitment and effort an individual is willing to exert in order to engage in a specific behavior [72]. Behavioral intention (BI) serves as a key precursor to actual behavior in theories such as reasoned action and planned behavior, thus holding significant importance within these frameworks. In the context of digital health, behavioral intentions refer to the individual's plans and intentions regarding the utilization of digital health solutions within a specific time frame.

4.6.2   Measuring Tools for Intention in Digital Health

Several theoretical models exist for assessing Behavioral Willingness (BW) and Behavioral Intention (BI). However, the choice of a specific measurement tool depends on the context and the strength of the available instruments. It is crucial to select a tool that aligns with a sound theoretical framework in order to effectively explain users' behavior towards the technology being investigated and address research questions.

The strength of a measurement tool is often evaluated based on its reliability and predictive values. In many constructs, including a greater number of multiple items in the tool leads to higher reliability and predictive validity. Therefore, the inclusion of multiple items can enhance the robustness and accuracy of the measurement tool [73].

Among various models, the Unified Theory of Acceptance and Use of Technology (UTAUT) stands out as a widely employed framework. This model encompasses key factors such as performance expectancy, social influence, effort expectancy, and facilitating conditions. Venkatesh et al. [74], the extended version of the UTAUT model incorporates three additional determinants: hedonic motivation, price value, and habit.

Further elaboration on the theoretical frameworks can be found in Chap. 1.

4.6.3   Why We Measure Intention?

In the realm of digital health, all stakeholders involved, including healthcare workers, administrative staff, patients, and the community, should possess key driving forces such as openness, motivation, confidence, and commitment to learn about digitalization within their respective roles. It would be ethically questionable to introduce new technology without ensuring that users are well-informed about its potential benefits and any associated challenges. Moreover, seeking their input, cooperation, consent, and assent, as necessary, becomes essential in this process.

Behavioral willingness and intention go beyond mere approval from digital health actors; they also serve as a means to evaluate the enabling environment prior to implementing a digital system. Taking this strategic step can help minimize resource wastage and ensure the effective and sustainable adoption of the intended system.

According to Fazio [75], An individual's attitude typically influences the way they engage in various activities. This study emphasizes the significance of attitude accessibility, the differentiation between controlled and automated information processing, and the biases that arise from automatically activated attitudes during information processing.

Similarly, the theories of reasoned action and planned behavior, have had a significant impact in this area [72, 76, 77]. Drawing from various theories, the immediate precursors of behavior, including specific attitudes, subjective norms, beliefs, perceptions of control, and intentions, are recognized as significant factors that drive the performance of that behavior.

In order to effectively adapt to digitalization, healthcare organizations should prioritize the social dynamics of the workplace and cultivate a supportive and positive work environment. Essential competencies related to digital health encompass basic ICT skills, digital proficiencies required for patient care, including relevant social

and communication skills, as well as ethical considerations regarding the implementation of digitalization in patient care [78].

4.6.4   eHealth Readiness

eHealth readiness can be defined as the readiness or preparedness of healthcare institutions or communities to embrace and adapt to anticipated changes resulting from programs associated with the utilization of information and communication technology [79]. Currently, there are still gaps in the capacity of instruments to comprehensively measure all aspects of eHealth readiness. Significant efforts are required to achieve a comprehensive assessment of eHealth readiness across entire systems.

The initial phase of a digital transformation journey involves assessing the organization's level of digital readiness using an established technology framework. This step is crucial as it significantly influences the subsequent stages of the process. After the preliminary evaluation, an exercise is undertaken to identify potential gaps in digital skills and talent. This stage may involve training sessions, seminars, or even additional recruitment measures to address the identified gaps. Establishing a digital talent repository can be advantageous, as it can provide ongoing support to the workforce throughout each phase of the deployment process.

A number of researchers classify the dimensions of eHealth readiness in various ways. According to Jennett et al. [80], Within rural communities, eHealth readiness for organizations can be classified into four types: core readiness, engagements, structural readiness, and non-readiness. Alternatively, some classifications categorize eHealth readiness into four categories: organizational readiness, technological/infrastructural readiness, societal readiness, and government readiness [81]. This book will be focusing on the three main dimensions-organizational, health professionals and public-patient readiness in which literatures are widely available [82].

4.6.4.1 Organizational Readiness

The majority of the available research focuses on the organizational readiness. Kruszyńska-Fischbach et al. [83] has summarized that organizational eHealth readiness can further classified in to seven dimensions including core, engagement, technological, societal, learning, policy, and acceptance readiness.

Core/Need Readiness

The core/need readiness component is commonly utilized in the evaluation of eHealth readiness. However, there is variation in how different authors have approached this dimension, resulting in diverse meanings and interpretations of this determinant. Many authors have expressed dissatisfaction with the existing state of affairs and circumstances while defining core readiness, with a focus on addressing demands or challenges [83, 84]. Core readiness comprises of:

- *Knowledge and experience of planners:* Evaluated the goals and functions, confirmed the issues the proposed solution would attempt to address, and made preparations for long-term business models [85].
- *Staff attitudes and perceptions:* Another crucial element cited was the attitudes and perspectives of the staff regarding the prospective usage of the technology [86].
- *Leadership*
- *Digital strategy, goals, vision:* A digital health innovation needs to be strongly integrated with the organizational vision and change roadmaps of the healthcare service to be successful [87].
- *Plans of change:* Giving greater importance to the planning phase of a potential eHealth program [88].
- *Appropriateness of technology:* Appropriateness of the technology and the integration of the technology with existing services [89].
- *Awareness and willingness to change* [90].
- *Realization of needs*: Need for change [90].
- *Dissatisfaction with status quo:* Dissatisfaction with manual systems [90].

- *Expectations of efficacy:* Before spending time and money to make a change, participants wanted to know if eHealth solutions would meet a functional requirement in their practice [91].

Engagement Readiness

Engagement involves introducing individuals to new ideas and actively involving them in the concept of eHealth. Throughout this process, individuals evaluate the perceived benefits and potential drawbacks of eHealth, assess risks, and actively question the chosen course of action. By engaging users, organizations enable them to express their hopes, anxieties, and concerns regarding the adoption of innovative digital tools, offering valuable understandings of the elements that can either support or hinder eHealth readiness. Individuals critically inquire to determine the cost-benefit ratio of adopting eHealth, both in the short term and in the long run. Within an organization, individuals' levels of readiness can range from outright rejection to cautious interest [84, 92].

The assessment of engagement readiness consists of factors.

- *Assessment of potential advantages and disadvantages:* Personal use of technology by employees, and employees' comfort with technology, health professionals' workload and confidence, concerns about data security [86].
- *Curiosity about the potential implications:* The willingness of medical professionals and hospital managers to make first expenditures demonstrates their readiness to engage with the concept of eHealth [93].
- *Expressing hopes, fears, and concerns:* were they genuinely interested, were there any frustration [80].
- *The cost benefit analysis:* Establishing efficient structure to facilitate eHealth implementations [94].

Technological Readiness

Technology readiness entails evaluating the affordability and availability of essential information and communication technology, the required information technology for implementing an innovative digital health technology. Assessing utilization status of the current available technology, the proficiency of IT support staff, the prior IT knowledge of healthcare professionals, the security and reliability of the digital infrastructure, the appropriateness of the technology, and ensuring adequate access to the necessary resources [80, 86, 88].

Recognizing the importance of guaranteeing physical access to technology, it was identified as a crucial element of technological readiness, along with promoting accessibility through factors such as affordability and capacity building. Additionally, key considerations include the performance and reliability of the network, speed requirements, compatibility of hardware and software, the presence of an ICT support team, and the availability and accessibility of the internet. All these factors play significant roles in ensuring comprehensive technological readiness [89]. To summarize, technological readiness encompasses the following elements:

• Assessment of the existing ICT infrastructure
• Availability of electronic resources
• Accounting for information technology availability and digital-divide
• Presence of technical assistance to information technology
• Evaluation of health workers' previous experience with information technology

Societal Readiness

Societal readiness refers to the level of preparedness of a healthcare facilities and health workers to engage in an interconnected domain. Societal readiness involves comprehending the current connections between the health facilities, relevant organizations and other healthcare entities. Sociocultural aspects of societal readiness are addressed through specific topics, which may also encompass considerations of gender and social class inequalities [84, 89]. The key aspects to be taken into account in terms of societal readiness include:

• Collaboration and cooperation with other entities
• Sharing of information
• Provision of care
• Sociocultural considerations of staff
• Socioeconomic and sociocultural positions

Learning Readiness

There are similarities between components of engagement readiness and certain aspects of eHealth adoption. Healthcare professionals may exhibit apprehension towards eHealth due to concerns that it could be used against them or potentially replace their roles in certain situations. However, the primary obstacle does not stem from fear of role replacement but rather from a lack of knowledge and expertise in eHealth, which significantly affects individuals' interaction with new technologies. Clinicians often feel overwhelmed by the rapid pace of technological advancements and struggle to keep up with emerging innovations. Therefore, when assessing learning readiness, it is important to evaluate training opportunities and how they align with professional responsibilities and identities.

One aspect of an organization's structural preparedness is the training provided to employees for utilizing eHealth in the workplace. This category addresses concerns related to the availability of resources and programs aimed at instructing healthcare professionals in the use of technology. This includes training sessions on procedures, access to resources, competent supervisors, and hands-on instruction. Specific elements of learning readiness address healthcare professionals' engagement in the planning process and factors promoting capacity building. Additionally, the value of investing time in learning new technologies is discussed, as well as the challenges faced by some healthcare professionals in convincing patients of the benefits associated with these advancements [80, 87]. In brief, learning readiness comprises the following components:

• Acquisition of eHealth-related knowledge and skills
• Alignment with professional roles and responsibilities

- Availability of training materials and resources
- Active engagement of healthcare providers in the planning process
- Utilization of technology for learning purposes
- Allocation of sufficient time for learning and skill development

Policy Readiness

The establishment of written policies can enhance an organization's readiness in terms of structure for the implementation of eHealth. While the importance of having appropriate policies is evident, there may be uncertainty regarding the responsibility for developing and enforcing these policies. Challenges related to accreditation, accountability, and compensation can be addressed through institutional and governmental policies. Specific elements of policy preparedness encompass factors related to accessibility, including the legal and regulatory framework and the presence of political will. This category assists in establishing the legislative framework, demonstrating national government commitment, providing sponsorship, facilitating regulation, and promoting eHealth and its various requirements [80, 89, 90]. In summary, policy readiness encompasses the following elements:

- Availing relevant strategic and working documents
- Considering accreditations and compensation mechanisms
- Establishing governance frameworks
- Managing uncertainty and establishing accountability frameworks
- Establishing validation and formal approval processes

Acceptance and Use Readiness

Acceptance and use readiness refers to individuals' expectations regarding effort and performance, which in turn influence their intention to adopt and utilize eHealth technology. Effort expectations may consider individual characteristics such as age, educational background, familiarity with networking technology, and the usability of the technology itself. On the other hand, performance expectancy encompasses factors that contribute to organizational awareness, satisfaction with the technology, and anticipated benefits.

Indicators used to assess this category may include attitudes towards using ICT in healthcare administration, perceived value of ICT, user-friendliness, social influence and facilitation, and the conditions for ICT use.

Diverse levels of digital access and literacy can pose significant challenges when implementing eHealth solutions. Research has shown that users vary, with younger individuals often being more proficient, confident, and eager to adopt digital tools, while older individuals may have limited prior knowledge or understanding of basic IT concepts. This applies to both healthcare professionals and patients. Despite reports of increasing usage of digital tablets and smartphones in the general population, many individuals still lack basic access to mobile devices. The high cost of technology, limited access to computer equipment, and lack of free internet services are common barriers preventing people from utilizing eHealth solutions [87, 90, 92, 94]. In general, acceptance and use readiness encompasses the following key aspects:

- Technology familiarity
- Support from vendors
- User-friendliness of eHealth solutions
- User satisfaction
- Anticipated benefits
- Quality of services
- Health workers' attitude in the use of information technology for health
- Perceived usefulness of digital health tools
- Perceived ease-of-use of digital health tools
- Social influence and facilitation
- Conditions for utilizing ICT

4.6.4.2 Health Professionals' Readiness

The influence of healthcare professionals' personal experiences, particularly their perceptions and reactions towards the utilization of eHealth technologies [95]. Healthcare professional readiness is a crucial aspect of eHealth readiness. While it is partly covered within organizational readiness, there are certain aspects that may not be fully addressed at the organizational level. Readiness can be understood through factors such as digital competency, perceived usefulness for both patients and healthcare workers, prior experience and attitudes, and the user-friendliness of the system. The digital competency of healthcare workers has been associated with various environmental factors.

- *Competency:* Competencies related to digitization encompass knowledge in areas such as telenursing, telephone triage, data utilization skills, and more. Factors influencing healthcare professionals' digital competency include their specific profession, workplace environment, team dynamics, and attitudes towards the use of digital devices [96].
- *Knowledge:* It is clear that healthcare professionals would be willing and open to digitalization as long as they believe that the new technology benefits patients and streamline workflows. A comprehensive understanding of the areas of expertise and experience of healthcare professionals in digitalization is required to increase the efficacy of digitalization [97]. According to reports, technology use may be hampered by a lack of knowledge of its function [96].
- *Experience:* The capacity to responsibly utilize technology can be influenced by previous experiences with technology. Past experiences can have either positive or negative effects on the adoption of digital health solutions [98, 99]. Insufficient expertise not only diminishes an individual's familiarity with technology but also decreases the frequency of its usage. Furthermore, there is a connection between dissatisfaction with the outcomes of technological adoption and negative past experiences. Prior negative attitudes and experiences can lead to frustration and reluctance in adopting new technologies.
- *Attitude towards digitalization:* The attitude of healthcare workers plays a crucial role in either facilitating (with a positive attitude) or impeding (with a negative attitude) individuals from carrying out their intended tasks. For

example, a study conducted by de Veer and Francke in 2010 demonstrated this relationship [100], highlighted that various factors influenced the attitudes of healthcare staff towards electronic patient records (EPRs). These factors included the type of healthcare organization they were employed in, their previous exposure to EPRs, the number of hours they worked per week, and their perception of the value of the digital application in enhancing the quality of care.

From the initial stages to the scaling up phase, establishing close collaboration among stakeholders is crucial. Significant progress can be made in adopting health information technologies in resource-limited countries through harnessing the knowledge and perspectives of a wide range of actors in the system, developers, policymakers, and program administrators in the health system. The scale-up process should be flexible and adaptable to accommodate changes in technological advancements and human requirements within the program's operational context. Depending on the healthcare regulatory landscape, the private sector plays a significant role in initiating and expanding digital health initiatives. In cases where governmental resources and expertise are limited, the private sector can contribute by offering financial support, expertise, and infrastructure assistance [101].

Continuous training and support are necessary for healthcare practitioners to effectively utilize technology, and this may include personalized one-on-one assistance. Adequate auditing and monitoring procedures should be in place to ensure proper oversight and assistance in using technology [99, 102]. Capability in ICT helps to enrich the proficiency of health professionals through introducing additional perspectives in developing own professional skills. It brings creativity, excitement, and motivation, helping individuals overcome their fears and uncertainties associated with new technologies. However, during the implementation of new technologies, healthcare personnel may encounter practical challenges such as limited availability of technical equipment or system failures [99, 103].

Several studies have demonstrated that technological proficiency has a direct impact on the frequency of technology usage. The attitudes of employees towards digital equipment and the utilization of technology in healthcare settings are influenced by their skill levels and previous experiences. Insufficient technological expertise hinders professionals from fully harnessing the advantages of technology. Therefore, technological proficiency is crucial for the effective and efficient use of technology [103, 104]. However, the degree of computer literacy does not always determine one's ability to use digital technology [105].

4.6.4.3 Customer/Public Readiness to eHealth

A number of scholars have contributed for the concept of patient engagement. Some of the definitions about patient engagement listed below.

- According to Carman et al. [106], Patient engagement encompasses a range of behaviors exhibited by patients, family members, and healthcare professionals, as well as organizational policies and procedures that promote the active involvement of patients and their families as integral members of the healthcare team. It emphasizes collaborative partnerships between patients, families, providers, and healthcare organizations, with the ultimate aim of enhancing the quality and safety of healthcare services.
- Graffigna et al. [107], Patient engagement can be described as a multi-dimensional psychosocial process that arises from the collective cognitive, emotional, and behavioral actions individuals undertake in relation to their health condition and its management.
- According to Gruman et al. [108], Patient engagement refers to the active and knowledgeable participation of individuals in their own healthcare, taking necessary actions to fully benefit from it.
- Hibbard et al. [109], Patient engagement involves individuals taking an active role in the management of their own health.

These definitions collectively emphasize that patient engagement is a complex and multifaceted process that extends beyond merely assessing a patient's ability to adhere to medical recommendations. In essence, patient engagement encompasses three dimensions [110]:

- *Cognitive:* This dimension pertains to the patient's knowledge, comprehension, and understanding of their condition, its treatments, possible advancements, and monitoring. It encompasses the patient's thoughts and awareness regarding their health.
- *Emotional:* This dimension involves the patient's emotional experiences. It encompasses the psychological and emotional responses that patients undergo as they navigate living with the illness and the changes it brings to their life.
- *Behavioral:* This dimension focuses on the patient's actions. It encompasses all the behaviors and actions taken by the patient to manage their illness and treatments.

It is widely acknowledged that involving patients in the responsible management of their own health is an effective strategy to enhance their well-being. Research has consistently demonstrated that patients who actively engage in their healthcare achieve superior clinical outcomes compared to those who adopt a passive and disengaged approach [111–113]. Additionally, there is growing consensus that patient engagement is a key element in raising quality of health care and patient safety [114].

How eHealth Facilitates Patient Engagement?

Deploying eHealth solutions can encounter significant challenges due to varying levels of digital access and literacy among users. Research indicates a wide range of user capabilities, with younger individuals generally being more adept, confident, and familiar with digital tools, while older individuals may possess limited or no prior knowledge of fundamental IT concepts. Furthermore, despite reports of increasing usage of digital tablets and smartphones among the general population, many individuals still lack basic access to mobile devices. Factors such as the high cost of technology, inadequate access to computer equipment, and limited availability of free internet services often hinder people from utilizing eHealth solutions effectively [87].

The readiness of customers to engage in a digital health system does not necessarily require them to be digitally equipped, whereas healthcare professionals should have the necessary digital competencies. Patients or the general public's readiness is often specific to a particular digital health intervention designed in a way that actively involves patients as key participants, primarily aimed at improving their own health [115]. The extent of patients' and the general public's awareness, accessibility, and affordability of eHealth services is a crucial factor to consider. Additionally, it involves assessing how their personal experiences have shaped their perceptions and responses to the utilization of eHealth technologies [95].

Practical ICT Solutions to Improve Patient Engagement

Evidence indicates a growing trend in the utilization of information and communication technologies to actively engage patients. These technologies have the potential to effectively convert patient-reported measurements into highly sophisticated information, leading to a fundamentally different interaction between patients and a new generation of healthcare professionals. Presented below are a few examples of digital interventions aimed at enhancing patient engagement, alongside numerous others.

Social Media

Use of social media platforms between healthcare professionals and patients to discuss for quality enhancement [116].

Online and Phone Care Management

Implementing a web-based online and phone care management approach facilitated by trained psychologists resulted in several positive outcomes. These included improved medication adherence, reduced depressive symptoms, enhanced access to information, and improved access to high-quality care [117].

Tele-Health System

The telehealth system serves as a self-monitoring tool that enables patients to electronically measure their blood pressure, upload data to a patient portal, and access a web-based dashboard. This system has successfully led to a substantial increase in the number of patients who are able to monitor and track their health status effectively [118].

Personal Health Records (PHRs)

PHR is tools for managing health information to store, retrieve, and manage individual health information and promote healthy behavior. It achieved significant improvement of positive interaction with healthcare providers and satisfaction with perceived care [119].

4.7   Major eHealth Initiatives

Digital health initiatives, including electronic health records (EHR), mobile health (mHealth), telehealth, and clinical decision support systems, have been undergoing pilot testing and scaling up in resource-limited settings. The primary objective of these initiatives is to improve both health system processes and health outcomes. As they progress beyond the pilot stage, there has been a shift in focus towards scalability, integration, and sustainability.

In resource-limited settings, the emphasis on scalability and sustainability stems from the willingness of local political leaders, donor organizations, the public-private partnership having impactful result in the implementation of healthcare programs. This focus ensures that digital health initiatives are not only effective during the pilot phase but also successfully integrated into the existing health system.

In practice, various digital health initiatives have been successfully scaled up and integrated into the health system in resource-limited settings. In the following section, we will discuss the primary initiatives adopted in these contexts.

4.7.1 District Health Information Software 2 (DHIS 2)

District Health Information Software 2 is a widely implemented digital health initiative in resource-limited settings. It serves as an open-source software platform specifically designed for the collection, management, analysis, and visualization of health data. Developed by the University of Oslo in 2006, DHIS-2 is a prominent example of an open-source digital health platform aimed at managing health management information systems (HMIS).

Since the inception of DHIS by the University of Oslo in 1994, the current version, DHIS-2 has been recognized for its flexibility, adaptability, and extensibility, as well as its web application program interfaces (APIs). These features offer significant advantages, enabling the development of software applications (apps) and allowing customization even for non-health programmes [120].

The initial implementation of DHIS took place in South Africa in 1998, followed by the development of DHIS 2. India adopted DHIS 2 in 2006, and the first national rollout of DHIS 2 occurred in Kenya in 2010. Subsequently, DHIS 2 has been widely embraced by low- and middle-income countries (LMICs) globally. The effectiveness of the DHIS 2 tool relies on several crucial factors that indicate a robust health information system (HIS). These factors include effective management and leadership, the establishment of policies and procedures, and the expertise of users of the DHIS 2 tool. Currently, DHIS 2 holds the distinction of being the largest health management information system (HMIS) platform worldwide, with more than 76 resource-limited countries having implemented the software, as of the report in April, 2023 [120].

4.7.1.1 Benefits
According to a review of literatures [121], DHIS 2 offers several key features that contribute to its usefulness as a tool:

- It is a web-based system, allowing users to access information from any location with computer and internet access. Additional features include the ability to send SMS messages, use the software offline, its open-source nature, and others features
- It facilitates integration and aggregation of information, streamlining data entry at the operational level of service provision.
- DHIS 2 enables the consolidation of previously separate systems within a country.
- The software ensures data quality by improving timeliness, completeness, and validity through assessment and feedback mechanisms.
- Its flexibility allows for the addition of new modules, enabling customization to meet local needs.
- DHIS 2 enhances efficiency and quality of reporting.
- It encourages the culture of using information for decision-making.
- The tool contributes to worker satisfaction by improving their ability to utilize data effectively.
- DHIS 2 fosters a sense of data and system ownership, increasing stakeholders' involvement and commitment

4.7.1.2 Challenges
In addition to the factors contributing to its success, the implementation of DHIS 2 in resource-limited countries has also faced operational challenges. These challenges predominantly pertain to system and infrastructure issues. Some of the notable challenges include:

- Inadequate health information system (HIS) infrastructure.
- Insufficient focus on staff training.
- Limited understanding and knowledge of the DHIS 2 software and its functionalities.
- Lack of technical expertise and knowledge required for effective utilization.

4.7.1.3 Lessons Learned
Collaboration: Collaboration has been a key success factor for DHIS 2. Universities, funders, governmental bodies, NGOs, and partners from around the world have come together to contribute to the successful implementation of DHIS 2.

The DHIS 2 business model: DHIS 2 operates on an open-source platform that allows for customization. It fosters a global community of users who can add new features, customize the software, and freely utilize it, even for non-health programs.

Sustainable funding: Securing sustainable funding is often a challenge, but DHIS 2 implementation has effectively managed this issue thus far.

Capacity building strategies: The University of Oslo, with available funding, has established a global HISP (Health Information Systems Program) network. This network provides training, assists with DHIS 2 installation, localization, and configuration, conducts local and regional training programs, and promotes DHIS 2 as a global public good.

Political commitment: Despite challenges, the engagement of political leaders and policy makers has played a significant role in the successful implementation of DHIS 2.

4.7.2 Electronic Community Health Information Systems (eCHIS)

While the development and implementation of digital-based community health information systems (CHIS) in low- and middle-income countries are still in their nascent stages, there has been a notable increase in their development and adoption to bolster community-based health services in LMICs. Pilot studies have shown that integrating digital technologies into existing CHIS has been both practical and resource-efficient in settings with limited resources [122].

The introduction of a mobile-based solution in Nigeria resulted in a significant improvement in the quality of information. The use of mobile technology made the data collection process simple, user-friendly, and efficient. This experience has demonstrated that mobile technology can enable the achievement of consistency, accuracy, and timeliness in data collection and submission processes [123].

In Kenya, technology offers a cost-effective alternative to traditional paper-based solutions.

The study revealed that mHealth systems have the potential for rapid user adoption, provided they align with the specific context's user and infrastructure requirements and promote user interaction [124].

The implementation of eCHIS applications in Ethiopia has brought about notable advancements in the functioning of the CHIS. This has allowed program administrators to easily access monthly data from each health post, resulting in timely and accurate data reporting. Overall, the use of eCHIS has been shown to enhance data quality, traceability, and transparency, while also serving as a source of motivation for community health workers in their daily tasks [125, 126].

4.7.2.1 Challenges
Despite the increasing interests, eCHIS implementation has been constrained various types of barriers in resource-limited settings [127–129]. Among others, some of the commonly reported challenges are listed below:

Poor HIS Infrastructure
There were several barriers related to infrastructure, including the shortage or inadequate specifications of tablets (such as low processing speed and storage capacity, limited power storage), unreliable connectivity and electricity supply, lack of maintenance services, and poor interoperability. As discussed earlier in this chapter, the infrastructure for digital health (info-structure) poses significant challenges, particularly in rural areas of resource-limited settings, where the situation is often worse compared to urban areas.

Inadequate Qualified Manpower
The implementation of eCHIS in resource-limited settings has faced obstacles due to insufficient skilled manpower, a shortage of dedicated community volunteers, and high staff turnover. These factors have been identified as significant bottlenecks for successful eCHIS implementation.

Poor Digital Literacy
In general, community health workers face challenges due to a lack of skills and prior exposure

to information technology. This lack of familiarity and expertise with IT poses a significant hurdle for them.

Fear of Losing Devices

In certain studies, community health workers expressed concerns about the risk of tablet robbery and theft during home visits and travels for outreach health services. Due to the high cost of computing devices like tablets, workers are often reluctant to take the risk of carrying such devices.

Policy Gaps

Policy directives that mandate the simultaneous recording of both the paper-based CHIS and eCHIS have hindered the implementation of eCHIS. This requirement increases workloads and creates challenges for effective adoption and integration of the digital system.

4.7.3   mHealth Apps

Following the increasing penetration of mobile phone in developing world, this opportunity brought mHealth that allows to use the potentials of the technology in public health. In LMICs, the adoption of mHealth technologies found to be promising; however, most of the mHealth initiatives in the resource-limited settings get perish on piloting stage. The most popular mHealth applications were SMS messages followed by smartphone/PDA apps. The health education, surveillance and health monitoring were the dominant areas of mHealth application [130].

In LMICs, mHealth has been applied in various health and health-related programmes. Some of the widely applied areas of mHealth to early screen and case identification of communicable and non-communicable illnesses, outbreak investigation, patient adherence support system, clinic-appointment reminder system, and others.

4.7.3.1 Screening Infectious Diseases

A number of studies identified that mobile health technology and applications may help with the screening of infectious diseases including COVID-19, Ebola, Severe Acute Respiratory

Syndrome (SARS), HIV, TB, Zika virus, in resource limited settings [131–135]. Mobile health applications have been employed for remote screening and identification of individuals suspected of having COVID-19. Frontline healthcare workers have utilized mHealth technologies for screening COVID-19, aiding an early detection. Similarly, mobile health apps served as a diagnostic tool for Ebola Virus Disease (EVD) and Zika virus outbreaks in West Africa and in South America, respectively. In Asia, mHealth applications have facilitated real-time detection of tuberculosis (TB). However, the utilization of mHealth applications for screening infectious diseases has been more prevalent in parts of Southern America and Asia compared to sub-Saharan Africa, primarily due to greater technological advancements in these regions.

4.7.3.2 Screening Non-Infectious Diseases

Applications for mobile health are being used to help with the screening for a number of non-infectious diseases such as diabetes, cancer, and hypertension [136–138]. Studies conducted in low- and middle-income countries have shown that mHealth applications have been instrumental in enabling rural communities to identify cancer symptoms, detect cardiovascular issues, and assist in diagnosing non-communicable diseases and cardio-metabolic disorders. Frontline healthcare professionals have utilized mHealth applications to make differential diagnoses based on patient circumstances. In India, mHealth applications have been particularly utilized for screening non-infectious disorders at a higher frequency.

4.7.3.3 Disease Surveillance

Due to logistical, financial, and infrastructure limitations, the surveillance of infectious and non-infectious illness outbreaks is unstable in LMICs [139–141]. The implementations of mHealth strategies have significantly reduced cost of healthcare particularly for case identification processes and has provided an efficient approach to conducting surveillance in countries with limited resources. mHealth initiatives are commonly utilized in low- and middle-income countries to support surveillance programs for both infectious and non-infectious diseases. For example, during the ongoing global COVID-19 outbreak, digital health Apps were used for case finding purposes that have significant contribution for reducing the transmission of the disease.

4.7.3.4 Medication and Treatment Support

Generally, research findings indicated that a phone-based messaging and medication and appointment reminders found to improve patient's engagement in the long-term treatments. Short message service (SMS) was generally found useful for reminding medications and healthcare services [142–146], providing health-tips and other educational messages [2, 3], and maintaining users' awareness of their health goals [20]. Audio messages were effective in transferring messages to support TB treatment as compared to other messaging types like text, graphics, however, it needs high bandwidth internet for data exchange [147]. Few studies demonstrated that text-based medication reminder systems showed promising effect on improving adherence to TB treatment [142, 144, 148, 149].

4.7.4 Electronic Health Records

Utilization of digital health systems offers several advantages, particularly in terms of patient and client-specific benefits. Electronic health records have the potential to facilitate the integration of socio-demographic data and maintaining the community's profile that in turn play a crucial role in the routine healthcare delivery. Moreover, EHRs can be utilized to detect and anticipate season-based epidemics, and risk areas. The use of EHRs for disease surveillance and monitoring systems has emerged as a critical element of public health strategies in Asia and other resource-limited settings [150]. Electronic health records have been demonstrated to be a crucial tool for enhancing patient information access and enhancing the standard of care. EHR has not, however, been widely used in Africa, especially in sub-Saharan Africa [151]. According to the review of

literatures [151], the key obstacles to EHR adoption were.

4.7.4.1 Unreliable Infrastructure

The lack of a reliable energy supply has been identified by numerous experts as a significant obstacle to the widespread adoption of electronic health records (EHR) in resource-limited settings. The challenges related to infrastructure, including inadequate power availability, unreliable internet connections, and inconsistent electricity supply, make it impractical to achieve broader EHR adoption in several Sub-Saharan countries. In general, limited power availability and inconsistent internet access are commonly cited as major barriers to the implementation of EHRs in resource-limited areas.

4.7.4.2 High Operational Cost

The high cost associated with implementing electronic health records (EHR) systems, including expenses related to hardware and software procurement, training, and support, is frequently cited as a significant barrier to EHR adoption. Furthermore, the maintenance and costs of additional accessories such as scanners, printers, paper, ink, and so on further contribute to the financial burden of EHR implementation.

4.7.4.3 Low Digital Literacy

Low computer literacy levels emerged as a significant barrier to the widespread adoption of EHR in sub-Saharan African nations. Physicians identified several skill-related characteristics that they believed would make using an EHR challenging. These included difficulties in typing while engaging with patients, limited or no computer proficiency, lack of awareness regarding EHR system usage, and poor typing skills.

4.7.4.4 Competing Priorities

Studies have revealed that developing nations often face a multitude of challenges, including disease epidemics, civil conflicts, and natural disasters. As a result, the implementation of EHRs may not be perceived as a top priority in such regions.

4.8 Adoption of Digital Health

4.8.1 What Is Digital Health Adoption?

Digital adoption in healthcare involves the transformation and enhancement of conventional healthcare practices through the integration of innovative technologies. It entails integrating and utilizing digital technologies within healthcare systems and practices to improve healthcare delivery, enhance patient outcomes, and reshape the healthcare landscape. It encompasses a range of elements, including incorporating electronic health records, telemedicine, mobile health applications, wearable devices, remote patient monitoring, health information systems, data analytics, and other digital tools that facilitate the collection, storage, analysis, and exchange of health-related information.

Digital health adoption not only entails implementing technology but also integrating these tools into existing healthcare workflows and practices. It necessitates training and education for healthcare professionals, ensuring data privacy and security, addressing interoperability challenges, and tailoring approaches to the unique needs and contexts of different healthcare settings.

4.8.2 Why Digital Health Adoption?

By investing in people and processes, in accordance with national strategies for digitizing the health sector, digital health has the potential to enhance care efficiency, cost-effectiveness, and enable the emergence of new service delivery models. The vision for digital health entails fostering research, development, innovation, and collaboration across various sectors. Sufficient investments in the leadership, organizational capacity, and skilled manpower enable the required transformations in health information system and data-informed healthcare practice progressively embraces digitalization.

Despite research highlighting the benefits of specific digital health solutions and policymakers expressing willingness in implementing these innovative solutions, the acceptability and scale-up of such solutions have not consistently aligned with healthcare practice, resulting in a delay in their implementation. The drive to adopt digital health technologies stems from their potential to enhance healthcare quality, promote patient engagement, optimize the delivery of healthcare services, lower costs, and increase access to care, facilitate data-driven decision-making, stimulate research and innovation, and bolster public health initiatives.

According to the WHO [2], adoption of digital health is about prioritizing accessible and fair access to high-quality healthcare services. Moreover, it should enhance the efficiency and sustainability of health systems by providing affordable and unbiased care.

Additionally, digital health needs to bolster health promotion, disease prevention, diagnosis, management, rehabilitation, and palliative care, even in times of epidemics or pandemics, while safeguarding patient privacy and the security of health information.

4.8.3 How to Measure Adoption of Digital Health

The adoption of digital health can be measured using various metrics and indicators. However, the specific metrics and methods of measuring digital health adoption may vary depending on the context, target population, and the specific digital health technologies being assessed. Here are some common approaches used to assess the adoption of digital health:

- Penetration rates
- Usage metrics
- Health records and data analysis
- Surveys and user feedback
- Clinical outcomes and quality indicators
- Cost and efficiency measures
- Interoperability and health information exchange

4.8.4 Digital Health Adoption in Resource-Limited Settings

In resource-limited settings, the adoption of digital health holds great promise for enhancing healthcare delivery and outcomes. The successful adoption and implementation of electronic medical record (EMR) systems in developing countries still face several challenges. There is frequently significant uncertainty surrounding the costs, implementation, and outcomes associated with e-health technology. One potential approach to address this uncertainty is to create comprehensive product comparisons of electronic medical records (EMRs). Government funding could support initiatives that compare different e-health technologies and conduct research to identify the complete range of financial, time, and quality outcomes associated with EMR adoption. These comparison projects would enable physicians to gain a clear understanding of how the adoption of e-health technology could impact their clinical practice [152].

Despite challenges posed by limited resources, including inadequate infrastructure and restricted technology access, digital health solutions have the capacity to surmount these obstacles and offer accessible and cost-effective healthcare services. Generally, positive results were reported, such as ease of use, infrastructure requirements, and the acceptability of the intervention. The studies also highlighted general benefits, including support for provider training and mentorship, communication among providers and clients, and improvement in data collection and management. However, there was a lack of studies evaluating individualized clinical outcomes, and the literature did not provide interventions targeting health system managers, despite the identified functionality of the surveyed systems for tasks like inventory management.

Therefore, by expediting the acceptance and integration of established digital health technologies into standard healthcare practices, there is a remarkable opportunity to transform human health. This can be achieved through enhanced effectiveness, reduced costs, and improved accessibility and capacity for delivering care.

4.9 Digital Health Maturity

During the year 2018, the World Health Assembly (WHA) [153] called upon Member States to evaluate their utilization of digital technologies in healthcare, specifically health information systems at both the national and subnational levels. The objective was to identify areas requiring improvement and prioritize the development, evaluation, implementation, scale-up, and enhanced utilization of digital technologies. The aim was to promote equitable, affordable, and universal access to healthcare for all individuals, including vulnerable groups, in the context of digital health.

4.9.1 Digital Health Assessment Approaches

There are three types of digital health assessment depending on the approach and types of indicators involved in the assessment.

4.9.1.1 Digital Health Landscape Profiling of Digital Health Systems

Digital Health Landscape profile (DHLP) is a set of indicators that includes fundamental sociodemographic data, the use of ICTs, the types of applications, and worker experience to the solutions.

4.9.1.2 Maturity Assessment of Digital Health Systems

A paradigm for measuring maturity in four areas including the info-structure, leadership, structural design & documents, application and analytical performances.

4.9.1.3 In-Depth Understanding of Digital Health Systems

To better comprehend some of the subjects covered, material from primary and secondary sources will be gathered.

- The DHLP is an overview of 50 items categorized into five groups with a complete picture of a nation's current state and the factors that support digital health. The indications provide context for the maturity rating tool's responses [154].

- The digital Health landscape profile indicators consist of sociodemographic and healthcare system basic information domains.
- The digital environment domain for digital Health landscape profile consists of:
  - eGovernment development index
  - Number of startups
  - Number of technology companies
- On the other hand, the infrastructure and communications domain for digital Health landscape profile consists of ICT development, access and use of digital technologies.
- The interventions and applications domain for digital Health landscape profile consists of the number of population, health organizations and the type of digital health technologies deployed and utilized.
- The workforce domain for digital Health landscape profile is about the IT specialists, size of young people on education, population with vocational/professional qualification

Overall, the main focus of this section of the book was on digital health maturity. Consequently, digital health maturity serves as the pathway towards the sustainable adoption of digital health systems.

4.9.2 What Is Digital Health Maturity

Digital maturity refers to the ability to effectively utilize digital technologies to achieve business objectives. It involves not only possessing the necessary technological tools and skills but also encompasses the attitudes, processes, and organizational structures required to leverage technology for optimal outcomes. A successful digital transformation can contribute to the growth of a business by enabling it to adapt to the connected digital world, addressing challenges, and seizing opportunities.

Likewise, a country's digital health profiles (DHPs), which encompass health priorities, technological advancements, and quality improvement initiatives, serve as indicators of digital health maturity that can be assessed over time. Analyzing data related to DHPs can provide valuable insights for evaluating the maturity of digital health technologies at subnational levels.

In order to make informed investments in digital health, whether through digital health initiatives or disruptive technologies, it is crucial to have a comprehensive understanding of the ecosystem, infrastructure, available resources, and the current state of the healthcare industry.

4.9.3 Digital Health Maturity Score

The digital maturity score of an organization reflects its effectiveness in utilizing digital technologies to achieve its objectives. This score is determined by considering various factors such as internet presence, site analytics, marketing automation, and customer service technologies. By assessing their digital maturity, companies can gain a better understanding of their current digital state and identify areas for improvement, enabling them to successfully navigate their digital transformation.

Maturity models place significant emphasis on people, processes, technology, and organizational skills. They facilitate an understanding of the current situation and help set future objectives. When maturity levels are low, there is room for investment and significant progress, while high maturity levels offer greater potential for successful disruptive interventions. Essentially, a maturity model describes the consistent and sustainable organizational behavior, practices, and overall processes that lead to desired results. It measures an organization's ability to progress steadily across various areas until it reaches an appropriate level of maturity. Assessment, and improving the quality of tools and methods are integral to the process of maturity assessment [155].

4.9.4 Digital Health Maturity Assessment Tools

According to World Bank Group of Health, Nutrition and Population Digital Health Assessment Toolkit Guide, [156], the tool for measuring digital health maturity: the indicators covering a wide range of subjects are offered within each category:

- ICT ecosystem: Measures the national approaches and digital health from a broad perspective.
- Architecture & Data: The metrics evaluate access to info-structure, information technology, initiative, eHealth Apps, including utilization of those technologies.
- Digital Apps: The metrics evaluate eHealth standpoints and interventions, using AI when appropriate. It also examines client satisfaction and acceptance.
- Analytical capabilities: This metrics include advanced tools, approaches used in healthcare data management and use of information in developing prediction models and algorithms.

In addition, several digital health maturity assessment tools have been reported such as,

- Global Digital Health Index (GDHI) with a national focus and with seven dimensions [157];
- Informatics Capability Maturity Model (ICMM) with organizational focus and with five dimensions [158];
- Health Information Systems Interoperability Maturity Toolkit (HISIMT) which focused on interoperability with three dimensions [159];
- Health Information System Stages of Continuous Improvement Toolkit (HISSCIT) with a focus on continuous improvement and with seven dimensions [160].

The characteristics of each assessment tool mentioned above are outlined in Fig. 4.1, providing a comprehensive overview.

4.9.5 Digital Health Maturity Assessment Toolkits and Processes

4.9.5.1 Toolkits

Currently, various digital maturity assessment toolkits available to aid a standardized methodology and instruments for the assessment process. Some of the toolkits are: Measure Evaluation HIS Framework, Global Observatory of eHealth, IS4H Maturity Assessment tool and others.

Digital health maturity assessment can be undertaken using a manual paper-based assessment and using software-assisted assessment. The use of software often simplifies the process and time saving, reduce computational errors, non- tedious.

4.9.5.2 Assessment Process

- Determine the need for an assessment: It is important to agree with the nation or organization on the assessment's goal at this step, which could include benchmarking, reviewing progress, or establishing a baseline.
- Determine the scope: The nation or organization should choose the assessment's scope based on its needs.
- Establish an oversight team: Obtaining support from the many stakeholders is crucial.
- Conduct a desk review: To comprehend the ecosystem and the stakeholders who ought to be considered in the assessment, secondary sources should also be examined.
- Assemble the assessment team: Contact both the assessment team and the list of stakeholders.
- Collect data: Determining the approach, methods, and instruments for gathering the information required to provide answers to all pertinent issues is crucial.
- Analyze data: Once data has been gathered, it must be organized and examined to produce preliminary findings.
- Action planning: It is the cyclic approach that all evaluation results are useful to inform the next step of the program. These processes continue following the same steps but using improved strategies and performances.

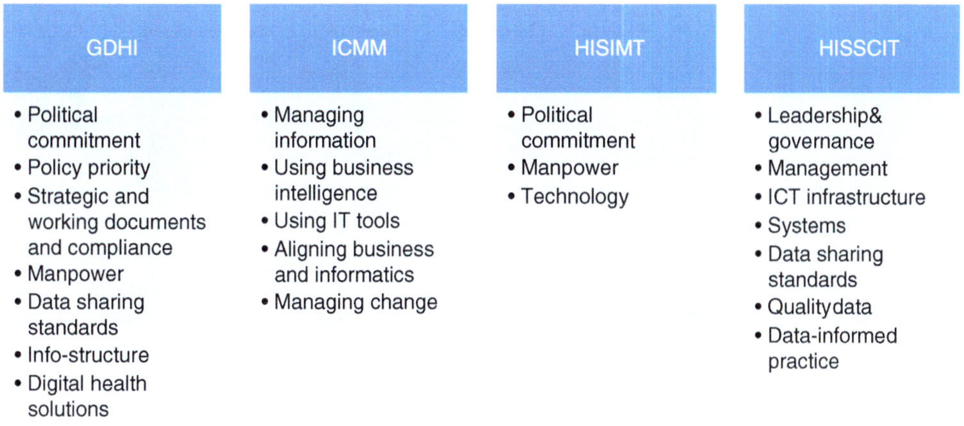

Fig. 4.1 Dimensions of GDHI, ICMM, HISIMT and HISSCIT maturity assessment tools

4.9.6 Digital Health Maturity Assessment Outcomes

Digital maturity can be assessed using various scales, with each scale consisting of a predefined set of process areas that correspond to different maturity levels. These levels represent the evolution of digital health domains and subdomains, progressing from lower to higher stages. They provide a framework for describing the performance and advancement of digital health.

The digital health maturity model commonly employs a five-point scale. Each point on the scale represents the level of digital health maturity achieved by an organization or country. The specific definitions of each level may vary across different scales. For instance, one scale may define the levels as follows:

- Level 1: "Very little digital progress"
- Level 2: "Underdeveloped and challenged"
- Level 3: "Developing rapidly with potential"
- Level 4: "Regional maturity and scaling"
- Level 5: "Sophisticated at a national scale"

These scales provide a standardized way to assess and communicate the degree of digital health maturity attained by an entity. The other five degrees of this concept of digital health interoperability maturity scale ranges from 1 to 5 including nascent, emergent, establishment, institutionalization and optimization, as indicated in the Fig. 4.2.

4.9.6.1 Level-I: Nascent

Indicates the digital health system lacks capabilities or does not adhere to procedures consistently. The digital health operations take place haphazardly or as one-off, sporadic attempts.

4.9.6.2 Level-II: Emerging

Although the nation has established digital health systems, they are not consistently documented. There is no official, continuous methodology for monitoring or measurement.

4.9.6.3 Level-III: Established

The nation's digital health structures are known to exist. The buildings are useful. Metrics are often used for performance evaluation, quality improvement, and monitoring.

4.9.6.4 Level-IV: Institutionalized

The government and other parties use the national digital health system and adhere to best practices.

4.9.6.5 Level-V: Optimized

Interoperability initiatives are periodically reviewed by the government and stakeholders, who change them as necessary to account for shifting circumstances.

Fig. 4.2 The five-levels
of maturity

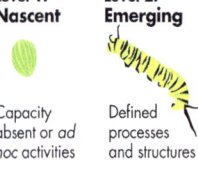
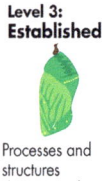
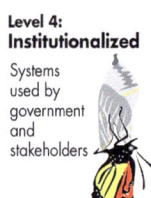
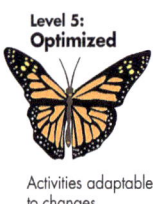

Level 1:
Nascent

Capacity
absent or *ad
hoc* activities

Level 2:
Emerging

Defined
processes
and structures

Level 3:
Established

Processes and
structures
documented and
functional

Level 4:
Institutionalized

Systems
used by
government
and
stakeholders

Level 5:
Optimized

Activities adaptable
to changes

4.9.7 Digital Health Maturity in Resource-Limited Settings

While there has been significant progress in achieving digital health maturity on a global scale, the pace of advancement varies across different nations. The scale-up of eHealth technologies are not straight forward in all settings, as each nation has its unique starting point on the path of digital transformation. Therefore, identifying leaders and laggards in terms of healthcare's digital maturity becomes crucial in determining the necessary actions for nations to advance.

Research has demonstrated a positive correlation between a nation's GDP per capita and its digital maturity score. This suggests that wealthier countries tend to perform better in digital health due to their strong cultural, political, economic, and regulatory foundations.

Conversely, complex contextual barriers hinder the development and maturity of digital health in resource-limited settings. As mentioned earlier, factors such as inadequate infrastructure, limited digital literacy, insufficient funding, and competing priorities pose challenges for the progress and maturity of digital health in these settings.

Despite the evident growth of digital health in developing countries, there remains a lack of sufficient evidence regarding the level and underlying determinants of digital health maturity in resource-limited settings.

4.9.8 How Countries Can Achieve Digital Health Maturity?

The concept of sustained digital growth holds great appeal as a means to improve healthcare efficiencies on a large scale, especially consider-

ing the increasing strain on healthcare systems and their limited resources. However, what truly excites people is the potential for improved community health management and ultimately better patient outcomes. To achieve these objectives, it is crucial to strive for digital maturity and closely monitor the progress of each nation. This presents an opportunity for developing countries to leapfrog towards advanced technology by adopting best practices from more developed nations [161].

There are various strategies to advance digital health maturity. It has been reported that successful digital health share some common features. These listed common features can be scaled-up for resource-limited countries.

4.9.8.1 Dedicated Digital Health Strategies

At the national level, it is crucial to have a well-defined vision and goals. Establishing a common understanding among all stakeholders ensures alignment and concerted efforts towards advancing digital health on a national scale. As organizations initiate specific digital health initiatives, having clear strategies becomes imperative for their success. However, these strategies must be practical and consider the contextual factors that influence their implementation. Developing feasible strategies for digital health is essential, taking into account the unique circumstances and influences at play.

4.9.8.2 Designated Funding

Having a dedicated funding strategy is essential for the sustainable adoption of digital health. Funding plays a central role in bridging the digital divide in low and middle-income nations by facilitating the development of digitally enhanced health systems. It is crucial to engage national governments, international donors, and the private sector to mobilize and enhance investments in this area.

However, securing dedicated and sustainable funding for digital health development poses significant challenges, particularly in resource-limited settings. Many digital health initiatives rely on donor-driven projects that often remain at the pilot stage, with only a few successfully transitioning to broader national-level scale-up and being locally owned by the government.

4.9.8.3 Well-Managed Data

Enabled access and use of data would facilitate data-informed decision-making in all aspects. As a result, the use of digital tools for data management would lead efficient and effective approaches in turn will motivate back the advancement to digital health.

4.9.8.4 National Electronic Health Records

The establishment and operation of a flexible digital national platform for health system records is crucial. Implementing digitalization in the healthcare system can be complex and challenging, but even in resource-limited settings, there are opportunities to be seized. The realization of an EHR system holds significant potential to facilitate digital health initiatives. EHR serves as a platform that enables seamless integration and smooth operation of various digital health applications.

4.9.8.5 Empowered Institutions

To promote innovation and advancements in the digital healthcare industry, it is crucial to ensure that data is transmitted and stored in accordance with current standards. By empowering healthcare practitioners and institutions to utilize the most advanced digital health technologies, we can foster an environment that encourages innovation and the development of new technologies in healthcare [162].

4.9.8.6 Emphasis on Interoperability

To achieve digital health maturity, it is essential to store and transmit data using contemporary standards. The lack of interoperability and integration among various digital health systems poses a significant obstacle. To successfully transition from fragmented applications to interconnected eHealth solutions, it is crucial to prioritize interoperability policies at the national level. This emphasis on interoperability is necessary because it enables healthcare institutions to exchange data, leading to improved patient safety, efficiency, cost-effectiveness, and quality of healthcare delivery, particularly in times of pandemics.

4.9.8.7 Innovation

Investing in the creation of new data sources to expand the scope of health data is crucial. Institutions should actively cultivate an innovative culture that recognizes and rewards experimentation and risk-taking. This can be achieved by fostering a culture of continuous learning, encouraging teamwork and effective communication, and providing employees with opportunities to explore novel concepts and technologies.

4.9.8.8 Experimentation

To enhance the development and maturity of digital health, it is important to initiate research and development projects through collaborative efforts, including frequent piloting and implementation science studies. Such strategies are essential for gaining valuable insights, refining digital health initiatives, and driving progress in this field.

References

1. World Health Organization. National eHealth strategy toolkit. Geneva: International Telecommunication Union, World Health Organization; 2012.
2. World Health Organization. Global strategy on digital health 2020–2025. Geneva: World Health Organization; 2021.
3. Broadband Commission and Working Group on Digital Health. The promise of digital health: addressing non-communicable diseases to accelerate Universal Health Coverage in LMICs. 2018. https://www.broadbandcommission.org/wp-content/uploads/2021/02/WGDigitalHealth_Report2018.pdf. Accessed 17 Apr 2023.
4. Singh HA. Digital health: a call for Government Leadership and Cooperation Between ICT and Health. Broadband Commission for Sustainable Development; 2017.

5. Carnicero J, Serra P. Governance for digital health: the art of health systems transformation. Washington, DC: Inter-American Development Bank; 2020.

6. World Health Organizatio. eHealth. World Health Organization: Geneva; 2005.

7. Källander K, et al. Mobile health (mHealth) approaches and lessons for increased performance and retention of community health workers in low- and middle-income countries: a review. J Med Internet Res. 2013;15(1):e17.

8. Akhlaq A, et al. Barriers and facilitators to health information exchange in low- and middle-income country settings: a systematic review. Health Policy Plan. 2016;31(9):1310–25.

9. Powell AC, Landman AB, Bates DW. In search of a few good apps. JAMA. 2014;311(18):1851–2.

10. Boulos MNK, et al. Mobile medical and health apps: state of the art, concerns, regulatory control and certification. Online J Public Health inform. 2014;5(3):229.

11. Labrique AB, et al. Best practices in scaling digital health in low and middle income countries. Glob Health. 2018;14(1):103.

12. Neha SS, et al. A tale of 'politics and stars aligning': analysing the sustainability of scaled up digital tools for front-line health workers in India. BMJ Glob Health. 2021;6(Suppl 5):e005041.

13. Rodgers A, et al. Do u smoke after txt? Results of a randomised trial of smoking cessation using mobile phone text messaging. Tob Control. 2005;14(4):255–61.

14. Gopinathan P, et al. Self-reported quit rates and quit attempts among subscribers of a mobile text messaging-based tobacco cessation programme in India. BMJ Innov. 2018;4(4):bmjinnov-2018-000285.

15. World Health Organization. International Telecommunication, Digital health platform handbook: building a digital information infrastructure (infostructure) for health. Geneva: World Health Organization; 2020.

16. Aklin M, et al. Factors affecting household satisfaction with electricity supply in rural India. Nat Energy. 2016;1:16170.

17. Times of India. Beyond access: the future of electricity in India. 19 October 2021. https://timesofindia.indiatimes.com/blogs/voices/beyond--access-the-future-of-electricity-in-india/. Accessed 13 Apr 2023.

18. Shah SAA, et al. Techno-economic analysis of solar PV electricity supply to rural areas of Balochistan, Pakistan. Energies. 2018;11(7):1777.

19. Rostam NEB, et al. Urban flood impact assessment for the electricity supply industry in Malaysia. Springer; 2019.

20. ITU. Digital trends in Africa, information and communication technology trends and developments in the Africa region 2017–2020. 2021. https://www.itu.int/dms_pub/itu-d/opb/ind/D-IND-DIG_TRENDS_AFR.01-2021-PDF-E.pdf. Accessed 17 Apr 2023.

21. ITU-WTDC. Digital trends in Africa. 2021. https://view.officeapps.live.com/op/view.aspx?src. Accessed 17 Apr 2023.

22. ITU. Nearly half of people with 4G network coverage remain offline, mainly due to high cost of Internet access. https://www.itu.int/en/mediacentre/Pages/pr02-2021-The-affordability-of-ICT-services-2020.aspx. Accessed 17 Apr 2023.

23. GSMA. The mobile economy Sub-Saharan Africa. 2020. https://www.gsma.com/mobileeconomy/wp-content/uploads/2020/09/GSMA_MobileEconomy2020_SSA_Eng.pdf. Accesses 17 Apr 2023.

24. ITU. Digital trends in Africa 2021: information and communication technology trends and developments in the Africa region 2017–2020. ITU Publications; 2021.

25. Griebel L, et al. A scoping review of cloud computing in healthcare. BMC Med Inform Decis Mak. 2015;15(1):17.

26. Kaboré SS, et al. Barriers and facilitators for the sustainability of digital health interventions in low and middle-income countries: a systematic review. Front Digit Health. 2022;4:1014375.

27. Hui CY, et al. Mapping national information and communication technology (ICT) infrastructure to the requirements of potential digital health interventions in low- and middle-income countries. J Glob Health. 2022;12:04094.

28. World Bank. Digital development. 2022. https://www.worldbank.org/en/topic/digitaldevelopment/overview#1. Accessed 18 Apr 2023.

29. e-Conomy-Africa. Africa's 180 billion internet economy. IFC and Google Report. 2020. https://www.ifc.org/wps/wcm/connect/publications_ext_content/ifc_external_publication_site/publications_listing_page/google-e-conomy. Accessed 18 Apr 2023.

30. Bogdan-Martin D. Accelerating digital connectivity in the wake of COVID-19: Building back better with broadband requires all stakeholders to work together. International Telecommunications Union, Geneva. 2020. https://www.itu.int/en/myitu/News/2020/09/16/19/22/UN75-Partnership-Dialogue-for-Connectivity-Doreen-Bogdan-Martin. Accessed 18 Apr 2023.

31. African Union. The digital transformation strategy for Africa (2020–2030). African Union, Addis Ababa. 2020. https://au.int/sites/default/files/documents/38507-doc-dts-english.pdf. Accessed 18 Apr 2023.

32. Laar AS, et al. Perspectives of health care professionals' on delivering mHealth sexual and reproductive health services in rural settings in low-and-middle-income countries: a qualitative systematic review. BMC Health Serv Res. 2022;22(1):1141.

33. African Development Bank. Digital connectivity and infrastructure. https://www.afdb.org/pt/topics-and-sectors/sectors/information--communication-technology/digital-connectivity-and-infrastructure#:~:text=There%20is%20

great%20disparity%20in,to%20attract%20pri-vate%20sector%20investment. Accessed 18 Apr 2023.

34. ITU. Recommendation ITU-T H.810: interoperability design guidelines for personal connected health systems. www.itu.int/rec/T-REC-H.810-201607-I/en/. Accessed 18 Apr 2023.

35. Sharma AK. Recent innovative trends in interdisciplinary research areas, vol. 2. Animesh Kumar Sharma; 2023.

36. Wilson K, et al. The journey to scale: moving together past digital health pilots. Seattle: Path; 2014.

37. World Health Organization. The World health report: 2000: Health systems: improving performance. Geneva: World Health Organization; 2000.

38. Almunawar M, Anshari M. Health Information Systems (HIS): concept and technology. IGI Global; 2012.

39. Gruman JA, Saks A. Performance management and employee engagement. Hum Resour Manag Rev. 2011;21:123–36.

40. Lemma S, et al. Improving quality and use of routine health information system data in low- and middle-income countries: a scoping review. PLoS One. 2020;15(10):e0239683.

41. Hersh W. Who are the informaticians? What we know and should know. J Am Med Inform Assoc. 2006;13(2):166–70.

42. Pavalko RM. Sociology of occupations and professions. Itasca, IL: FE Peacock; 1971.

43. Hersh W. The health information technology workforce: estimations of demands and a framework for requirements. Appl Clin Inform. 2010;1(2):197–212.

44. Goldzweig CL, et al. Costs and benefits of health information technology: new trends from the literature: since 2005, patient-focused applications have proliferated, but data on their costs and benefits remain sparse. Health Aff. 2009;28(Suppl2):w282–93.

45. Damiani G, et al. The effectiveness of computerized clinical guidelines in the process of care: a systematic review. BMC Health Serv Res. 2010;10(1):2.

46. Eardley T. NHS informatics workforce survey. London: ASSIST; 2006.

47. Legg M, Lovelock B. A review of the Australian Health Informatics Workforce. Melbourne: Health Informatics Society of Australia; 2009.

48. O'Grady J. Health informatics and health information management: human resources report. Toronto: Prism Economics and Analysis; 2009.

49. Hersh W, et al. Building a health informatics workforce in developing countries. Health Aff (Millwood). 2010;29(2):274–7.

50. Mon DT. Further defining e-HIM. J AHIMA. 2004;75(2):54–6.

51. Tilahun B, Endehabtu BF. Current and future needs for human resources for Ethiopia's National Health Information System: survey and forecasting study. JMIR Med Educ. 2022;8(2):e28965.

52. Building A. Health informatics workforce in developing countries. Health Aff. 2010;29(2):274–7.

53. Giri K, et al. Keeping up to date: continuing professional development for health workers in developing countries. Intra Health International; 2012.

54. Bertman V, et al. Health worker text messaging for blended learning, peer support, and mentoring in pediatric and adolescent HIV/AIDS care: a case study in Zimbabwe. Hum Resour Health. 2019;17(1):41.

55. Feldacker C, et al. Experiences and perceptions of online continuing professional development among clinicians in sub-Saharan Africa. Hum Resour Health. 2017;15(1):89.

56. Norman CD, Skinner HA. eHealth literacy: essential skills for consumer health in a networked world. J Med Internet Res. 2006;8(2):e9.

57. Pooryaghob M, et al. Assesse the health literacy in multiple sclerosis patients. J Health Literacy. 2018;2(4):266–74.

58. Bailey SC, et al. The progress and promise of health literacy research. J Health Commun. 2013;18(Suppl 1):5–8.

59. Neter E, Brainin E. eHealth literacy: extending the digital divide to the realm of health information. J Med Internet Res. 2012;14(1):e19.

60. Loomis GA, et al. If electronic medical records are so great, why aren't family physicians using them? J Fam Pract. 2002;51(7):636–41.

61. Boonstra A, Broekhuis M. Barriers to the acceptance of electronic medical records by physicians from systematic review to taxonomy and interventions. BMC Health Serv Res. 2010;10:231.

62. Lee J, Lee EH. eHealth literacy instruments: systematic review of measurement properties. J Med Internet Res. 2021;23(11):e30644.

63. Norman CD, Skinner HA. eHEALS: the eHealth literacy scale. J Med Internet Res. 2006;8(4):e27.

64. Petrič G, Atanasova S, Kamin T. Ill literates or illiterates? Investigating the eHealth literacy of users of online health communities. J Med Internet Res. 2017;19(10):e331.

65. Seçkin G, et al. Being an informed consumer of health information and assessment of electronic health literacy in a national sample of internet users: validity and reliability of the e-HLS instrument. J Med Internet Res. 2016;18(7):e161.

66. Van Der Vaart R, Drossaert C. Development of the digital health literacy instrument: measuring a broad spectrum of health 1.0 and health 2.0 skills. J Med Internet Res. 2017;19(1):e27.

67. Karnoe A, et al. Assessing competencies needed to engage with digital health services: development of the eHealth literacy assessment toolkit. J Med Internet Res. 2018;20(5):e178.

68. Kayser L, et al. A multidimensional tool based on the eHealth literacy framework: development and initial validity testing of the eHealth liter-

acy questionnaire (eHLQ). J Med Internet Res. 2018;20(2):e36.

69. Paige SR, et al. Transactional eHealth literacy: developing and testing a multi-dimensional instrument. J Health Commun. 2019;24(10):737–48.

70. Sørensen K, et al. Health literacy and public health: a systematic review and integration of definitions and models. BMC Public Health. 2012;12:80.

71. Idemudia EC. Handbook of research on technology integration in the global world. IGI Global; 2018.

72. Ajzen I. The theory of planned behavior. Organ Behav Hum Decis Process. 1991;50(2):179–211.

73. Ajzen I, Fishbein M. The influence of attitudes on behavior. In: Albarracín D, Johnson BT, Zanna MP, editors. The handbook of attitudes. Lawrence Erlbaum Associates Publishers; 2005. p. 173–221.

74. Venkatesh V, Thong JY, Xu X. Consumer acceptance and use of information technology: extending the unified theory of acceptance and use of technology. MIS Q. 2012;36:157–78.

75. Fazio RH. Multiple processes by which attitudes guide behavior: the MODE model as an integrative framework. In: Advances in experimental social psychology. Elsevier; 1990. p. 75–109.

76. Ajzen I. Handbook of theories of social psychology, vol. 1. Sage: London; 2012.

77. Fishbein M, Ajzen I. Belief, attitude, intention, and behavior: an introduction to theory and research. Addison-Wesley; 1977.

78. Konttila J, et al. Healthcare professionals' competence in digitalisation: a systematic review. J Clin Nurs. 2019;28(5–6):745–61.

79. Khoja S, et al. e-Health readiness assessment tools for healthcare institutions in developing countries. Telemed J E Health. 2007;13(4):425–31.

80. Jennett P, et al. The essence of telehealth readiness in rural communities: an organizational perspective. Telemed J e-Health. 2005;11(2):137–45.

81. Mauco KL, Scott RE, Mars M. Critical analysis of e-health readiness assessment frameworks: suitability for application in developing countries. J Telemed Telecare. 2018;24(2):110–7.

82. Lennon MR, Bouamrane MM. Readiness for delivering digital health at scale: lessons from a Longitudinal Qualitative Evaluation of a National Digital Health Innovation Program in the United Kingdom. J Med Internet Res. 2017;19(2):e42.

83. Kruszyńska-Fischbach A, et al. Organizational e-Health readiness: how to prepare the primary healthcare providers'; services for digital transformation. Int J Environ Res Public Health. 2022;19(7):3973.

84. Rezai-Rad M, Vaezi R, Nattagh F. E-health readiness assessment framework in Iran. Iran J Public Health. 2012;41(10):43.

85. Overhage JM, Evans L, Marchibroda J. Communities' readiness for health information exchange: the National Landscape in 2004. J Am Med Inform Assoc. 2005;12(2):107–12.

86. Parker Oliver DR, Demiris G. An assessment of the readiness of hospice organizations to accept technological innovation. J Telemed Telecare. 2004;10(3):170–4.

87. Lennon MR, et al. Readiness for delivering digital health at scale: lessons from a longitudinal qualitative evaluation of a national digital health innovation program in the United Kingdom. J Med Internet Res. 2017;19(2):e6900.

88. Khoja S, et al. e-Health readiness assessment tools for healthcare institutions in developing countries. Telemed e-Health. 2007;13(4):425–32.

89. Jennett P, et al. Organizational readiness for telemedicine: implications for success and failure. J Telemed Telecare. 2003;9(2_suppl):27–30.

90. Kgasi M, Kalema B. Assessment E-health readiness for rural South African areas. J Ind Intell Inf. 2014;2(2):131–5.

91. Campbell JD, Harris KD, Hodge R. Introducing telemedicine technology to rural physicians and settings. J Fam Pract. 2001;50(5):419.

92. Ojo S, et al. Formal model for e-healthcare readiness assessment in developing country context. In: 2007 innovations in information technologies (IIT). IEEE; 2007.

93. Coleman A, Coleman MF. Activity theory framework: a basis for e-health readiness assessment in health institutions. J Commun. 2013;4(2):95–100.

94. Justice EO. E-healthcare/telemedicine readiness assessment of some selected states in Western Nigeria. Int J Eng Technol. 2012;2(2):195–201.

95. Mauco KL, Scott RE, Mars M. Validation of an e-health readiness assessment framework for developing countries. BMC Health Serv Res. 2020;20(1):575.

96. Garred P, et al. Mannan-binding protein—levels in plasma and upper-airways secretions and frequency of genotypes in children with recurrence of otitis media. Clin Exp Immunol. 1993;94(1):99–104.

97. Buntin MB, et al. The benefits of health information technology: a review of the recent literature shows predominantly positive results. Health Aff. 2011;30(3):464–71.

98. Jain S, Tiwari RV, Tiwari HD. Digitalized versus non digitalized doctors-emergence of digital medical care via tech savvy doctors: a systemic review. J Positive School Psychol. 2022;6(8):8430–47.

99. Zuzelo PR, et al. Describing the influence of technologies on registered nurses' work. Clin Nurse Spec. 2008;22(3):132–40.

100. de Veer AJ, Francke AL. Attitudes of nursing staff towards electronic patient records: a questionnaire survey. Int J Nurs Stud. 2010;47(7):846–54.

101. Baylies C. The meaning of health in Africa. Rev Afr Polit Econ. 1986;13(36):62–73.

102. Secginli S, Erdogan S, Monsen KA. Attitudes of health professionals towards electronic health records in primary health care settings: a questionnaire survey. Inform Health Soc Care. 2014;39(1):15–32.

103. Anttila M, Koivunen M, Välimäki M. Information technology-based standardized patient education in psychiatric inpatient care. J Adv Nurs. 2008;64(2):147–56.
104. Garavand A, et al. Factors influencing the adoption of health information technologies: a systematic review. Electron Physician. 2016;8(8):2713–8.
105. O'Connell MB, Reid B, O'Loughlin K. An exploration of the education and training experiences of ICU nurses in using computerised equipment. Aust J Adv Nurs. 2007;25:46.
106. Carman KL, et al. Patient and family engagement: a framework for understanding the elements and developing interventions and policies. Health Aff. 2013;32(2):223–31.
107. Graffigna G, Barello S, Riva G. How to make health information technology effective: the challenge of patient engagement. Arch Phys Med Rehabil. 2013;94(10):2034–5.
108. Gruman J, et al. From patient education to patient engagement: implications for the field of patient education. Patient Educ Couns. 2010;78(3):350–6.
109. Hibbard JH, et al. Development of the patient activation measure (PAM): conceptualizing and measuring activation in patients and consumers. Health Services Res. 2004;39(4p1):1005–26.
110. Barello S, et al. eHealth for patient engagement: a systematic review. Front Psychol. 2015;6:2013.
111. Hibbard JH, et al. Do increases in patient activation result in improved self-management behaviors? Health Serv Res. 2007;42(4):1443–63.
112. Frosch DL, Elwyn G. I believe, therefore I do. Springer; 2011.
113. Barello S, et al. 'Engage me in taking care of my heart': a grounded theory study on patient–cardiologist relationship in the hospital management of heart failure. BMJ Open. 2015;5(3):e005582.
114. Schwappach DL. Engaging patients as vigilant partners in safety: a systematic review. Med Care Res Rev. 2010;67(2):119–48.
115. Greenhalgh T, et al. Adoption, non-adoption, and abandonment of a personal electronic health record: case study of HealthSpace. BMJ. 2010;341:c5814.
116. Bornkessel A, Furberg R, Lefebvre RC. Social media: opportunities for quality improvement and lessons for providers—a networked model for patient-centered care through digital engagement. Curr Cardiol Rep. 2014;16(7):504.
117. Meglic M, et al. Feasibility of an eHealth service to support collaborative depression care: results of a pilot study. J Med Internet Res. 2010;12(5):e63.
118. Aberger EW, et al. Enhancing patient engagement and blood pressure management for renal transplant recipients via home electronic monitoring and web-enabled collaborative care. Telemed e-Health. 2014;20(9):850–4.
119. Agarwal R, et al. If we offer it, will they accept? Factors affecting patient use intentions of personal health records and secure messaging. J Med Internet Res. 2013;15(2):e2243.
120. UiO, DHIS2 overview. https://dhis2.org/about/#:~:text=DHIS2%20is%20an%20open%20source,countries%20where%20DHIS2%20is%20used. Accessed 23 Apr 2023.
121. Dehnavieh R, et al. The District Health Information System (DHIS2): a literature review and meta-synthesis of its strengths and operational challenges based on the experiences of 11 countries. Health Inform Manage J. 2019;48(2):62–75.
122. Mekonnen ZA, et al. Lessons and implementation challenges of community health information system in LMICs: a scoping review of literature. Online J Public Health Inform. 2022;14(1):e5.
123. Asangansi I, et al. Improving the routine HMIS in Nigeria through mobile technology for community data collection. J Health Inform Dev Countries. 2013;7(1):76–87.
124. Kagiri MM. Enhancing community based health information system CBHIS reporting through open source short message service based tool. University of Nairobi; 2014.
125. Hirvonen K, Berhane G, Assefa TW. Assessing community health information systems: evidence from child health records in food insecure areas of the Ethiopian Highlands. Matern Child Health J. 2020;24:1028–37.
126. Medhanyie AA, et al. Health workers' experiences, barriers, preferences and motivating factors in using mHealth forms in Ethiopia. Hum Resour Health. 2015;13(1):2.
127. Odhiambo-Otieno GW. Implementing a community-based health management information system in Bungoma district, Kenya. Health Policy Dev. 2005;3(2):170–7.
128. Jeremie N, et al. Utilization of community-based health information systems in decision making and health action in Nyalenda, Kisumu County, Kenya. Univ J Med Sci. 2014;2(4):37–42.
129. Chewicha K, Azim T. Community health information system for family centered health care: scale-up in Southern Nations Nationalities and People's Region. Ethiop Ministry Health Q Health Bull. 2013;5(1):49–51.
130. Abaza H, Marschollek M. mHealth application areas and technology combinations*. A comparison of literature from high and low/middle income countries. Methods Inf Med. 2017;56(7):e105–22.
131. Yahya H. Healthcare-related smartphone use among doctors in hospitals in Kaduna, Nigeria-a survey. Niger J Clin Pract. 2019;22(7):897–905.
132. Sutcliffe CG, et al. Use of mobile phones and text messaging to decrease the turnaround time for early infant HIV diagnosis and notification in rural Zambia: an observational study. BMC Pediatr. 2017;17(1):66.
133. Udugama B, et al. Diagnosing COVID-19: the disease and tools for detection. ACS Nano. 2020;14(4):3822–35.
134. Bassi A, et al. An overview of mobile applications (apps) to support the coronavirus dis-

ease 2019 response in India. Indian J Med Res. 2020;151(5):468–73.

135. Ahmadi S, et al. The role of digital technologies in tackling the Zika outbreak: a scoping review. J Public Health Emerg. 2018;2(6):20.

136. Zhang D, et al. Mobile technologies and cervical cancer screening in low- and middle-income countries: a systematic review. JCO Glob Oncol. 2020;6:617–27.

137. Bhatt S, Evans J, Gupta S. Barriers to scale of digital health systems for cancer care and control in last-mile settings. J Glob Oncol. 2018;4:1–3.

138. Bhatt S, et al. Mobile technology and cancer screening: Lessons from rural India. J Glob Health. 2018;8(2):020421.

139. Gökalp MO, et al. Current and emerging mhealth technologies adoption, implementation, and use. Springer; 2018.

140. Vokinger KN, et al. Digital health and the COVID-19 epidemic: an assessment framework for apps from an epidemiological and legal perspective. Swiss Med Wkly. 2020;150:w20282.

141. Watkins JA, et al. mHealth text and voice communication for monitoring people with chronic diseases in low-resource settings: a realist review. BMJ Glob Health. 2018;3(2):e000543.

142. Iribarren S, et al. TextTB: a mixed method pilot study evaluating acceptance, feasibility, and exploring initial efficacy of a text messaging intervention to support TB treatment adherence. Tuberc Res Treat. 2013;2013:349394.

143. Mohammed S, et al. User engagement with and attitudes towards an interactive SMS reminder system for patients with tuberculosis. J Telemed Telecare. 2012;18(7):404–8.

144. Mohammed S, Glennerster R, Khan AJ. Impact of a daily SMS medication reminder system on tuberculosis treatment outcomes: a randomized controlled trial. PLoS One. 2016;11(11):e0162944.

145. Leong KC, et al. The use of text messaging to improve attendance in primary care: a randomized controlled trial. Fam Pract. 2006;23(6):699–705.

146. Liu Q, et al. Reminder systems to improve patient adherence to tuberculosis clinic appointments for diagnosis and treatment. Cochrane Database Syst Rev. 2014;11:CD006594.

147. Daftary A, et al. A qualitative evaluation of the acceptability of an interactive voice response system to enhance adherence to isoniazid preventive therapy among people living with HIV in Ethiopia. AIDS Behav. 2017;21:3057–67.

148. Liu X, et al. Effectiveness of electronic reminders to improve medication adherence in tuberculosis patients: a cluster-randomised trial. PLoS Med. 2015;12(9):e1001876.

149. Hoffman JA, et al. Mobile direct observation treatment for tuberculosis patients: a technical feasibility pilot using mobile phones in Nairobi, Kenya. Am J Prev Med. 2010;39(1):78–80.

150. Dornan L, et al. Utilisation of electronic health records for public health in Asia: a review of success factors and potential challenges. Biomed Res Int. 2019;2019:7341841.

151. Odekunle FF, Odekunle RO, Shankar S. Why sub-Saharan Africa lags in electronic health record adoption and possible strategies to increase its adoption in this region. Int J Health Sci (Qassim). 2017;11(4):59–64.

152. de Grood C, et al. Adoption of e-health technology by physicians: a scoping review. J Multidiscip Healthc. 2016;9:335–44.

153. World Health Organization. Seventy-first world health assembly: digital health. Geneva: WHO; 2018.

154. Liaw ST, et al. A digital health profile & maturity assessment toolkit: cocreation and testing in the Pacific Islands. J Am Med Inform Assoc. 2021;28(3):494–503.

155. Carvalho JV, Rocha Á, Abreu A. Maturity models of healthcare information systems and technologies: a literature review. J Med Syst. 2016;40:1–10.

156. World Bank. Digital health assessment toolkit guide. 2021.

157. Global Digital Health Index consortium. Global Digital Health Index Indicator guide. 2016.

158. Liaw S-T, et al. The informatics capability maturity of integrated primary care centres in Australia. Int J Med Inform. 2017;105:89–97.

159. Measure Evaluation. Health information systems interoperability maturity toolkit: assessment tool. 2017. https://www.measureevaluation.org/tools/health-information-systems-interoperability-toolkit.html. Accesses 26 April 2023.

160. Measure Evaluation. HIS Stages of Continuous Improvement Toolkit. 2019. https://measureevaluation.org/resources/publications/cl-19-022.html. Accesses 26 April 2023.

161. We Forum. How can countries achieve digital maturity in healthcare? 2022. https://www.weforum.org/agenda/2022/08/countries-achieve-digital-maturity-healthcare/. Accessed 28 Apr 2023.

162. Empowering Health Care Providers in the Digital Era: Digital Health Care Market Study, Part 3. 2022. Competition Bureau Canada = Bureau de la concurrence Canada.

Implementation Status of Public Health Informatics

5

Moges Asressie Chanyalew

Abstract

This chapter provides an overview of Public Health Informatics (PHI) in the context of developing countries. It highlights the use of computer technology, specifically eHealth apps, to improve public health outcomes and addresses the challenges and opportunities associated with implementing these technologies. The chapter emphasizes the significant role of digital devices and eHealth apps in improving long-term health services and healthcare for the general population. These technologies are essential for disease monitoring, disease prevention, preparedness for health issues, and promoting overall population health. It covers a range of factors that influence the feasibility, adoption, cost, penetration, acceptability, and fidelity of eHealth implementation in developing countries. These factors can include technological infrastructure, human resource capacity, funding availability, cultural considerations, and policy support. Understanding these enablers and barriers is crucial for successful implementation and long-term sustainability of eHealth initiatives. It briefly explores the opportunities for future development and the prospects of eHealth in developing countries. This may include discussions on potential advancements in technology, policy changes, capacity-building initiatives, and collaborations that can drive the further adoption and utilization of eHealth apps in these settings.

Keywords

Implementation status · e-Health applications Digital health solutions · Low- and middle-income countries

5.1 Introduction

Information and communication technologies (ICTs) have revolutionized the healthcare industry and are providing numerous benefits to individuals, healthcare professionals, and organizations worldwide. ICTs encompass various technologies such as electronic health records (EHRs), telemedicine, mobile health (mHealth) applications, data analytics, and other digital tools that facilitate the collection, storage, and exchange of health information. One of the significant advantages of ICTs in healthcare is the improvement in healthcare quality. Electronic health records (EHRs) and digital health systems have revolutionized the way healthcare profes-

M. A. Chanyalew (✉)
Planning, Monitoring, and Evaluation Directorate, Amhara National Regional State Health Bureau, Bahir Dar, Ethiopia

SMART Health, Research and Publication Department, Bahir Dar, Ethiopia

sional's access and manage patient information, leading to numerous benefits for both patients and healthcare providers. ICTs, including EHRs and digital health systems, have transformed healthcare by improving access to patient information, enabling care coordination, reducing medical errors, facilitating remote care, and leveraging data for population health management. These technologies have the potential to enhance healthcare delivery, improve patient outcomes, and drive advancements in public health [1].

Furthermore, ICTs play a crucial role in addressing healthcare disparities, particularly in rural and isolated regions and developing nations. Telemedicine and mHealth applications allow individuals in remote areas to access healthcare services, receive consultations from specialists, and monitor their health conditions without the need for extensive travel. This helps overcome geographical barriers and improves healthcare access and outcomes for underserved populations. National learning health and care systems are made possible by health information technology as well. These systems leverage data-enabled infrastructure to collect and analyze health information on a large scale [2]. Policymakers and public health professionals can get important insights to guide decision-making, policy creation, and resource allocation by integrating data from many sources, including electronic health records, health registries, and public health databases [3]. Additionally, personalized services can be delivered based on the analysis of individual health data, leading to more targeted interventions and improved patient care. ICTs have transformed healthcare by providing data-driven solutions, enhancing healthcare quality, improving access to care, and enabling the development of national learning health and care systems. These technologies have the potential to drive significant advancements in public health, policy, and personalized healthcare services, benefiting individuals and healthcare systems globally.

In fact, public health informatics (PHI) is the methodical use of technology, computer science, and information to public health areas [4]. It involves the use of data, information systems,

and technology to support public health activities such as health promotion, prevention, monitoring, and research. The primary goals of PHI are twofold. First, it aims to enhance community health, recognizing that improving the health of the population as a whole ultimately leads to better individual health outcomes. By leveraging information and technology, PHI can help identify health trends, assess the health needs of communities, and develop targeted interventions to address specific health issues. Second, PHI focuses on preventing illnesses and injuries by modifying factors that contribute to population-level risks. This involves using data and technology to identify risk factors, monitor disease outbreaks, track the spread of infectious diseases, and implement interventions to mitigate those risks. By applying informatics principles to public health, PHI enables more effective surveillance, early detection, and response to public health threats. Overall, PHI plays a crucial role in improving public health by harnessing the power of information, computer science, and technology to enhance community well-being and prevent disease in populations [5].

5.1.1 ICT4Health

As part of ICT for development (ICT4D), the concept of ICT for health (ICT4Health) is now widely used to indicate the contribution of information technology in advancing the health system.

Public health informatics (PHI), which was founded in 1995, has developed into a separate field with unique research goals, specific expertise, and technological know-how. It focuses on the application of information and communication technologies (ICTs) to public health domains, aiming to improve health outcomes and enhance the efficiency of healthcare systems [6]. Digital technologies, including ICTs, play a crucial role in enabling universal healthcare and sustainable health systems. These technologies provide the tools and infrastructure necessary for efficient data management, health information exchange, telemedicine, and other digital health solutions. They facilitate access to healthcare services, enable remote consultations, enhance care coordination, and support evidence-based decision-making.

To fully capitalize on the potential of digital health initiatives, a robust strategy is essential. This strategy should integrate organizational, financial, human, and technological resources, ensuring that all necessary components are aligned and effectively utilized. Leadership is a critical factor in guiding and driving the implementation of digital health initiatives, fostering collaboration among stakeholders and promoting innovation. Additionally, the strategy should form the basis for a costed action plan that outlines the necessary steps, resources, and timelines for implementation. This action plan should facilitate coordination among various stakeholders, including government agencies, healthcare providers, technology vendors, and patient advocates. Collaboration and cooperation among these stakeholders are crucial to ensure seamless integration, interoperability, and sustainability of digital health solutions. By adopting a comprehensive strategy and action plan, healthcare systems can harness the potential of digital technologies to transform healthcare delivery, improve health outcomes, and achieve universal health coverage. The effective integration of organizational, financial, human, and technological resources, along with strong leadership, will be instrumental in realizing the full potential of digital health initiatives [7].

5.1.2 Why ICT in Healthcare?

Indeed, ICT equipment and goods have been instrumental in the development and advancement of the healthcare industry worldwide. Over the years, the healthcare sector has increasingly adopted digital technologies to improve patient care, enhance operational efficiency, and optimize clinical procedures. One notable aspect of ICT in healthcare is the use of digital apps, which has emerged as a valuable tool, particularly in underdeveloped nations. These apps have the potential to raise the standard of healthcare by overcoming geographical barriers, improving access to information, and providing remote consultations and health monitoring. Mobile health (mHealth) applications, for example, enable individuals to access healthcare services, receive health education, and track their health conditions using their smartphones or other mobile devices.

Mathur et al. [8] have highlighted several advantages of ICT in the provision of healthcare:

(a) Smoother Exchange of Information: Modern information technologies facilitate seamless communication and exchange of patient information among healthcare professionals. Electronic health records (EHRs) and health information exchange systems enable the secure sharing of patient data, ensuring that healthcare providers have access to accurate and up-to-date information, leading to more informed decision-making and improved patient care.

(b) Real-time Access to Patient Data: ICTs enable healthcare professionals to access patient data in real-time at the point of care. This immediate access to critical information, such as medical history, diagnostic test results, and medication records, enhances clinical decision-making and enables timely interventions. It can lead to more efficient and personalized care delivery.

(c) Transformation of Paper-based Records: Advanced information technologies, such as computer-based patient records and expert information systems, have transformed the documentation of patients' receipt of healthcare services. Moving from paper-based records to digital systems improves data accuracy, reduces administrative burden, and enhances the overall efficiency of healthcare processes. It also enables data analytics and population health management.

(d) Cost Reduction and Increased Productivity: Implementing ICT solutions in healthcare has the potential to reduce traditional costs and increase the productivity of medical professionals. Streamlining workflows, automating administrative duties, and digitizing processes can all help to maximize resource use, cut down on paperwork, and improve operational effectiveness. This enables healthcare providers to more efficiently deploy resources and concentrate on patient care.

By leveraging ICTs, healthcare organizations can improve efficiency, enhance patient care, and reduce costs. The adoption of digital technologies in healthcare has the potential to transform healthcare delivery, particularly in underdeveloped nations, by leveraging the advantages of real-time data access, streamlined processes, and increased productivity of healthcare professionals.

In order to effectively embrace digital applications and enhance their use in the healthcare system, it is imperative to analyze and understand the cost-benefit of e-Health apps both before and after deployment. This will provide full knowledge to program implementers and policymakers, enabling them to make the best decisions. Among the financial advantages of e-Health are [9]:

Bandwidth and mobility: Both communications traffic and bandwidth capacity have been growing rapidly in recent years. The expansion of digital technologies, internet connectivity, and the increasing demand for data-intensive applications have contributed to this trend. Funding and development efforts have indeed been focused on broadband and networking technologies to meet the growing need for faster and more reliable communication infrastructure. Overall, the rapid expansion of communications traffic and bandwidth capacity, coupled with the continuous improvement of computer capacity, plays a crucial role in supporting the growth of digital technologies, enabling faster and more efficient data transmission, and facilitating the development of innovative applications and services.

Internet: Estimating the exact number of internet users can be challenging due to various factors, including variations in internet penetration across regions and countries, multiple devices per user, and the dynamic nature of internet usage. However, the number of hosts, which represents unique addresses posted online, can provide an indication of the growth and expansion of internet connectivity. The number of hosts has indeed experienced significant growth in recent years. This growth can be attributed to several factors, including the increasing global internet penetration, the proliferation of internet-connected devices, and the expanding reach of internet infrastructure. While estimating the exact number of internet users can be challenging, the significant growth in the number of hosts reflects the expanding reach and impact of the internet globally. The increasing availability and accessibility of internet connectivity continue to shape various aspects of society, including communication, commerce, education, and access to information.

Miniaturizations: the development and proliferation of micro-electromechanical systems (MEMS) have the potential to contribute to further miniaturization of medical instruments and equipment. This miniaturization can lead to several anticipated outcomes and advancements in healthcare. While the miniaturization of medical instruments and equipment through MEMS technology holds significant promise, challenges remain. These include ensuring the accuracy and reliability of miniaturized devices, addressing regulatory considerations, and integrating data from multiple devices into comprehensive healthcare systems. However, with ongoing advancements and research in MEMS technology, the anticipated outcomes of improved health outcomes, increased mobility, and expanded care options are within reach.

Imaging technologies: Document imaging, which involves capturing images of paper forms, scanning them, and storing them electronically, offers various benefits in the healthcare sector. The ease of sharing and accessing electronic images allows clinicians and administrators located in different regions to collaborate more effectively. Additionally, advancements in materials science have the potential to fuel new trends and enhance the cost-effectiveness of various medical imaging, remote diagnostic, and therapeutic technologies. Overall, the combination of document imaging, ICT integration, advancements in medical devices, and materials science contributes to the enhancement and cost reduction of various healthcare technologies. These advancements enable improved collaboration, efficiency, and accessibility of medical information, supporting better patient care and outcomes.

Data handling: The expansion of data storage capacity has been a long-term trend, and there have been recent developments that promise to sustain and even accelerate this growth. Some of the examples are: increasing disk driver density, growing deployed storage capacity, optical storage advancement, and solid-state drive (SSD). The rapid growth in data storage capacity, including the tripling of disk drive density and advancements in optical storage, reflects the ongoing efforts to meet the increasing demand for data storage. The development of new technologies, such as SSDs and emerging storage solutions, further contributes to expanding storage capacities and addressing the evolving needs of data-intensive applications and services.

Converging technologies: Convergence is a significant mega-trend that has been observed in recent years, particularly in the intersection of information technology and the biological sciences. This convergence has been driven by advancements in biotechnology, medicine, and the increasing integration of embedded computers, wireless tracking, and ubiquitous computing. The convergence of information technology and the biological sciences is a transformative mega-trend that holds immense potential for advancements in biotechnology, medicine, and the overall improvement of human health. The integration of embedded computers, wireless tracking, and ubiquitous computing, along with the increasing programmability and intelligence of matter, is driving innovation and enabling groundbreaking discoveries in these fields.

Digital health technologies are used by nations to enhance the quality of health information. The availability of high-quality information is vital for informed medical judgments and decision-making, as it provides real-time insights from service delivery locations. Consequently, healthcare systems have developed digital solutions to improve the quality of information. However, data indicates that various pressures, such as administrative, financial, regulatory, or donor-related factors, have resulted in a disorganized and fragmented evolution of health information systems [10]. Despite, the healthcare community acknowledges the need for coordinated actions to address these challenges. By fostering collaboration and implementing standardized approaches, health systems can work towards achieving organized and cohesive health information systems that enhance the quality of information and support improved medical judgments and decision-making.

The use of information and communication technology (ICT) in the healthcare industry has shown promise in developing countries. However, it is true that there has been relatively limited research and study conducted specifically on the development and use of technology platforms for health applications in Sub-Saharan Africa (SSA) [11]. Efforts are being made by governments, international organizations, and research institutions to increase research and investment in ICT for healthcare in SSA. By gaining a better understanding of the local context and conducting rigorous studies, it is possible to develop sustainable and effective technology platforms that address the unique healthcare challenges faced by the region. Moreover, there is a dearth of comprehensive documentation regarding the state of ICT implementation, particularly with regard to e-Health applications, challenges, and potential, in developing nations. This chapter discusses the opportunities and problems associated with the current state of e-Health app or digital solution implementation in low- and middle-income countries.

5.2 Implementation Science

5.2.1 What Is Implementation Science?

Implementation Science (IS) is an academic discipline that centers on the process of converting research outcomes into practical applications. In order to make it easier for research results and evidence to be incorporated into healthcare policy and practice, it entails looking into and assessing the most effective ways to change or enhance processes and systems. Implementation Science is concerned with bridging the gap between research and practice by studying how to effectively implement evidence-based interventions, programs, and policies in real-world settings. It seeks to understand the factors that influence successful implementation, dissemination, and sustainability of evidence-based practices, and to develop strategies to optimize these processes [12, 13].

Implementation Science encompasses a range of disciplines and methodologies. It involves studying various factors related to the implementation process, such as the characteristics of the intervention, the individuals and organizations involved, the context in which the implementation occurs, and the strategies used to promote adoption and sustained use. It also involves evaluating the impact and outcomes of implementation efforts. It is crucial in healthcare because research evidence often does not automatically translate into changes in practice. The acceptance and use of evidence-based approaches can be hampered by a variety of obstacles, including organizational limitations, opposition to change, a lack of resources, and a lack of understanding. Researchers and practitioners can find practical solutions to get beyond these obstacles and encourage the adoption of evidence-based interventions, which will eventually improve patient outcomes, by researching implementation techniques.

Implementation Science employs a range of research methods and approaches. These may include qualitative and quantitative research, mixed-methods designs, implementation frameworks and models, and participatory approaches that involve stakeholders at various levels. The field also emphasizes the importance of iterative learning, continuous improvement, and ongoing evaluation to refine implementation strategies and to enhance the sustainability of interventions. Its findings have implications for healthcare policy and practice. By identifying effective implementation strategies, policymakers and healthcare leaders can make informed decisions about resource allocation, quality improvement efforts, and the scaling up of evidence-based practices. Implementation Science also helps practitioners understand how to effectively integrate research findings into their daily practice, improving the quality and effectiveness of healthcare delivery. Implementation Science is a multidisciplinary field that focuses on the process of translating research into practice. It aims to identify and evaluate strategies that promote the integration of evidence-based interventions into healthcare policy and practice. By studying implementation processes, barriers, and facilitators, Implementation Science contributes to improving the delivery and outcomes of healthcare services.

5.2.2 Taxonomy of Implementation Outcomes

The success of applying evidence-based innovations in real-world settings can be assessed through implementation outcomes. These outcomes help us understand the complex implementation process and identify intermediary outcomes that may influence the effectiveness of an intervention in a specific setting. To ensure the precision of implementation research, it is essential to rigorously conceptualize and measure these outcomes. Implementation outcomes are important for assessing the success of applying evidence-based innovations. For accurate implementation research, these outcomes must be conceptualized and measured with great care. Through the comprehension and assessment of implementation outcomes, scholars can discern variables that influence the efficiency of implementation tactics and render well-informed determinations to refine the implementation procedure and, in turn, augment the influence of evidence-based interventions in practical contexts.

Proctor et al. [14] define implementation outcomes as distinct from service system and clinical outcomes. Implementation outcomes refer to the specific results or effects of the implementation process, including acceptability, uptake, reach, adoption, fidelity, implementation cost, and sustainability. These outcomes focus on evaluating the implementation strategies, processes, and contextual factors that influence the successful implementation of an intervention [14]. According to Proctor et al., implementation outcomes play a crucial role in implementation assessment. They serve as intermediate indicators that help assess the effectiveness of implementation strategies and elucidate the mechanisms by which these strategies produce desired changes. By focusing on implementation outcomes, researchers and practitioners can establish a valid conclusion about the success of implementation efforts and avoid unnecessary waste of resources.

The paradigm developed by Proctor and colleagues illustrates the rational correlation among implementation outcomes, service outcomes, and client outcomes. It implies that the attainment of service and client outcomes comes after implementation outcomes. In other words, it is important to first assess whether an intervention has been successfully implemented before expecting it to have an impact on service quality or client outcomes. By considering implementation outcomes before dealing with service and client outcomes, researchers and practitioners can establish a valid conclusion about the effectiveness and impact of an intervention. This approach helps minimize unnecessary resource waste by ensuring that implementation challenges are addressed and resolved before investing further resources in assessing service and client outcomes.

By prioritizing the assessment of implementation outcomes, stakeholders can identify barriers and facilitators to successful implementation, make necessary adjustments, and optimize the delivery of evidence-based interventions. This approach increases the likelihood of achieving desired service and client outcomes while minimizing the risk of investing resources in interventions that have not been effectively implemented. Overall, the framework presented by Proctor et al. highlights the importance of considering implementation outcomes as a critical step in the evaluation and implementation of interventions. By focusing on these outcomes first, stakeholders

can ensure the validity of their conclusions and optimize resource allocation during the implementation phase.

5.2.2.1 Acceptability

The belief that a particular treatment, service, practice, or innovation is agreeable, palatable, or satisfying among implementation stakeholders (such as healthcare professionals, organizations, and patients) is known as acceptability, and it is a crucial implementation outcome. It expresses how much the intervention is thought to be suitable, workable, and appropriate for the particular implementation situation [15]. It has been acknowledged that a major obstacle to implementation attempts is the lack of acceptability. It might be difficult for an intervention to be successfully adopted and implemented if the stakeholders do not think it is acceptable. Acceptability is a personal opinion that varies depending on the stakeholders. The implementation process considers the viewpoints, convictions, principles, and inclinations of the persons or groups concerned.

Divergent perspectives may exist among stakeholders on the intervention's applicability, degree of ease of use, compatibility with current procedures, and possible advantages. It is essential to comprehend and handle these varied viewpoints in order to advance acceptability. The acceptability of an intervention can be influenced by a number of things. These comprise the features of the intervention itself, such as its complexity, evidence foundation, and adaptability; the organizational context, such as its resources, culture, and leadership support; and the specific end-users, such as their attitudes, knowledge, and abilities. It is essential to consider these factors when assessing and addressing acceptability challenges. Acceptability is a critical determinant of implementation success. If an intervention is not perceived as acceptable, stakeholders may resist its adoption, engage in selective implementation, or discontinue its use altogether. Lack of acceptability can lead to poor engagement, low adherence, and limited sustainability of the intervention, ultimately affecting its effectiveness and the desired outcomes.

To address acceptability challenges, implementation efforts should involve active engagement and collaboration with stakeholders from the early stages. It is important to understand their perspectives, concerns, and needs, and to actively involve them in decision-making processes. Adapting interventions to fit the local context, providing training and support, and addressing potential barriers and misconceptions can also enhance acceptability. Valid and reliable measurement tools are needed to assess acceptability. Various qualitative and quantitative approaches can be used to capture stakeholders' perceptions and experiences. This may include surveys, interviews, focus groups, and observation. These assessments can provide insights into the specific aspects of the intervention that stakeholders find acceptable or unacceptable, informing targeted strategies for improvement. Acceptability plays a crucial role in implementation efforts. Addressing the lack of acceptability is essential to overcome implementation challenges and promote the successful integration and adoption of evidence-based interventions. Implementation practitioners and researchers can improve the acceptability of interventions and raise the possibility of attaining targeted implementation results by comprehending stakeholders' viewpoints, involving them in the process, and actively resolving their concerns.

5.2.2.2 Adoption

Adoption, sometimes called "uptake," is the desire, first choice, or action to use or test a new idea or evidence-based practice. It is a crucial implementation result that shows how much people, organizations, or systems are using or implementing an intervention [16, 17]. Adoption can be measured from various angles, such as the supplier's or the organization's perspective. Various approaches are used by researchers and practitioners to evaluate adoption, depending on the intervention and particular situation under study [18].

Adoption is often considered alongside other implementation outcomes, such as acceptability, fidelity, reach, sustainability, and implementation cost. These outcomes are interconnected and collectively contribute to the overall success of implementation efforts. Adoption is a critical implementation outcome that reflects the intention, initial decision, or action to try or employ an innovation or evidence-based practice. It can be measured from various perspectives, including the supplier's or organization's point of view. Measuring adoption provides valuable information about the implementation process, helping researchers and practitioners identify areas for improvement and optimize the adoption and utilization of evidence-based interventions.

Adoption is frequently taken into account in conjunction with other implementation outcomes, including cost, reach, sustainability, and acceptability. All of these results are related to one another and help make implementation efforts successful overall. An innovation or evidence-based practice's adoption is a crucial implementation outcome that represents the goal, first choice, or action to test or use it. It can be evaluated from a number of angles, such as the viewpoint of the business or the provider. Adoption measurement yields important insights into the implementation process, assisting practitioners and academics in pinpointing areas that require improvement in order to maximize the uptake and use of evidence-based interventions.

5.2.2.3 Appropriateness

An innovation or evidence-based approach's perceived fit, relevance, or compatibility within a particular practice context, for a provider or for a customer, is referred to as appropriateness, a concept that is crucial to implementation science. It also includes how well the idea is thought to fit into solving a certain issue or problem. Acceptability and appropriateness share conceptual similarities, and the terms are frequently used synonymously in academic literature. Both models place emphasis on stakeholders' subjective assessments of an intervention's appropriateness and congruence in a particular setting. It is crucial to remember that many scholars may define and utilize these terms slightly differently from one another, resulting in some discrepancies.

Assessing and addressing appropriateness is crucial for successful implementation. When an intervention is perceived as appropriate, it is more likely to be accepted, adopted, and integrated into practice. On the other hand, if an innovation is perceived as inappropriate or incompatible, it can hinder its implementation and reduce the likelihood of achieving desired outcomes. Appropriateness is highly context-dependent and may vary across different settings, populations, or stages of implementation. Factors such as organizational culture, resources, policies, and the unique needs and preferences of stakeholders influence the perceived appropriateness of an intervention. It is imperative to take these contextual elements into account when evaluating and advocating for the suitability of an intervention. An innovation or evidence-based practice's perceived fit, relevance, or compatibility within a particular context is reflected in the construct of appropriateness, which is critical to implementation science. It shares conceptual similarities with acceptability, and the phrases may be used interchangeably in the literature. Since appropriateness affects stakeholders' acceptance, adoption, and integration of the intervention into practice, evaluating and resolving it is crucial for a successful implementation.

5.2.2.4 Cost (Incremental or Implementation Cost)

Cost, specifically incremental or implementation cost, refers to the financial impact associated with implementing an intervention or carrying out an implementation effort. It reflects the expenses incurred in delivering a treatment or intervention within a specific context. There are several factors that contribute to the variation in implementation costs: complexity of the treatment, complexity of the implementation, setting and overheads, and location. Measuring and understanding the implementation costs is essential for assessing the feasibility, sustainability, and scalability of interventions. It helps decision-makers allocate resources effectively and make informed choices regarding the implementation of evidence-based practices. Economic evaluations and cost-effectiveness analyses are often

conducted to estimate and compare the costs and benefits of different implementation strategies or interventions. Understanding and considering implementation costs are important for effective resource allocation and decision-making in implementation efforts.

5.2.2.5 Feasibility

The degree to which a novel therapy, innovation, or intervention may be successfully used or carried out within a particular agency, organization, or place is referred to as feasibility in the area of implementation science. It evaluates a program or intervention's viability and practicality in light of a number of variables. Retrospective evaluations of feasibility are common in order to ascertain why a project was successful or unsuccessful, based on metrics such as participation, retention, recruiting, or other pertinent outcomes [18]. Feasibility examines whether an intervention can be effectively implemented in real-world settings. It focuses on practical considerations, such as the availability of resources (e.g., funding, personnel, and infrastructure), organizational capacity, and the fit between the intervention and the existing context. Feasibility is an important determinant of the potential success and sustainability of an intervention. Feasibility is assessed within the specific agency, organization, or setting where the intervention is being implemented. Different settings may have unique characteristics, resources, and constraints that can influence the feasibility of implementation. Therefore, feasibility assessments should consider the specific context and its potential impact on implementation success.

Feasibility is often evaluated retrospectively, looking back at the implementation process to understand the factors that influenced success or failure. This analysis may involve examining participation rates, retention rates, recruitment challenges, or other outcomes that reflect the practicality and effectiveness of the implementation effort. Feasibility assessments typically involve evaluating multiple dimensions, such as acceptability, appropriateness, resources, organizational capacity, and stakeholder readiness. These dimensions collectively provide insights into the potential barriers and facilitators to successful implementation. It inform decision-making during the planning and implementation stages. If an intervention is found to be infeasible or faces significant challenges, adaptations may be necessary to enhance its fit and viability within the specific context. Flexibility and adaptation strategies can help address potential barriers and increase the likelihood of successful implementation. Researchers often conduct feasibility studies to systematically evaluate the practicality and potential success of an intervention before proceeding to larger-scale implementation or research studies. Feasibility studies help identify potential challenges, refine implementation strategies, and inform the design of subsequent implementation efforts.

5.2.2.6 Fidelity

The degree to which an intervention is carried out according to its original design, as directed by the intervention protocol, or as intended by the program architects is referred to as fidelity in the field of implementation science. It evaluates the degree to which the planned or intended implementation and the actual implementation match [16, 19]. Fidelity examines whether an intervention is delivered and implemented as it was originally designed or prescribed. It focuses on adhering to the program protocol, procedures, and core components outlined in the intervention manual or guidelines. Fidelity assessment helps ensure that the intervention is delivered as intended, maximizing the likelihood of achieving the desired outcomes.

Fidelity is often assessed by comparing the disseminated or implemented intervention to the original evidence-based intervention. This comparison involves evaluating three main aspects:

(a) Dose or Amount of Program Delivered: Fidelity examines whether the intervention is delivered with the intended intensity, duration, and frequency. It assesses whether participants receive the recommended number of sessions, interventions, or dosage as specified in the protocol.

(b) Quality of Program Delivery: Fidelity assesses the quality of program delivery by evaluating the competence, skills, and adherence of intervention providers or practitioners. It examines whether the intervention is delivered with appropriate techniques, strategies, and fidelity to the intervention model.

(c) Adherence to the Program Protocol: Fidelity also evaluates the extent to which the implementation adheres to the program protocol, including the sequence of activities, content delivery, and key components. It assesses whether there are deviations or modifications made during the implementation process.

Fidelity is crucial for ensuring intervention effectiveness and achieving desired outcomes. When an intervention is implemented with high fidelity, it increases the likelihood of replicating the conditions under which the intervention was originally shown to be effective. Fidelity assessment helps identify potential challenges or areas of improvement to enhance implementation quality and increase the chances of achieving positive outcomes. While fidelity aims to ensure adherence to the original intervention, it is important to note that some adaptations may be necessary or appropriate in certain contexts. Adaptations should be made in a thoughtful and deliberate manner, considering the core components and principles of the intervention. Fidelity assessments can help monitor and guide adaptation processes to maintain the integrity of the intervention while addressing the needs of the specific context.

5.2.2.7 Penetration

The process of incorporating a practice, intervention, or evidence-based program into a service setting and its subsystems is referred to as penetration in the area of implementation science. It evaluates how far the practice integrates and becomes part of the setting's established procedures, institutions, and culture. The degree of integration of a practice within an organization or service setting is the main focus of penetration. It examines how the practice becomes a part of the routine operations, policies, and procedures of the setting, rather than being seen as a separate or isolated activity. Penetration also considers the integration of the practice within the various subsystems or components of the service setting. This includes the organizational structure, staffing, communication channels, information systems, and other elements that make up the setting. Penetration assesses how the practice becomes embedded and influences these subsystems [16, 19].

The notion of service penetration, as described by Stiles et al. [16], and niche saturation, as described by Rabin et al., are similar concepts to penetration. They highlight the process by which a practice or intervention becomes widely adopted and utilized within a service setting, reaching a point where there is a saturation or high level of implementation. Penetration is not a one-time event but an ongoing process. It involves sustained efforts to integrate the practice within the setting, promote its acceptance and utilization, and address any barriers or challenges that may arise. To guarantee that the practice stays ingrained and productive throughout time, penetration calls for constant observation, assessment, and modification. Factors Influencing Penetration: Penetration can be influenced by various factors, including organizational readiness, leadership support, staff engagement, resource allocation, and the fit between the practice and the setting's values, culture, and priorities. Understanding these factors and addressing them effectively can facilitate successful penetration [6].

5.2.2.8 Sustainability

It might be described as the degree to which the continuous, stable operations of a service setting sustain or institutionalize a recently established treatment. According to Rabin et al., institutionalization occurs in three stages and is determined by how rules and practices integrate a program into an organization's culture: (1) passage, which refers to a single event like moving from temporary to permanent funding; (2) cycle or routine, which is the process of repeatedly reinforcing the value of the evidence-based intervention by incorporating it into routine organizational or community behaviors and procedures like the

annual budget and evaluation standards; and (3) niche saturation, which is the degree to which an evidence-based intervention is built into all organizational subsystems [16].

According to Rabin et al., institutionalization occurs in three stages:

(a) Passage: Passage refers to a single event or milestone that signals a transition from temporary or pilot implementation to permanent adoption. Examples of passage events include securing long-term funding, formal policy or program approval, or establishing dedicated resources for the program.

(b) Cycle or Routine: The cycle or routine stage involves repeatedly reinforcing the value and importance of the evidence-based intervention within the organization's behaviors, procedures, and practices. This integration occurs through incorporating the program into routine organizational processes, such as budgeting, evaluation standards, performance metrics, staff training, and other established practices.

(c) Niche Saturation: Niche saturation is the highest level of institutionalization, where the evidence-based intervention is built into all organizational subsystems. It permeates the organizational culture, policies, and practices across various levels and functions, becoming deeply embedded within the organization.

Sustainability involves integrating the program into the organization's culture, values, and identity. It requires aligning the program with the organization's mission, goals, and strategic priorities. The program should fit seamlessly into the existing organizational structure, processes, and routines, rather than being seen as an external or separate entity. Several factors can influence the sustainability of an implemented program, including leadership support, staff buy-in and engagement, resource availability, ongoing training and support, stakeholder collaboration, adaptability to changing needs, and the program's demonstrated effectiveness and impact. Addressing these factors can enhance the likelihood of sustained implementation and institutionalization. Sustainability requires ongoing evaluation and monitoring to assess the continued effectiveness and impact of the program, identify areas for improvement, and make necessary adaptations. Regular assessments help ensure that the program remains aligned with the organization's evolving needs and maintains its relevance and value over time.

5.2.3 Why Implementation Fidelity?

The degree to which a program or intervention is carried out in conformity with its intended aims, protocols, and guidelines is known as implementation fidelity (IF). It includes the degree to which the program is carried out in accordance with the program developers' or researchers' original plans or intentions. Expectations about how programs will be implemented are often present during the design and development process. One common expectation is that programs will be executed with a high degree of fidelity. Stated differently, the program's goals, components, and processes are expected to be adhered to faithfully, and the program will be provided as intended [16, 19].

High implementation fidelity is important for several reasons:

(a) Consistency: Fidelity ensures that the program is consistently delivered across different settings and contexts. This consistency allows for accurate replication of the program's intended effects and increases the likelihood of achieving the desired outcomes.

(b) Program Integrity: Fidelity helps maintain the integrity of the program by ensuring that its core components and principles are preserved during implementation. It ensures that the program's essential elements are not compromised or diluted, which is crucial for achieving the intended results.

(c) Validity of Research Findings: High fidelity implementation is essential for research studies evaluating program effectiveness. It allows researchers to accurately assess the impact of the program and draw valid conclusions based on the implemented intervention. Deviations from fidelity can introduce confounding variables and affect the validity of research findings.

(d) Program Improvement: Monitoring fidelity during program implementation provides valuable feedback for program improvement. It allows program developers and implementers to identify areas where fidelity may be compromised and make necessary adjustments to enhance program delivery and effectiveness.

5.2.3.1 Purpose of Implementation Fidelity

Implementation fidelity measures how closely a program was carried out in accordance with its intended goals in order to guarantee that evaluation results fairly represent a program's efficacy. Data on implementation fidelity sheds light on how closely the intended program and the actual program are aligned.

Here are the key purposes of assessing implementation fidelity:

- Accurate Evaluation: Assessing implementation fidelity helps avoid making incorrect assumptions about a program's effectiveness based solely on evaluation results. By gathering fidelity data, evaluators can determine whether the program was implemented as intended, and whether any deviations or variations from the original plan may have influenced the evaluation outcomes. This allows for a more accurate interpretation of the evaluation results.

- Program Improvement: Fidelity data can inform program improvement efforts. By identifying areas where the program deviated from the original plan, implementers can pinpoint potential challenges, barriers, or gaps in implementation. This information can be used to make targeted improvements and adjustments to enhance program delivery and effectiveness.

- Replication and Scaling: Comprehending implementation fidelity is essential for duplicating and expanding efficacious initiatives. If a program shows promising results, fidelity data can assist in guaranteeing that the program is appropriately replicated in various contexts and settings. Guidance on preserving program integrity during replication is provided via fidelity assessment, enabling consistent and dependable results.

- Accountability and Transparency: Assessing implementation fidelity promotes accountability and transparency in program delivery. It provides evidence of whether the program was implemented as intended, and stakeholders can make informed decisions based on this information. Fidelity data can be used to address concerns or discrepancies and ensure that programs are implemented with integrity and fidelity.
- Research Validity: In order to guarantee the validity and reliability of study findings, implementation fidelity assessment is crucial for research studies analyzing program efficacy. Researcher comprehension of the program's implementation context and circumstances is facilitated by fidelity data, which enables accurate interpretation and broad applicability of study findings.

5.2.3.2 When to Gather Data on Implementation Fidelity

Gathering data on implementation fidelity can be done in conjunction with or prior to collecting data on program outcomes. This approach helps ensure that resources are used efficiently and that any concerns related to program implementation are addressed before investing in outcome evaluation.

Here are two common approaches to gathering data on implementation fidelity:

(a) Pretest-Implementation Fidelity-Posttest: This method uses pretest and posttest measurements to evaluate the program's results. Before the posttest data are analyzed, however, implementation fidelity data is gathered using fidelity checklists, observations, or other pertinent metrics. This makes it possible to investigate how program outcomes and

implementation fidelity relate to one another. It assists in determining whether changes in fidelity may have affected the outcomes or whether faithful execution is the sole reason for the program's efficacy.

(b) Implementation Fidelity Prior to Outcome Evaluation: Alternatively, implementation fidelity data can be gathered before conducting outcome evaluations. This approach involves assessing the level of fidelity in program delivery using fidelity checklists, observations, or other methods. By analyzing implementation fidelity data first, any concerns or challenges related to program implementation can be identified and addressed before investing resources in outcome evaluation. This ensures that the evaluation focuses on a program that has been implemented as intended and maximizes the likelihood of obtaining accurate and meaningful outcome data.

By prioritizing implementation fidelity data collection, organizations can make informed decisions about the readiness of the program for outcome evaluation. It helps allocate resources effectively and ensures that evaluation efforts are conducted on programs that have been implemented with fidelity.

The degree to which an intervention is delivered in accordance with the requirements and guidelines established by the program designers is referred to as implementation fidelity. Usually, it is measured in multiple categories, such as time, content, frequency, and coverage (dosage) [20]. Implementation fidelity can be influenced by various factors, such as participant response, delivery quality, intervention complexity, and facilitation techniques.

(a) Coverage (dose): Refers to the extent to which the intervention is delivered to the intended target population or participants. It measures the proportion of individuals who receive the intervention as planned.
(b) Frequency: Refers to the regularity or number of intervention sessions or activities delivered to participants. It measures how

often the intervention is implemented as prescribed.

(c) Content: Refers to the fidelity of the intervention components, procedures, and materials. It assesses whether the intervention is delivered with the intended content and follows the recommended practices.

(d) Duration: Refers to the length of time over which the intervention is implemented. It measures whether the intervention is delivered for the intended duration as specified by the program designers.

Regarding implementation fidelity and intervention outcomes, it is critical to realize that fidelity is not the only factor that influences the relationship between an intervention and its results. The relationship between the intervention's results and degree of fidelity, however, may vary. Conducting an outcome analysis can assist in determining the components of the intervention that are vital to its success. By pinpointing these essential components, it becomes possible to define the minimal standards for high implementation fidelity, ensuring that these critical elements are carried out effectively. By defining the minimal standards for fidelity, the evaluation of the intervention can also provide guidance for the intervention's content. It helps in determining which aspects of the intervention are essential and need to be prioritized in order to achieve the desired outcomes.

The role of moderators needs to be taken into consideration in order to give a more thorough picture of the interactions and dynamics involved. Moderators are factors that can modify or influence the relationship between implementation fidelity and intervention outcomes. These factors can include participant characteristics, contextual factors, or other variables that may interact with fidelity to affect the outcomes. Understanding the function of each aspect, such as implementation fidelity, essential intervention components, and the influence of moderators, is crucial for designing and implementing effective interventions. By examining these relationships and considering examples from research, it becomes possible to gain insights into how fidelity, essential compo-

nents, and moderators interact to shape intervention outcomes.

Adherence

One essential metric for evaluating implementation fidelity is adherence. It describes how closely an intervention is carried out in relation to the coverage, frequency, content, and duration that its designers planned. Measurement of the degree to which the intervention is carried out according to plan makes adherence a crucial component of implementation fidelity. Examining whether the intervention is presented in line with the planned content—that is, if the intervention's main ideas, tactics, or procedures are faithfully carried out—allows evaluators to determine adherence. This ensures that the intervention's active components, such as medication, therapy, abilities, or information, are delivered as intended to the recipients. Additionally, adherence also includes considerations of the frequency, duration, and coverage of the intervention. Frequency refers to how often the intervention is delivered, duration refers to the length of each session or episode, and coverage refers to the extent to which the intervention is implemented across the target population or settings. These subcategories of adherence provide insights into the consistency and completeness of the intervention delivery [16, 19].

Evaluators can ascertain whether the intervention's active components are successfully administered to the recipients and the degree to which it is being implemented as intended by evaluating adherence. It makes it more likely that the intended results will be achieved and helps guarantee that the intervention is carried out faithfully. It is important to remember that adherence is not the sole aspect of implementation fidelity assessment, even though it is an essential one. Depending on the particular intervention or program under review, other aspects of fidelity, such as delivery quality, participant responsiveness, and program differentiation, may also be pertinent.

To measure adherence, assessments can be conducted to determine the quantity, frequency, and duration of the intervention's prescribed content. This helps evaluate whether the intervention is being delivered as intended in terms of its specific components and their planned implementation. However, it's important to note that adherence does not necessarily mean using every single component of the intervention. In some cases, only the essential elements of the intervention, as defined by the underlying model or theory, need to be implemented to achieve the desired impact. Identifying these essential elements is crucial for ensuring effective and meaningful implementation.

Performance outcomes from several trials of the same intervention and implementation fidelity data can be used to do a sensitivity analysis or component analysis to identify the key elements. This analysis assists in determining the precise component or components that must be present in order for the intervention to have the intended effect. Through analyzing the correlation between fidelity and results in various implementations, the essential components that lead to program efficacy can be identified. Nonetheless, adherence to the intervention as a whole becomes required in circumstances when the intervention's fundamental components are ambiguous or poorly defined.

Moderators
It might be difficult to attain a high level of fidelity or devotion to an intervention or its core components. Numerous variables can influence or lessen the degree of fidelity with which an intervention is carried out.

5.2.3.3 How Complexity of an Intervention Can Influence Fidelity?
The complexity of an intervention can influence fidelity. Intervention complexity refers to the level of intricacy or sophistication involved in delivering the intervention. Simple interventions are typically easier to understand and implement, while complex interventions involve multiple components, steps, or interactions. The complexity of an intervention can influence fidelity levels in several ways:

(a) Fidelity and Clarity of Intervention Description: Implementing the intervention with high fidelity is more likely when it is described in clear and precise terms. Implementers are better able to understand what needs to be done when intervention guidelines are well-documented and offer detailed instructions. Variability in implementation and reduced fidelity can result from ambiguity or vagueness in the description of the intervention.

(b) Response Barriers: Complex interventions may have more "response barriers" or challenges that hinder implementation fidelity. With multiple components or steps, there is a greater likelihood of at least one element not being carried out correctly. These barriers can include logistical challenges, resource constraints, technical difficulties, or a lack of understanding of certain components. Simple interventions, on the other hand, have fewer response barriers, making it easier to achieve high fidelity.

(c) Variability in Delivery: Complex interventions are more susceptible to variability in their delivery. Different implementers may interpret and implement the various components differently, leading to variations in fidelity. In contrast, simpler interventions tend to have a more standardized and consistent delivery, making it easier to achieve high fidelity across different implementers and settings.

To address the challenges associated with complex interventions, there have been calls for enhancing the documentation and reporting of intricate interventions. This includes providing detailed descriptions of each component, specifying implementation procedures, and outlining potential challenges or adaptations. By improving the clarity and comprehensiveness of intervention descriptions, it becomes easier to identify and address potential causes of implementation variability, ultimately supporting higher fidelity.

5.2.3.4 Facilitation Strategies to Improve Fidelity
Facilitation strategies, such as manuals, guidelines, training, supervision, and feedback, are commonly employed to promote standardized implementation and improve fidelity. These strat-

egies provide support and guidance to intervention providers, ensuring that the intervention is administered consistently to all participants. The sufficiency of facilitation techniques can vary depending on the complexity of the intervention. Simple interventions may require minimal training or teaching to achieve high fidelity. The intervention components and procedures are straightforward, and implementers can easily understand and follow the guidelines without extensive support measures. In contrast, complex interventions often necessitate a range of support measures to ensure fidelity. The multiple components, interactions, or steps involved in the intervention may require more comprehensive training, ongoing supervision, and feedback to ensure that all aspects are implemented correctly.

The issue of sufficiency arises when determining the appropriate level of facilitation for a given intervention. Understanding the relationship between the complexity of the intervention and the effectiveness of facilitation techniques can help establish the optimal level of support required. While observational research cannot definitively establish a direct causal relationship between facilitation approaches and the quality or severity of intervention execution, it is considered a plausible mediator. Observational studies can examine the association between the use of facilitation strategies and implementation fidelity, shedding light on whether certain techniques are associated with higher fidelity levels. By examining the relationship between facilitation techniques and the complexity of the intervention description, researchers can gain insights into the effectiveness of specific support measures. This understanding can inform the development and refinement of facilitation strategies to enhance fidelity and improve the overall quality of intervention implementation.

Delivering an intervention with high quality is a clear way to potentially moderate the link between fidelity and implementation. This pertains to the suitability of an intervention's implementation for attaining its desired outcomes. If an intervention is presented in an ineffective manner, it may not have the full impact on its intended audience. The quality of delivery is a crucial factor that can moderate the relationship between fidelity and implementation and ultimately impact the effectiveness of an intervention.

The quality of delivery refers to how well the intervention is presented and implemented, taking into account factors such as the skills, competence, and proficiency of the intervention providers. When an intervention is delivered with high quality, it increases the likelihood of achieving the desired outcomes. If an intervention is presented in an ineffective manner, it may not have the desired impact on the intended audience. Poor delivery can result in miscommunication, confusion, or a lack of engagement among participants. This can undermine the fidelity of the intervention and lead to suboptimal outcomes. On the other hand, high-quality delivery ensures that the intervention is implemented as intended, with fidelity to the prescribed components and procedures. Effective delivery involves clear communication, appropriate timing, engaging presentation techniques, and the ability to adapt and respond to participant needs. It also requires the intervention providers to have the necessary knowledge, skills, and competence to deliver the intervention effectively.

The quality of delivery is closely linked to fidelity. When the intervention is delivered with fidelity, it increases the chances of achieving the intended outcomes. However, fidelity alone may not be sufficient if the delivery quality is poor. By focusing on both fidelity and the quality of delivery, intervention implementers can maximize the impact of the intervention and improve the overall effectiveness of the program. To ensure high-quality delivery, ongoing training, supervision, and feedback are important. These measures can help intervention providers enhance their skills, address any challenges or gaps in delivery, and continuously improve the quality of implementation.

If participants believe an intervention is unimportant to them, it may not be implemented with high fidelity and this might contribute significantly to its low coverage or failure. This idea: the adoption of a new mediation depends on its acceptance and suitability for the parties receiving it. Participant response may thus be a key factor in any process assessing implementation fidelity.

Participant responsiveness refers to the engagement, acceptance, and perceived relevance of the intervention by the individuals receiving it. If participants do not perceive the intervention as important or suitable for their needs, it can have a significant impact on fidelity and the overall effectiveness of the intervention. When participants are responsive to an intervention, they are more likely to actively engage with the intervention components, follow the prescribed procedures, and adhere to the intervention guidelines. This, in turn, increases the fidelity of implementation and maximizes the potential benefits of the intervention. On the other hand, if participants perceive the intervention as irrelevant or unimportant to them, it can hinder their motivation to fully engage with the intervention or follow the recommended practices. This can result in lower fidelity, reduced participation, and limited impact on the desired outcomes.

Understanding participant responsiveness is crucial when assessing implementation fidelity. It is important to consider participants' perspectives, needs, and preferences when designing and implementing interventions. By involving participants in the process, seeking their input, and tailoring the intervention to their specific context, the likelihood of participant responsiveness and high fidelity increases. To enhance participant responsiveness, it is important to communicate the purpose and benefits of the intervention clearly. Engaging participants in the intervention design phase, providing opportunities for input and feedback, and addressing their concerns and preferences can foster a sense of ownership and increase their motivation to engage with the intervention. Regular monitoring of participant responsiveness throughout the implementation process is also important. Collecting participant feedback, assessing their satisfaction, and addressing any barriers or challenges they might face can help maintain and enhance their engagement and responsiveness to the intervention.

5.2.4 Implementation Frameworks

Implementation Science (IS) encompasses a wide range of theories, models, and frameworks that are used to investigate and address the challenges faced by practitioners in implementing new scientific findings into real-world settings. These theories and frameworks provide guidance and support for the implementation process. One crucial distinction in implementation science is the contrast between efficacy and effectiveness, which is relevant to all IS frameworks. Efficacy refers to how well an intervention performs in a controlled research setting or under ideal conditions. It assesses the intervention's impact under controlled circumstances to determine its potential benefits. On the other hand, effectiveness refers to how well an intervention performs in real-world settings, considering the practical constraints, limited resources, and complex contextual factors that may exist. Effectiveness evaluates the intervention's impact when implemented in the context of public clinics, community-based programs, or other real-world settings. The idea of scale-up is also integral to IS frameworks. Scale-up refers to the process of expanding the implementation of an intervention from a small-scale pilot phase to a larger population or broader context. It involves assessing the intervention's efficacy in controlled settings, piloting it locally to evaluate its effectiveness, and then scaling it up to assess its impact at the population level [21].

An intervention is considered effective when it is applied in a real-world context and shows results. This phrase recognizes the difficulties and limitations associated with putting treatments into practice in real-world situations where resources and support may be scarce. On the other hand, the performance of an intervention in a study or ideal context—where conditions are closely monitored and resources may be more plentiful—is referred to as efficacious. It recognizes that the outcomes observed in controlled research settings may not always be replicated in real-world implementation due to various factors such as resource constraints, organizational barriers, or contextual challenges. Understanding the distinction between efficacy and effectiveness is crucial in implementation science, as it helps researchers and practitioners evaluate and adapt interventions for real-world contexts. It recognizes the importance of considering the practical implementation challenges and the need to assess the intervention's impact in diverse settings.

After reviewing the scientific literature on IS, Moulin and colleagues categorize the frameworks and models used in the area based on the framework's comprehensiveness and ability to target innovation. They establish fundamental elements and provide a general framework that expands upon those fundamental elements [22]. These fundamental elements provide a foundation for understanding and guiding the implementation of interventions in implementation science. The fundamental elements that are commonly considered in implementation science frameworks often taken into account when designing and implementing interventions include:

- Implementation Process: This element focuses on the steps and strategies involved in planning, executing, and monitoring the implementation of an intervention. It includes activities such as assessing readiness for implementation, engaging key stakeholders, and developing an implementation plan.
- Innovation: This element refers to the specific intervention or practice being implemented. It involves understanding the evidence base supporting the innovation, its core components, and how it is expected to bring about the desired change.
- Setting: The setting element considers the context in which the intervention is being implemented. It includes factors such as the organizational culture, resources available, and infrastructure that may influence the implementation process and outcomes.
- Influencing Factors: These are the factors that can impact the implementation process and outcomes. They can include individual-level factors (e.g., knowledge, attitudes), organizational factors (e.g., leadership support, staff turnover), and external factors (e.g., policy environment, funding).
- Tactics: Tactics refer to the specific strategies and approaches used to facilitate the implementation process. These can include training and education, providing ongoing support and supervision, adapting the intervention to fit the local context, and using implementation frameworks or models.

- Assessment: This element focuses on evaluating the implementation process and outcomes. It involves measuring fidelity (adherence to the intervention), assessing the reach and engagement of the intervention, and evaluating the effectiveness and sustainability of the implemented intervention.

The Diffusion of Innovations Theory by E. Rogers is indeed a foundational theory that explains how ideas spread and innovations are disseminated from research to end consumers [23]. The identification of 61 models for dissemination and/or implementation research by Tabak and colleagues highlights the diversity and richness of approaches in this field. These models can be applied at different levels, such as the community or organizational level, to facilitate the dissemination and implementation of innovations [13]. The classification of these models, as described by Tabak and colleagues, is valuable for understanding the scope and focus of each model. It indicates the extent to which a specific implementation science (IS) model addresses different levels within the social-ecological model, which is a framework that recognizes the influence of multiple levels of factors on behavior change and implementation outcomes. This classification helps researchers and practitioners select appropriate models based on their implementation goals and target populations.

Additionally, the flexibility rating reflects the continuum of constructs within each model, ranging from broad and malleable concepts to more fixed and operational elements. This rating can inform decision-making regarding the suitability of a particular model for a given implementation context. Models with greater flexibility may allow for adaptation and customization to fit specific settings, whereas models with more fixed constructs may provide a standardized approach. By offering this comprehensive analysis and classification, Tabak and colleagues contribute to the knowledge base of dissemination and implementation research in the field of health. Researchers and practitioners can benefit from their work by gaining a better understanding of the available models and their applicability to different levels and contexts.

The models shown here serve as illustrations of popular IS frameworks and incorporate strategies to improve communication between researchers and end users. Some of the models among others are:

- Generic Implementation Framework (GIF): The GIF is a broad framework that provides a systematic process for implementing evidence-based interventions. It emphasizes the importance of adaptation to fit the local context and encourages collaboration between researchers and end-users throughout the implementation process.
- Framework for Reach, Effectiveness, Adoption, Implementation, and Maintenance (RE-AIM): RE-AIM is a widely used framework that focuses on evaluating the impact and sustainability of interventions. It considers multiple dimensions, including reach (the proportion of the target population that participates), effectiveness, adoption (the extent to which organizations or systems implement the intervention), implementation (the fidelity and quality of implementation), and maintenance (the long-term sustainment of the intervention).
- Consolidated Framework for Implementation Research (CFIR): This all-encompassing framework incorporates a number of components and variables that affect the success of implementation. It is composed of several areas, including person traits, inner and exterior surroundings, intervention features, and the implementation process. CFIR looks for important elements that help or impede implementation and offers suggestions for how to deal with them.
- Dynamic Sustainability Framework (DSF): The DSF focuses on sustaining interventions and their benefits over time. It considers both internal and external factors that influence sustainability and provides a framework for planning and evaluating sustainability efforts. The DSF recognizes that sustainability is an ongoing process that requires continuous adaptation.

- Precede-Proceed, Dynamic Sustainability, Practical, and Robust Implementation Sustainability Model (PRISM): PRISM is a model that combines several frameworks and models to address implementation sustainability. It emphasizes the importance of assessing readiness for implementation, engaging stakeholders, using evidence-based practices, and considering the socio-political context. PRISM provides practical guidance for implementing and sustaining interventions.

These frameworks, among others, offer valuable guidance for researchers and practitioners in planning, implementing, and sustaining evidence-based interventions. They consider various factors, such as intervention characteristics, context, and stakeholder engagement, to enhance the effectiveness and sustainability of implementation efforts.

5.2.4.1 The Generic Implementation Framework (GIF)

Indeed, the Generic Implementation Framework (GIF) can be a useful tool for conceptualizing interventions and understanding the core components of implementation science (IS). It provides a high-level overview of the essential elements and their relationships within the implementation process. The GIF helps researchers and practitioners organize their thinking and consider key components when planning and implementing interventions. It typically includes elements such as:

- Intervention: This refers to the evidence-based practice or innovation being implemented. It involves understanding the intervention's key components, theory of change, and the evidence supporting its effectiveness.
- Fidelity: Fidelity refers to the extent to which an intervention is implemented as intended. It involves ensuring that the intervention is delivered with fidelity to its core components and that any adaptations are made with careful consideration.
- Context: The context refers to the broader setting or environment in which the intervention

is implemented. It includes factors such as the organizational culture, resources, policies, and external influences that can impact implementation success.

- Stakeholder Engagement: This component emphasizes the importance of involving relevant stakeholders throughout the implementation process. Stakeholders can include researchers, practitioners, policymakers, and individuals or groups affected by the intervention. Engaging stakeholders helps build support, gather input, and address potential barriers or facilitators to implementation.
- Capacity Building: Capacity building involves strengthening the skills, knowledge, and resources of individuals and organizations involved in the implementation. It may include training, education, technical assistance, and infrastructure development to support successful implementation.
- Evaluation: Evaluation focuses on assessing the implementation process and outcomes. It involves collecting data to monitor fidelity, measure reach and uptake, and evaluate the effectiveness and sustainability of the intervention.

By visualizing these core concepts and their relationships, the GIF provides a framework for understanding how these components interact and influence each other throughout the implementation process. It helps identify areas that may require additional attention or strategies to enhance implementation success. Additionally, the GIF can be used in conjunction with other models or frameworks that have a deeper literature base. Combining the GIF with more specific or specialized frameworks allows for a more comprehensive and nuanced understanding of implementation processes within a specific context or field. It's important to note that while the GIF offers a valuable starting point, the selection of additional models or frameworks should be based on the specific research question, context, and needs of the implementation project.

The suggestion of a generic implementation framework (GIF) to illustrate the fundamental ideas of implementation is valuable in providing guidance to researchers, legislators, health administrators, and practitioners. While different implementation frameworks may have specific models and variables, having a high-level depiction of the key implementation principles can help establish a common understanding across diverse implementation efforts. The non-linear and recursive structure depicted in the GIF, with double arrows and overlapping circles, recognizes the iterative nature of the implementation process. Implementation is often a dynamic and complex process that involves feedback loops, interactions between different components, and the need for ongoing adjustments and adaptations.

By illustrating the recursive nature of implementation, the GIF acknowledges that implementation is not a linear process with discrete phases or steps. Instead, it highlights the interdependencies and interactions between different elements, allowing for flexibility and adaptation as needed throughout the implementation journey. While the GIF provides a high-level depiction of the key implementation principles, it is important to note that the specific phases and steps of the implementation process may vary depending on the context, intervention, and framework being used. The GIF serves as a foundational framework that can be complemented by more specific models or frameworks that address the unique needs and considerations of a particular implementation effort. The use of a generic implementation framework can help stakeholders gain a better understanding of the fundamental concepts and principles that underpin successful implementation efforts. It provides a common language and visual representation that can facilitate communication, collaboration, and knowledge sharing among different stakeholders involved in the implementation process.

The innovation to be implemented is at the core of the structure, and the contextual domains or degrees of impact surround it. A path of implementation will be influenced by many aspects, methods, and assessments that need to be taken into account at every step and for every domain of the implementation process. It is crucial to understand that the GIF is a combination of the elements found in the most, if not all, other frameworks rather than a brand-new one. Making use of the GIF as a guide or checklist guarantees that the framework(s) selected address the fundamentals of implementation.

The GIF serves as a comprehensive framework that combines elements found in various other implementation frameworks. By using the GIF as a guide or checklist, stakeholders can ensure that the selected framework(s) address the fundamental principles of implementation. This approach helps to ensure that essential elements are not overlooked and that the implementation efforts are grounded in evidence-based practices. By considering the various aspects, methods, and assessments at each step and for each domain of the implementation process, stakeholders can make informed decisions and adapt their strategies as needed. It helps to align the implementation efforts with the specific context, stakeholders' needs and resources, and the evidence supporting the intervention.

Using the GIF as a guide or checklist can also facilitate collaboration and communication among stakeholders. It provides a common reference point and language, allowing for shared understanding and discussions about the implementation process. This can enhance coordination and alignment among stakeholders and increase the likelihood of successful implementation outcomes. It's important to note that while the GIF incorporates elements from various frameworks, stakeholders should still consider the specific needs and characteristics of their implementation context. They may need to supplement the GIF with additional frameworks or models that address unique aspects of their implementation effort.

5.2.4.2 RE-AIM Framework

The RE-AIM Framework, offers a comprehensive perspective on the public health impact of an intervention. It considers five key factors: reach, effectiveness, adoption, implementation, and maintenance. These factors collectively influence the overall impact of an intervention on the target population and the broader public health context [21, 24].

- Reach: The percentage of the target population that takes part in the intervention is referred to as "reach." It highlights how crucial it is to involve a varied and representative set of people in order to guarantee the intervention's potential influence on public health.
- Effectiveness: Effectiveness assesses the impact of the intervention on relevant outcomes. It evaluates whether the intervention achieves the desired health outcomes and its overall efficacy in real-world settings.
- Adoption: Adoption focuses on the extent to which organizations or systems implement the intervention. It examines the uptake of the intervention by organizations, institutions, or communities and considers factors that facilitate or hinder its adoption.
- Implementation: The integrity and caliber of delivering the intervention are referred to as implementation. It evaluates the effectiveness of the intervention's execution, taking into account compliance with the intervention protocol, the skill of the intervention providers, and the process of implementation as a whole.
- Maintenance: Maintenance examines the long-term sustainment of the intervention and its effects. It considers the durability and continued impact of the intervention after the initial implementation phase, including factors that contribute to its ongoing sustainability.

The RE-AIM Framework aligns with systems-based methodologies and the social-ecological model. It recognizes that interventions occur within complex systems and are influenced by multiple levels of influence, including individual, interpersonal, organizational, community, and societal factors. By considering these factors, the RE-AIM Framework provides a more comprehensive and holistic understanding of the implementation and impact of interventions. The RE-AIM Framework is particularly useful when evaluating interventions that target multiple causes and holistic systems. It allows for a more nuanced assessment of the intervention's reach, effectiveness, adoption, implementation, and maintenance in relation to the complex health issues being addressed. By incorporating both implementation and distribution difficulties, the RE-AIM Framework offers a practical and operational approach to implementation science. It provides a framework for evaluating interventions that goes beyond isolated efficacy studies and considers the real-world challenges and implications of implementing interventions on a larger scale.

The RE-AIM paradigm was developed over 20 years ago in response to the need for improving the application of scientific knowledge to practice and policy. It has since become one of the most widely utilized planning and assessment frameworks in the domains of behavioral science, public health, and implementation science [21]. One of the key features of the RE-AIM framework is its emphasis on transparency of reporting. It encourages researchers and practitioners to provide detailed information across all dimensions of RE-AIM, including reach, effectiveness, adoption, implementation, and maintenance. This transparency facilitates the replication and dissemination of interventions, enabling others to better understand and evaluate their potential impact. In addition to internal validity, which focuses on the rigor of the study design and internal consistency, RE-AIM also highlights the importance of external validity. External validity, or generalizability, considers the extent to which findings from an intervention study can be applied to other populations, settings, or contexts. By considering both internal and external validity, RE-AIM provides a more comprehensive perspective on the transferability and real-world applicability of interventions.

The wide range of applications for the RE-AIM framework demonstrates its adaptability. It has been applied to the assessment of interventions aimed at changing the environment and policy, as well as interventions addressing different health issues in community, clinical, and corporate settings. This adaptability makes interventions more useful in a variety of implementation scenarios by enabling evaluation across a range of people, locations, and health contexts. The popularity and versatility of the RE-AIM framework attest to its usefulness as a planning, evaluating, and reporting tool for interventions. It advances implementation science and facilitates the efficient translation of research into practice and policy by emphasizing external validity and open reporting.

Initially, there may have been a focus on individual and organizational levels when providing examples of RE-AIM applications. This could be due to the fact that the A, I, and M domains (adoption, implementation, and maintenance) were primarily utilized at the organizational level, while the R and E domains (reach and effectiveness) were specifically applied at the patient level. However, it is crucial to note that the intention of the RE-AIM framework was never to restrict its applications to only these two categories. In recent years, there has been a growing recognition and utilization of RE-AIM across multiple levels of the socioecological framework. This expansion acknowledges that interventions and their implementation occur within complex systems that encompass individual, interpersonal, organizational, community, and societal levels. By deploying RE-AIM domains at three or more levels, researchers and practitioners can better capture the interplay and impact of interventions across different levels of the socioecological model. This broader perspective allows for a more comprehensive understanding of implementation and its potential outcomes in diverse contexts.

Considering multiple levels within the RE-AIM framework enables a more holistic assessment of interventions and their implications. It recognizes that the success and sustainability of interventions are influenced by factors operating at various levels, including individual behaviors, social dynamics, organizational structures, community norms, and policy environments. Expanding the application of RE-AIM to multiple levels promotes a systems-oriented approach to implementation science. It encourages stakeholders to consider the complex and interconnected factors that influence the implementation and effectiveness of interventions, thereby enhancing the potential for successful and sustainable outcomes.

5.2.4.3 Consolidated Framework for Implementation Research (CFIR)

The Consolidated Framework for Implementation Research (CFIR), was introduced in 2009 by

Damschroder et al. with the aim of providing a more comprehensive and inclusive framework by integrating components from earlier implementation theories [25]. The goal of the CFIR framework is to make it easier to develop theories and cross-context validate the efficiency of interventions or therapies. It provides a typology that includes several areas and notions that are pertinent to study on implementation. These domains include intervention characteristics, outer setting, inner setting, characteristics of individuals, and the implementation process.

Researchers and practitioners can use both qualitative and quantitative methods to apply the CFIR framework. This flexibility allows for a comprehensive exploration of the factors influencing the implementation and effectiveness of interventions. Qualitative methods, such as interviews and focus groups, can help capture in-depth insights and rich contextual information. Quantitative methods, such as surveys and statistical analyses, can provide broader perspectives and support hypothesis testing. The CFIR framework can be particularly valuable when formulating hypotheses about intervention effectiveness and analyzing the factors contributing to success or failure. By systematically considering the various domains and constructs within CFIR, researchers can identify potential facilitators and barriers to implementation and draw conclusions about the factors that influence intervention outcomes.

Additionally, CFIR encourages academics to think about how many domains and constructs interact with one another. It acknowledges that implementation is a dynamic, intricate process that is impacted by many different things at different times. This all-encompassing method advances knowledge of the dynamics of implementation and aids in the creation of evidence-based implementation strategies. For researchers and practitioners engaged in implementation research, the CFIR framework is a useful resource overall. Its thorough typology and incorporation of past ideas offer a strong framework for investigating implementation challenges and comprehending the elements that influence the success or failure of interventions.

(a) *Intervention:* The intervention refers to the essential elements of the intended execution, which are the core components of the intervention that are not tailored to a specific setting. These elements represent the strategies or activities designed to bring about the desired change or outcome.

(b) *Inner and Outer Settings*: There are particular situations in which the implementation process takes place, both inside and outside the setting. The institutions or environments—such as clinics, hospitals, or health centers—where the intervention is applied are sometimes referred to as the inner setting. Conversely, the external setting comprises the wider social, political, and economic contexts that impact the context of implementation.

(c) *Change Agents*: Involved parties in the implementation process are known as change agents. They have the power and aptitude to look for, evaluate, test, build, or innovate interventions. The community people who drive implementation initiatives can be change agents, as can healthcare professionals, organizational leaders, and legislators.

(d) *Implementation Process*: The implementation process outlines the active sequence of actions and steps undertaken by individuals or organizations to achieve the intended goals of the intervention. It involves planning, executing, and monitoring the implementation activities to ensure fidelity and success.

Within each of these five domains, the CFIR framework further breaks down the components into more manageable parts. This breakdown helps in the preparation and implementation of the intervention by providing a structured approach to understanding and addressing the various factors and influences at play. By considering these different domains and their subcomponents, the CFIR framework provides a comprehensive and systematic approach to implementation research. It allows researchers and practitioners to assess and address the multiple factors that can influence the success or failure of an intervention in a specific context.

CFIR falls under the category of determinant frameworks, aiming to understand and explain the organizational and individual factors that influence implementation outcomes. It was developed by consolidating ideas from 19 different theories, primarily focused on healthcare. By incorporating these theories, CFIR offers a comprehensive list of constructs that can act as barriers or enablers to implementation efforts. One of the key strengths of CFIR is its flexibility in adapting to various contexts and circumstances. It has been widely applied in a diverse range of investigations, demonstrating its utility across different fields and settings. CFIR takes a systematic and thorough approach by systematically assessing the potential contextual and intervention factors that impact implementation and effectiveness. It recognizes that implementation is influenced by multiple layers of factors, including individual-level, organizational-level, and environmental-level constructs.

A notable feature of CFIR is its emphasis on the effects of changing organizational processes. It recognizes that implementing interventions often involves modifying existing organizational procedures and practices. CFIR considers the dynamic interaction between individuals and their organizations, as well as how this relationship influences behavioral changes and implementation outcomes. By investigating the barriers and facilitators to the implementation of a specific intervention, CFIR aims to enhance implementation efforts. It provides a framework for systematically examining the various factors that can influence implementation success and effectiveness, helping researchers and practitioners identify areas for improvement and develop strategies to overcome implementation challenges. Overall, CFIR serves as a valuable tool for understanding the complexities of implementation and identifying factors that contribute to successful implementation efforts. Its comprehensive approach and focus on organizational and individual elements make it a robust framework for implementation research.

5.2.4.4 Dynamic Sustainability Framework

The Dynamic Sustainability Framework (DSF) was developed in 2013 by Chambers et al. to address the growing interest in examining the sustainability of implemented initiatives [12]. The framework is designed to guide the exploration and understanding of sustainability factors in various contexts. The DSF is built on seven empirically supported tenets or principles:

- Contextual Relevance: It is not reasonable to expect that data gathered in one particular environment would always hold true in drastically other contexts. As a result, treatments shouldn't be completely optimized before being put into practice because modifications can be required to make them appropriate for the particular setting in which they are used.
- Continuous Improvement: Interventions are not static, and there is room for ongoing improvement. This principle emphasizes the importance of continually refining interventions based on feedback, evaluation, and new knowledge to enhance their effectiveness and sustainability.
- Outcome Relevance: Assessment metrics must to be pertinent to patient results and cognizant of how well the intervention fits into the particular setting. This principle emphasizes the necessity of outcome measures that account for context-specific elements that may affect outcomes and quantify the impact of the intervention on the intended beneficiaries.
- Voltage Drop: Voltage drop refers to the inevitable decline in intervention fidelity or effectiveness over time when interventions are implemented in real-world settings. This principle recognizes that challenges may arise during implementation, leading to deviations from optimal implementation. It emphasizes the need to address and mitigate these challenges to maintain intervention effectiveness.
- Fit between Setting and Intervention: The fit between the intervention and the setting in which it is implemented is crucial for sustainability. This principle recognizes that the alignment between the intervention and the specific context, including the organizational and environmental factors, is essential for successful implementation and long-term sustainability.
- Organizational Learning: Organizational learning plays a vital role in embracing contextual changes and adapting interventions. This principle emphasizes that organizations

need to be adaptable and responsive to changes in the context to ensure ongoing sustainability. Learning from implementation experiences and incorporating feedback is essential for continuous improvement.

- Stakeholder Involvement: Better results can only be attained by ongoing stakeholder interaction. This principle emphasizes the significance of incorporating and including patients, healthcare professionals, organizational leaders, and community members throughout the implementation process. Their opinions and contributions help the intervention be successful and long-lasting.

These seven tenets provide a framework for understanding and promoting sustainability in the implementation of interventions. The DSF recognizes the dynamic and context-dependent nature of sustainability and provides guidance for optimizing interventions, engaging stakeholders, and adapting to changes over time. The DSF likely provides a structured approach to investigating sustainability by considering multiple dimensions and factors that contribute to the long-term success and viability of initiatives. By using the DSF, researchers and practitioners can gain insights into the complex dynamics of sustainability and identify strategies to foster and maintain the continued success of implemented initiatives.

5.2.4.5 The Practical, Robust Implementation and Sustainability Model (PRISM)

The Practical, Robust Implementation and Sustainability Model (PRISM) is a theoretical model that serves as a foundation for understanding and promoting effective implementation and sustainability of interventions. It consists of multiple components, including context, infrastructure, beneficiaries, and intervention [26].

- Context: The context refers to the broader environment in which the intervention is implemented. This may include organizational, social, political, and economic factors that can influence the implementation process and outcomes. Understanding the context is crucial for tailoring the intervention to fit the

specific circumstances and addressing potential barriers or facilitators to implementation.

- Infrastructure: The infrastructure component of PRISM focuses on the necessary structures, resources, and support systems needed for successful implementation and sustainability. This may include organizational structures, policies, leadership support, training programs, and other elements that enable the intervention to be effectively implemented and maintained over time.
- Beneficiaries: The people or groups who are supposed to gain from the intervention are included in the beneficiary component. To implement an intervention that fulfills the target population's specific requirements and maximizes the possibility for good outcomes, it is imperative to have a thorough understanding of their traits, needs, and preferences.
- Intervention: The intervention component refers to the specific strategies, activities, or techniques designed to bring about the desired change or outcome. This could include clinical interventions, behavior change programs, policy changes, or other approaches aimed at addressing a particular problem or achieving a specific goal.

Together, these elements form the PRISM model, which offers a thorough grasp of the variables affecting implementation and sustainability. Through an examination of the infrastructure, beneficiaries, context, and intervention, the model seeks to provide guidance to academics and practitioners in the development, implementation, and maintenance of interventions that provide long-term effects.

5.3 eHealth Implementation Status: Integrating e-Health Research in to Practice and Policy

5.3.1 Feasibility

Throughout the healthcare system, there are several uses for digital health apps. A digital health intervention that enables the tracking and alerting of patients who are at risk in accordance with an established treatment regimen is one example. Technological monitoring of patient data, including vital signs and symptoms, is probably used in this intervention. When particular risk indicators are found, notifications or alerts are sent out. This can assist medical professionals in taking proactive measures to assist patients in need and in providing prompt care. Using electronic Clinical Decision Support Systems (eCDSS) to issue cautions or reminders regarding adherence to clinical guideline recommendations and expected standards is another use for these tools. By analyzing patient data and comparing it with predetermined parameters, these systems use digital technology to deliver alerts or recommendations for healthcare providers. By ensuring that medical professionals have access to current information and direction at the point of care, this helps to improve patient outcomes and the standard of care [4].

Digital apps are also used for quality assessment, diagnostic process design, and remote diagnostic tracking. Digital microscopy pictures can be captured, explored, analyzed, interpreted, and reported with the help of these programs. These apps make it easier to remotely analyze and diagnose a variety of medical issues by utilizing cutting-edge algorithms and digital imaging technology. Additionally, they aid in quality assessment by offering instruments for uniform picture analysis and reporting, which improves the precision and uniformity of diagnostic procedures [27]. Overall, the usage of digital health apps in these situations shows how technology may help assist clinical decision-making, improve patient monitoring and management, improve healthcare delivery, and expedite diagnostic procedures. These technological advancements hold promise for bettering patient outcomes, boosting productivity, and facilitating more easily accessible and individualized healthcare.

Implementation feasibility of digital solutions in healthcare can be hindered by several factors [28–30]. Here are some reasons that have been identified:

- Cost: The cost of digital equipment and solutions can be a significant barrier to implementation feasibility. Healthcare organizations and providers may face financial constraints when acquiring and maintaining the necessary technology infrastructure. The affordability and sustainability of digital solutions play a crucial role in determining their viability for widespread adoption.
- User-Friendly Design: To enhance implementation feasibility, digital solutions should be user-friendly and accessible. This includes using plain language and uncomplicated images to ensure that users, including healthcare professionals and patients, can easily navigate and understand the technology. Intuitive and user-centered design principles can help overcome usability barriers and promote successful implementation.
- Time Efficiency: Digital solutions, such as eHealth applications, have the potential to streamline healthcare services and reduce the time it takes to access and deliver care. For example, eHealth solutions can facilitate faster access to maternity and child health services, improving efficiency and patient satisfaction. By optimizing workflows and reducing administrative burden, digital solutions can enhance implementation feasibility.
- Lack of Awareness and Mistrust: Although eHealth apps are helpful in resolving health-related issues, potential users' lack of knowledge and mistrust may make deployment and acceptance difficult. Implementation may be hampered by worries about how user data will be managed, preserved, and safeguarded. Promoting the viability of implementing digital solutions requires fostering trust, increasing knowledge of data privacy and security precautions, and resolving user concerns.

A complete strategy that takes into account budgetary constraints, user experience design, efficiency improvements, and efforts to foster trust is needed to overcome these obstacles. Policymakers, healthcare providers, technology developers, and users must work together to ensure that digital solutions are successfully implemented and used in the healthcare industry.

The deployment of e-health in rural areas presents unique challenges, and several factors have been identified as either encouraging or impeding its adoption. The three critical themes that emerged in the implementation of e-health in rural areas are geographic isolation, targeting disadvantaged populations, and ownership changes [31]. Let's explore these themes in more detail:

- Geographic Isolation: Rural areas often face challenges related to geographic isolation, including limited access to healthcare facilities and healthcare professionals. The implementation of e-health solutions can help bridge this gap by providing remote access to healthcare services, reducing the need for patients to travel long distances for medical consultations or follow-ups. E-health interventions such as telemedicine can enable remote consultations, diagnosis, and monitoring, improving healthcare accessibility for rural populations.
- Targeting Disadvantaged Populations: Rural areas are more likely to have populations that are disadvantaged in terms of socioeconomic status, education, and healthcare access. Successful implementation of e-health in rural areas requires a focus on addressing the specific needs and challenges faced by these populations. E-health initiatives should be designed to be inclusive, culturally sensitive, and tailored to the unique requirements of disadvantaged rural communities. This may involve providing educational resources, ensuring language accessibility, and considering the digital literacy levels and preferences of the target population.
- Ownership Changes for Sustained Adoption: Implementing e-health solutions in rural areas may require changes in ownership and governance structures. This involves establishing collaborations between different stakeholders, such as healthcare providers, government agencies, community organizations, and technology vendors. Sustainable adoption of e-health in rural areas often necessitates shared ownership and collective decision-making processes. Engaging local communi-

ties and involving them in the planning, design, and implementation of e-health initiatives can foster a sense of ownership and increase the likelihood of sustained adoption.

These themes emphasize how crucial it is to take into account the unique requirements, circumstances, and difficulties of rural areas when putting e-health treatments into practice. Enhancing the acceptance and sustainability of e-health solutions in rural areas can be achieved through addressing geographic isolation, targeting underprivileged people, and easing ownership transitions. It's important to remember that other aspects of e-health deployment in rural areas, like infrastructure development, connectivity, healthcare professional training and support, and handling privacy and security concerns, must also be taken into consideration for the program to be implemented successfully.

5.3.2 Adoption

Utilizing e-health solutions has created new opportunities for self-management training, social and medical therapy, and health information access. The use of e-health solutions by a variety of stakeholders, including members of the public, patients, healthcare providers, and medical professionals, has significantly increased during the last 10 years. When it comes to e-health, adoption is the deliberate decision or action made to test or apply an innovation or evidence-based practice. Another name for it is "uptake" [16, 17]. This concept is consistent with the definitions offered by Rabin et al. and Rye and Kimberly. As previously noted, "uptake" is another word for adoption [18].

5.3.3 Factors Facilitating the Successful Adoption of e-Health

The adoption of ICT in the healthcare sector is influenced by various internal and external factors, which contribute to the provision of services using ICT tools. These factors can be categorized into elements that support better outcomes, effectiveness, and technology management. Scholars have identified several motivations for the adoption of eHealth applications by practitioners [32]. Some of these motivations include:

- Better Quality Services: eHealth applications can help medical professionals give patients with better services. Healthcare workers may obtain evidence-based information, follow established procedures, and use decision support systems by utilizing digital tools, which will improve patient care and clinical results.
- High-Quality Information Delivery: ICT technologies make it easier to transmit information in healthcare settings accurately and efficiently. In order to guarantee that correct and current information is available for decision-making and care delivery, healthcare providers can access patient data, clinical guidelines, and medical literature through the use of electronic health records, telemedicine platforms, and health information systems.
- Easy Access: Geographical barriers are removed and the necessity for in-person visits is decreased with the use of digital applications that facilitate quick access to healthcare services and information. The utilization of telemedicine and mobile health applications facilitates distant patient-provider communication, hence augmenting accessibility and convenience of care.
- Enhanced Communication Efficiency: ICT tools improve communication and coordination among healthcare teams. Secure messaging platforms, teleconferencing, and collaborative tools enable real-time communication, facilitating care coordination, interdisciplinary collaboration, and remote consultations.
- Improved Clinical Flow and Performance: Applications for eHealth improve the efficiency of clinical workflows and the delivery of healthcare as a whole. Digital tools help to streamline procedures, lower errors, and increase productivity in duties like treatment planning and drug management. Examples of

these tools are electronic prescribing systems and clinical decision support systems.
- Improved Information Delivery: ICT solutions enhance the timeliness and accuracy of information delivery. Real-time data exchange, alerts, and notifications enable healthcare providers to receive critical information promptly, leading to improved patient safety and more informed decision-making.
- Improved Public Image: The adoption of eHealth applications can enhance the public image and reputation of healthcare organizations. Embracing digital solutions demonstrates a commitment to leveraging technology for improved patient care, which can positively impact public perception and trust.
- Increased Patient Contact Time: ICT tools can increase the amount of time healthcare providers spend with patients. By automating administrative tasks and improving efficiency, digital applications free up more time for direct patient interaction, enabling better patient-provider communication and relationship building.
- Decreased Inaccuracies and Medical Errors: eHealth applications have the potential to reduce inaccuracies and medical errors. Through standardized documentation, decision support systems, and automated alerts, healthcare providers can minimize errors in medication administration, diagnosis, and treatment planning.
- Decreased Overall Costs: The adoption of ICT in healthcare can lead to cost savings. By optimizing resource utilization, reducing redundant procedures, and improving efficiency, eHealth applications can contribute to overall cost reduction in healthcare delivery.
- Saved Effort and Time: Digital tools streamline processes and reduce manual effort, leading to time savings for healthcare professionals. Automation of administrative tasks, electronic health records, and digital communication platforms save time, allowing healthcare providers to focus on clinical care.
- Reduced Workload: ICT solutions can alleviate the workload burden on healthcare professionals. Through automation and improved

efficiency, digital applications help manage and prioritize tasks, reducing the overall workload and improving work-life balance.

These motivations highlight the potential benefits of adopting eHealth applications in the healthcare sector. However, it's important to consider the specific context, challenges, and implementation strategies when incorporating ICT solutions to ensure their successful adoption and integration into healthcare workflows.

The desire to embrace digital health solutions is one of the many reasons influencing the adoption of apps in developing country healthcare systems. Specifically, the involvement of medical professionals in the creation, layout, and implementation of clinical decision support systems (CDSS) has the potential to increase the system's adoption rate. Physicians are more likely to adopt and use the technology when they are actively involved in the process and believe that the CDSS will improve their performance at work [33]. The adoption of digital health systems in developing countries can be positively impacted by a number of additional factors in addition to physician engagement [34]:

- Leadership Team: Adoption of digital health solutions is largely dependent on effective leadership. An atmosphere that is favorable to the adoption and use of apps and other digital health technologies can be created by a strong leadership team that understands the importance of technology, establishes clear goals, and offers assistance and resources.
- IT-Friendly Workplace: Creating an IT-friendly workplace environment is essential for successful adoption. This includes having the necessary infrastructure, such as reliable internet connectivity and hardware, as well as IT support services to address technical issues and ensure smooth functioning of the digital health systems.
- Effective Communication: Clear and effective communication is vital to promoting understanding, acceptance, and adoption of digital health solutions. Stakeholders, including healthcare providers, administrators, and patients, need to be well-informed about the

benefits, functionalities, and potential impact of the apps or systems. Communication strategies should address any concerns, provide training and support, and encourage feedback and collaboration.
- User Attitude and Skill Set: The attitude and skill set of healthcare professionals towards digital health technologies can significantly influence adoption. A positive attitude towards technology, coupled with the necessary digital literacy and training, enhances the likelihood of successful adoption and effective utilization of digital health systems.

It's important to note that these factors may interact and influence each other. For example, effective communication can help foster a positive user attitude, while a supportive leadership team can create an IT-friendly workplace environment. Moreover, the specific context and cultural factors of the developing nation should be taken into account when implementing digital health solutions, as they may influence the readiness and acceptance of these technologies. By considering these factors and addressing any barriers or challenges, healthcare systems in developing nations can improve the adoption and utilization of apps and other digital health solutions. This, in turn, can contribute to enhancing healthcare access, quality, and outcomes.

Indeed, the adoption of e-health applications is influenced by various factors that can have either positive or negative effects. These factors can be broadly categorized into technology-related, human-related, and organizational-related factors [35]. Here are some key adoption factors within each category:

Technology-related factors:
- Ease of Use: The ease of use of e-health applications is an important factor in their adoption. User-friendly interfaces, intuitive navigation, and simple workflows contribute to a positive user experience and encourage uptake.
- System Usefulness: The perceived usefulness of e-health applications is crucial. If users perceive that the technology will bring benefits, such as improved efficiency, better patient

outcomes, or enhanced communication, they are more likely to adopt it.

- System Flexibility: The flexibility of e-health applications to adapt to different contexts and user needs is important. Customizable features and the ability to integrate with existing systems can increase adoption rates.
- Time Efficiency: E-health applications that save time and streamline processes are more likely to be adopted. The technology should be able to deliver information and perform tasks efficiently, reducing the burden on healthcare professionals.
- Information Accessibility and Relevancy: Easy access to relevant and up-to-date information is critical. E-health applications that provide timely and accurate data support decision-making, leading to improved adoption.

Human-related factors:

- User Training: Adequate training and support for users are essential for successful adoption. Training programs should address the specific needs and skill levels of healthcare professionals to ensure they are proficient in using the e-health applications.
- User Perception: User perception of the benefits, risks, and impact of e-health applications influences adoption. Clear communication about the advantages, potential challenges, and expected outcomes can shape positive perceptions and increase acceptance.
- User Roles and Skills: The alignment of e-health applications with users' roles and skills is important. The technology should support and enhance their existing tasks and responsibilities, rather than creating additional burden or complexity.
- Clarity of System Purpose: Users need a clear understanding of the purpose and objectives of the e-health applications. When they see the value and relevance of the technology to their work, they are more likely to adopt it.
- User Involvement: Adoption rates are raised and a sense of ownership is fostered when end users are involved in the creation and development of e-health apps. It is important to get user input and feedback at every stage of the development process.

Organizational-related factors:

- Leadership and Support: Strong leadership support and commitment are crucial for successful adoption. Leaders should advocate for the adoption of e-health applications, allocate resources, and create a supportive environment for implementation.
- Clinical Process: Aligning e-health applications with existing clinical processes and workflows is important for integration. The technology should complement and enhance the existing care delivery processes, rather than disrupting them.
- User Involvement: Adoption rates can rise when users are included in the decision-making and implementation phases. Successful collaborative models involve healthcare experts in the technology's design and implementation.
- Internal Communication: Effective communication within the organization promotes understanding, acceptance, and adoption of e-health applications. Clear and transparent communication channels should be established to disseminate information and address concerns.
- Interorganizational System: The integration and interoperability of e-health applications with other healthcare systems and organizations are crucial. Seamless information exchange and collaboration between different stakeholders facilitate adoption and use.

The fit between these factors is important, as they are interconnected and can influence each other. A comprehensive understanding of these factors and their interplay is essential for successful adoption and utilization of e-health applications.

5.3.4 Factors Hindering Successful Adoption of e-Health

The adoption of platforms in the healthcare industry can face challenges and barriers that impede their widespread use [11]. To address the challenges and promote the broad adoption of eHealth, further research is necessary. Exploring new avenues and conducting studies can help identify potential solutions, best practices, and strategies to overcome barriers and encourage wider adoption of eHealth technologies [36]. Certainly, obstacles to eHealth adoption in underdeveloped nations can be categorized into various categories [37]. Here are some common categories that researchers have identified:

Financial: Sufficient funding is essential for the effective deployment and utilization of digital health apps. However, there are hurdles that prevent the adoption of eHealth solutions, including high initial and recurring expenses, uncertainty regarding return on investment, and a lack of funding.

Technical: Lack of computers or hardware; lack of technical support and training; lack of standards or interoperability; lack of customization; lack of staff or doctor expertise; and lack of technical training. In addition, differences in employment, a break in the continuity of care, the impact on consultation duration, and a reminder system. Patient inactivity, patient confidence in physicians, and the paternalistic attitude of healthcare professionals all have an impact on the implementation of digital health solutions. Lack of treatment continuity can present problems for medical practitioners [38].

Time: Time is needed for the system's selection, acquisition, and implementation; it is also needed for system training; data entry; the requirement for additional time for each patient; and data conversion for patients. Moreover, results from earlier research showed that the largest constraints for users were technological and time-related, including poor loading times, firewalls that prevent cloud-based apps, system compatibility issues, certain state requirements, and device interoperability [39]. The general deployment of eHealth apps was also hampered by unexpected negative outcomes, timing and illness progression, concern about technology, system failures, the digital divide, and a lack of understanding or access to IT [40].

Social: Uncertainty over the vendor, a lack of outside support, disruptions to the patient-provider relationship, a lack of support from colleagues, and a lack of support from higher management are examples of societal barriers that are commonly mentioned. Moreover, evidence suggests several specific technological and socio-cultural issues that can complicate the adoption of digital health solutions in poor countries. These problems include insufficient network coverage in remote locations, computer illiteracy, unstable energy supplies, and technology that is not "fit" culturally with low resource situations [41]. Le PTD et al. claim that important barriers also appear in domains that are more challenging to change or intervene in. These comprise elements in the client characteristics as well as structural and broader social levels of influence (i.e., the organizational and mental health system domains) [42].

Resource and infrastructure limitation: With more healthcare professionals possessing basic IT abilities, e-Health solutions have a great chance of being utilized. However, the most significant barriers to the eHealth solution's adoption were found to be poverty, cultural attitudes, organizational problems, a lack of human resources, and connection [29]. Implementation was further hampered by stakeholders' inability to agree on sustainable HR information systems, their inability to gather baseline data, their lack of computer skills, and their poor infrastructure for information and communication technologies [43].

Change process: More often mentioned obstacles were a lack of support from company culture, incentives, involvement, and leadership.

Lack of a trained workforce: Everyone agrees that if continuous growth is to be made, having a workforce with the right training is essential. Evidence, however, indicates that there are insufficient numbers of highly qualified medical informaticians and that their geographic dispersion is insufficient to fulfill the demands and level of skill required for the deployment of health IT [44].

Development of health IT agenda: In underdeveloped nations, e-Health agendas have suffered from a lack of proper focus and prioritized targets. Few of them have an HIS that is robust and efficient enough to fulfill all of their various demands [45].

Regional integration: Research revealed that interoperable mHealth apps and eRecord systems were crucial in the context of national eHealth Strategies as well as in the health sectors of different countries. However, the data indicates that in many countries, the current method does not address integrating mHealth apps to eRecord systems. Many countries' health sectors frequently use application programming interfaces and global interoperability standards. Institutions that are public and private can work together within them, but not outside of them. Additionally, a range of open-source and commercial solutions that make use of relational database systems and associated data formats are available to support eRecord systems. Following the discovery and categorization of problems with integrating mHealth apps and eRecord systems, a set of guidelines was developed to enhance the National eHealth Strategy [3].

results showed that EHR systems enhanced system quality by supporting the clinical responsibilities and workflows of healthcare providers. Moreover, users' performance was improved by increased knowledge quality, indicating that appropriate and pertinent information access is essential for the efficient use of digital health systems [47].

These studies emphasize how crucial it is to take into account knowledge quality as well as system compatibility when assessing the suitability and efficacy of digital health solutions. It is crucial to comprehend how effectively the technology fits user requirements, workflows, and the environment of healthcare practice in order to encourage adoption and maximize user output. It's important to keep in mind that the terms "acceptability" and "appropriateness" are occasionally employed in the literature inconsistently or with overlapping meanings. As such, it is crucial to take into account the precise meanings and settings in which these terms are employed in each given research or conversation.

5.3.5 Appropriateness

The concept of "appropriateness" describes how well an innovation or evidence-based strategy fits within a certain practice context, provider, or client, as well as how well it solves a specific issue or problem. Because of their close relationship to the idea of "acceptability," these concepts are occasionally used interchangeably or with overlapping meanings in the literature [14]. According to Mosa et al., medical professionals, nursing students, and medical professionals thought that some applications were very useful when it came to digital health solutions. These users specifically named the medical calculator, drug reference, and disease diagnostic applications as the most useful features [46]. System compatibility was shown to be the most important system quality factor in predicting the effectiveness of electronic health record (EHR) systems in a different study conducted by Salleh et al. Furthermore, when it came to forecasting user performance, knowledge quality received the highest score and the biggest impact size. The

5.3.6 Acceptability

The perception among implementation stakeholders that a specific intervention, service, process, or idea is agreeable, appetizing, or fulfilling is known as acceptance. It is crucial to the effective execution of healthcare interventions, and implementation difficulties are frequently linked to a lack of acceptability [15]. Studies on eHealth apps have revealed that a number of factors affect healthcare workers' intents to use and use these apps. Adoption decisions are greatly impacted by performance expectations, which are related to the apps' perceived utility and advantages [48]. Acceptance is also influenced by the accessibility of cloud-based health knowledge, which gives users access to current medical resources and information. The adoption of the apps is also influenced by the strength and caliber of the IT infrastructure that powers them. Furthermore, the attitudes and adoption intentions of healthcare professionals towards eHealth apps might be shaped by social influence, which can originate from peers, professional networks, or opinion leaders [49].

Clinical decision support is among the digital application kinds that are tested the most often in health systems in developing nations. Large academic hospitals and clinics that are not located in hospitals frequently use these apps. In an effort to enhance patient outcomes and treatment quality, it appears that an emphasis is being placed on utilizing digital tools to support clinical decision-making processes in these contexts. These results emphasize how critical it is to address acceptance when introducing eHealth apps and to take into account various elements, including social impact, cloud-based health knowledge, performance expectations, and IT infrastructure. Gaining insight into and taking action on these variables can aid in resolving implementation issues and encourage the effective uptake and application of digital health solutions.

The majority of healthcare professionals had good opinions about the electronic health record (EHR) system, believing it to be beneficial and able to improve the quality of medical care (Alzghaibi & Hutchings et al.). The effectiveness and usability of the EHR system were largely praised by users. They did, however, voice discontent with a few organizational facets, such as user engagement, training, and support. According to these results, system usability and efficiency are crucial enablers for the effective deployment of an EHR system in Saudi primary healthcare facilities [50]. A positive opinion of a digital device was held by participants in another study conducted by Bentley et al. They discovered it to be user-friendly, likable, appropriate, and inspiring. These favorable opinions imply that consumers gave the digital device a favorable reception, demonstrating a high degree of acceptance and contentment with its features and capabilities [51]. These studies demonstrate the importance of user engagement, support, training, system efficiency, and usability in the adoption and deployment of digital health solutions, such as electronic health record systems and mobile devices. A more effective and fruitful deployment of such technologies in healthcare settings can be achieved by addressing these issues, offer-

ing sufficient assistance and training, and guaranteeing user-friendly interfaces.

The deployment of digital technology is indeed crucial for promoting the use of eHealth in the healthcare system due to its potential benefits and viability. In the context of Uganda, the Tuuka application, which is a mobile-based solution, was found to be acceptable and sustainable by healthcare practitioners [52]. The Tuuka application provided several advantages to healthcare practitioners in Uganda. Firstly, it improved case notification, allowing healthcare providers to receive timely information about new cases and facilitate efficient coordination of care. Additionally, the platform facilitated collaboration among hospitals and enhanced communication between healthcare specialists, enabling them to exchange knowledge and expertise more easily. It also contributed to quicker medical decision-making, enabling healthcare practitioners to make informed decisions promptly. This feature can be particularly valuable in situations where timely decisions are critical for patient outcomes. Furthermore, the platform was seen as beneficial for improving patient-centered care. It helped notify healthcare staff at public hospitals about referred patients, ensuring that they were prepared for their arrival and could provide appropriate care. The application also played a role in reminding referred patients to keep their appointments, promoting adherence to scheduled healthcare visits. Additionally, the platform streamlined communication across different healthcare institutions, facilitating seamless information exchange and collaboration. These findings highlight the positive impact of the Tuuka application on healthcare delivery in Uganda. By leveraging digital technology, the platform addressed various challenges and facilitated improved case management, collaboration, communication, and patient-centered care.

5.3.7   Implementation Cost

Cost, in the context of implementation, refers to the monetary impact associated with the implementation attempt. There are three key factors that contribute to the variation in implementation costs.

Firstly, the complexity of the intervention being implemented influences its cost. More complex interventions may involve additional resources, equipment, or specialized training, which can increase the overall cost of implementation. Secondly, the choice of implementation technique also affects the cost. Different implementation techniques may require varying levels of planning, training, infrastructure setup, and ongoing support. These factors can impact the overall cost of implementing the intervention. Lastly, the total costs of delivery are influenced by the context in which the treatment is provided. Different healthcare settings, such as tertiary care centers or individual practitioners' offices, have varying overhead costs and levels of complexity. These differences in context can result in variations in the overall cost of executing a therapy. As a result, the location of service delivery, the mode of implementation that is selected, and the costs related to the particular intervention all affect how much it actually costs to administer a therapy. When organizing and allocating funds for the execution of a healthcare intervention, several elements must be taken into account.

The cost of an eHealth deployment in healthcare is influenced by various factors. Here are five significant factors that affect the overall cost:

- Hardware: The cost of hardware includes devices such as servers, laptops, tablets, printers, and scanners. The selection and quantity of hardware required for the eHealth deployment impact the cost.
- Software: The cost of software includes the purchase of the eHealth software itself, including interface modules and eHealth apps. The cost can also be influenced by any necessary software upgrades. The deployment strategy chosen can also impact the cost of purchasing the software.
- Implementation: The implementation phase involves a multidisciplinary team responsible for the deployment. The cost of implementation may include expenses related to the redesign of workflows or processes to accommodate the new eHealth system. These costs are typically covered by the implementation fees.
- Training: The implementation of a new system requires extensive training for personnel.

This includes training for clinical experts, staff members in the workplace, and healthcare providers. The cost of training is an important consideration to ensure optimal results from the eHealth deployment.
- Ongoing costs: Ongoing costs include support services, internet connectivity fees, and maintenance charges. These costs are associated with the continuous operation and maintenance of the eHealth system after deployment.

Budgeting and planning for an eHealth deployment in healthcare require careful consideration of these aspects. The effective deployment and long-term viability of the eHealth system can be ensured by being aware of and budgeting for these expenses. Automation has, in fact, proven to be a cost-effective and strategically valuable move for public sector hospitals [2]. Hospitals have had positive outcomes from automation in a number of areas, including:

- Cost-effectiveness: Automation can lead to cost savings by streamlining processes, reducing manual labor, and minimizing errors. Automated systems can optimize resource allocation, improve efficiency, and minimize unnecessary expenses. By reducing administrative burdens and automating routine tasks, hospitals can allocate resources more effectively and focus on providing quality patient care.
- Patient experience: Automation can enhance the overall patient experience by reducing waiting times, improving scheduling efficiency, and enhancing communication. Automated systems can facilitate online appointment booking, patient registration, and electronic health record management, leading to smoother and more convenient interactions for patients. This can contribute to increased patient satisfaction and improved healthcare outcomes.
- Workflow improvements for hospital employees: Automation can alleviate administrative burdens for hospital employees, freeing up their time to focus on essential tasks and

patient care. By automating repetitive and time-consuming processes such as documentation, data entry, and inventory management, healthcare professionals can devote more time to delivering quality care, leading to improved workflow efficiency.

- Workplace morale: Automation can contribute to improved workplace morale by reducing the burden of repetitive and mundane tasks. Healthcare professionals can benefit from automated systems that simplify administrative processes, allowing them to spend more time on meaningful patient interactions and professional development. This can enhance job satisfaction, engagement, and overall workplace morale among hospital employees.

These positive outcomes demonstrate the value of automation in public sector hospitals. By leveraging technology and automation, hospitals can achieve cost savings, improve patient experiences, enhance workflow efficiency, and boost workplace morale, ultimately leading to better healthcare delivery and outcomes.

5.3.8 Penetration

Global understanding of the significance of health informatics (HI) has grown since the WHO Health Metrics Network (HMN) was founded in 2005. Developing nations have been greatly aided by the HMN in embracing HI and starting eHealth projects [53]. First-world nations, with their more advanced healthcare systems, have implemented numerous public and commercial initiatives to promote the growth and utilization of health informatics. These initiatives have provided substantial evidence of the advantages and benefits of HI technology. They have demonstrated improvements in healthcare delivery, patient outcomes, data management, and decision-making processes through the effective use of health informatics. However, developing nations have faced more significant challenges in integrating health informatics into their healthcare systems. These challenges can include limited resources, inadequate infrastructure, lack of

technical expertise, and socioeconomic constraints. Developing nations often face difficulties in implementing and adopting HI solutions due to these barriers.

Despite the challenges, there is a growing recognition of the potential benefits of health informatics in developing nations. Efforts are being made to address the barriers and promote the integration of HI technology in these settings. International organizations, governments, and stakeholders are working together to provide support, resources, and capacity-building initiatives to facilitate the adoption of health informatics in developing countries [54]. The goal is to ensure that all nations, regardless of their level of development, can harness the potential of health informatics to improve healthcare delivery, enhance data management, and ultimately contribute to better health outcomes for their populations.

5.3.9 Sustainability

In the context of putting interventions into practice, sustainability is the degree to which a recently introduced intervention is institutionalized and integrated into the continuing operations of a service environment. There are many different ways to interpret the complex idea of sustainability. A viewpoint on sustainability that is highlighted by Rabin et al. [16] stresses how policies and practices can be used to integrate a program into an organization's culture. This involves the incorporation of the intervention into the routine procedures and behaviors of the organization or community. Rabin et al. propose three stages that determine the institutionalization of an intervention:

- Passage: This stage refers to a significant event that marks the transition from temporary to permanent funding or support for the intervention. It could include securing long-term financial resources or establishing policies that ensure the ongoing availability of necessary resources.
- Cycle or routine: In this stage, the intervention becomes part of the regular organizational or

community procedures and behaviors. It is consistently reinforced and recognized as an evidence-based practice. For example, the intervention may be included in the annual budget, evaluation criteria, or standard operating procedures, ensuring its continuous presence and importance in the organization.

• Niche saturation: This level shows how well the evidence-based intervention has been incorporated into each of the organization's or community's smaller subsystems. It penetrates every aspect of the system, not just particular departments or initiatives. The intervention is supported by all organizational levels and functions and becomes firmly ingrained in the organizational culture.

These stages represent a progression towards sustainability, with each stage contributing to the long-term institutionalization of the intervention within the service environment. Understanding and implementing strategies to support sustainability are crucial for ensuring the long-term effectiveness and impact of interventions. By integrating evidence-based practices into the organizational culture and systems, interventions are more likely to endure and continue to benefit the target population.

Scenario analysis and a deep comprehension of the ground reality are, in fact, essential for closing the "design-reality gap" and guaranteeing the creation of sustainable systems that are easy to use. Systems can be better designed and implemented to better address the demands and difficulties of target users and stakeholders by taking into account their unique context. Social factors are often found to be of great importance in the successful implementation of healthcare systems. These factors encompass the attitudes, beliefs, behaviors, and interactions of individuals and communities within the healthcare environment. Understanding and addressing these social factors are key to overcoming barriers and ensuring the adoption and sustainability of the implemented systems.

While specific manuals and implementation toolkits were not mentioned in the statement, they can indeed be valuable resources for electronic medical record (EMR) implementers.

Summative manuals and implementation toolkits can provide comprehensive guidance, best practices, and step-by-step instructions for the design, implementation, and maintenance of EMR systems. They can help implementers navigate through the complexities of the implementation process, address technical and operational challenges, and ensure effective system utilization [55]. These resources can offer practical insights, standardized approaches, and lessons learned from previous implementations, enabling implementers to make informed decisions and overcome common pitfalls. They can serve as a reference and support tool throughout the implementation journey, enhancing the chances of successful adoption and long-term sustainability of EMR systems.

Digital health technologies hold immense potential in strengthening health systems to support Universal Health Coverage (UHC) and achieve the health-related Sustainable Development Goals (SDGs). To maximize their impact, it is crucial to shift the focus from donor-led initiatives to building resilient, sustainable, and country-owned digital health solutions. A people-centered strategy is essential in this shift, where the emphasis is on meeting the needs and demands of individuals, communities, and healthcare providers. By adopting a demand-driven approach, precious time can be saved by avoiding unnecessary interventions, eliminating duplication of efforts, and preventing the wastage of limited health resources.

In the Nigerian context, it has been recognized that government ownership and leadership are vital for ensuring long-term funding and successful expansion of digital health projects. When the government takes ownership of digital health initiatives, it demonstrates commitment, provides sustained funding, and creates an enabling environment for the implementation and scaling up of digital health technologies [56]. Government ownership facilitates the integration of digital health technologies into existing health systems, enabling seamless coordination and collaboration among various stakeholders. It also helps overcome potential challenges such as interoperability, data privacy, and security concerns.

Digital health projects can be in line with national health priorities, strategies, and policies by giving the government control over the matter. The possibility of sustainability and the assimilation of digital health technology into standard healthcare delivery are both increased by this connection. Additionally, government ownership promotes collaborations with other stakeholders, such as development partners, the commercial sector, and civil society organizations. These partnerships can help with the execution and growth of digital health projects by utilizing knowledge, assets, and creative solutions. In general, attaining long-term funding, scalability, and sustainability in digital health depends on acknowledging the significance of government ownership and leadership in this field. By adopting a people-centered, demand-driven approach, countries can optimize the potential of digital health technologies to strengthen health systems, advance UHC, and contribute to the attainment of the health-related SDGs.

5.4   Implementation Barriers, Facilitators and Opportunities

5.4.1   Barriers

The potential of e-health technologies to improve the quality of healthcare services has sparked significant interest in both developed and developing countries regarding their adoption and utilization. It's crucial to remember, nevertheless, that e-health programs don't always succeed in their implementation. Significant failure rates in the adoption of e-health have been reported by both industrialized and developing countries. Several barriers have been noted in the context of developing countries that impede the adoption of e-health applications. These barriers can be categorized into several domains, as illustrated in Fig. 5.1:

- Patient-related barriers: These include factors such as patient knowledge, attitudes, skills, and compliance with using e-health technolo-

gies. Patients may lack awareness or understanding of the benefits and functionalities of e-health solutions, or they may face challenges in using the technology effectively.
- Social context barriers: The social context encompasses collaboration, leadership, the opinion of colleagues, and the culture of the network. Resistance to change, lack of buy-in from healthcare professionals, and inadequate collaboration among stakeholders can hinder the successful adoption and implementation of e-health initiatives.
- Economic and political context barriers: This domain includes policies, regulations, and financial arrangements. Insufficient policy support, unclear regulations, and inadequate funding can impede the implementation and sustainability of e-health projects in developing nations.
- Organizational context barriers: These barriers are related to resources, organizational structure, the organization of care processes, capacities, and staff. Limited resources, inadequate infrastructure, and the absence of clear strategies for integrating e-health technologies into existing healthcare systems can pose significant challenges.
- Individual professional barriers: These barriers pertain to healthcare professionals and their individual characteristics such as awareness, motivation to change, knowledge, behavioral routines, and attitudes towards e-health. Resistance to change, lack of awareness or training, and skepticism towards technology can hinder the successful adoption of e-health solutions.
- Innovation barriers: These barriers are associated with the e-health technology itself, including its feasibility, relative advantages in practice, accessibility, and attractiveness to end-users. If the technology is not user-friendly, lacks interoperability, or does not offer clear advantages over existing practices, it may face resistance and limited adoption.

In order to overcome these obstacles, a multifaceted strategy involving legislators, medical professionals, patients, technology developers, and

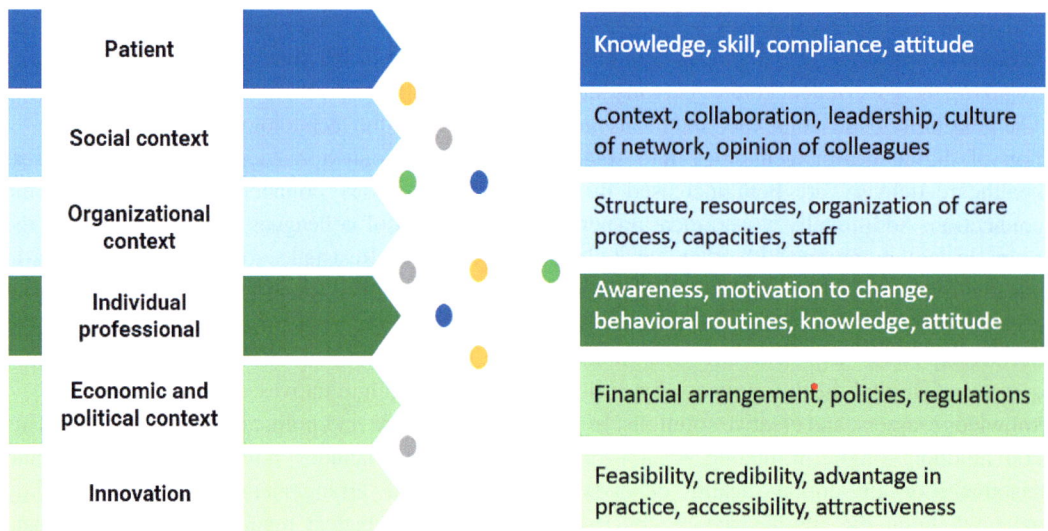

Fig. 5.1 Categories of implementation barriers of eHealth

communities is needed. A few strategies may be educating the public about e-health, encouraging leadership and teamwork, creating laws and rules that support the industry, providing sufficient funding, and guaranteeing that e-health technologies are acceptable and easy to use. Developing countries may overcome implementation problems and leverage the promise of e-health to enhance healthcare delivery and outcomes by comprehending and mitigating these hurdles.

5.4.2 Facilitators

There were several obstacles to overcome while implementing e-Health apps in developing countries. Nonetheless, the salient features that significantly contributed to the actualization of program utilization in resource-constrained environments were delineated. The entire implementation of e-Health was supported by the following factors: the use of local specialists for system development; user engagement; good attitudes among users; emphasis on the everyday activities of system users; and provision of operations and data use trainings [43]. Additionally, development capacities boost people's ability to share knowledge, which results in the formulation and implementation of more eHealth laws [57]. Additionally, empirical data shows that distinct

roles for the health professionals have enabled cooperative application adoption that yields fruitful outcomes [38].

Financial resources were determined to be the facilitator that had the most impact on helping to overcome certain obstacles, such software selection. The second factor that contributed to the effective adoption was the size of the primary health care facilities. According to reports, another factor that helps ensure the effective adoption of digital applications is perceived utility [50]. System quality, on the other hand, was mentioned as a significant contributing element. A person's education and professional background, for example, were observed to be related to the successful use of e-Health solutions [58]. As demonstrated, the most common facilitators were found to be provider and intervention attributes [42].

Implementation is often influenced by organizational and individual capacities (e.g., patient and provider computer literacy), data analytics, expanding care, and opportunities for health systems to advance e-health care adoption (e.g., intersectoral research, rapid testing cycles, and sustainable funding). Implementation and workflow, patient empowerment, EMR integration, credibility, knowledge, intersectoral networks, and sustainable financing were found to be highly correlated [59].

Personalized training and co-designed solutions, the engagement of all important stakeholders, simplicity of use and support, and cultural relevance were recognized and reported by Saigí-Rubió F et al. as the main motivators for the deployment and acceptance of digital applications [40]. The variable with the most explanatory power for telemedicine use was also found to be the physician's degree of personal information and communication technology (ICT) use. For example, in the Spanish sample, telemedicine usage was driven by two additional variables: the physicians' perceived ease of use of ICTs in clinical practice and their willingness to innovate; in the Colombian and Bolivian samples, the determining factor was their degree of optimism about ICTs [60].

Labrique et al. identified five critical emphasis areas that are necessary for the effective implementation of digital health apps. The program's or initiative's core features must, first and foremost, provide particular benefits to answer an unmet need and allow for early end-user input. The technological profile of the project ought to prioritize ease of use, compatibility, and adaptability. Third, in order to embark on a new project, all stakeholders must be motivated, educated, and involved. The legal framework that the digital healthcare program is intended to operate under is the fourth and most important element. Here, long-term funding that, when necessary, incorporates private sector participation as well as alignment with broader healthcare policies are essential. Finally, the external environment must be taken into account, encompassing the presence of suitable infrastructure to facilitate the implementation of extensive digital projects. The leadership needed to enable innovative solutions to reach medical staff and patients in low- and middle-income countries (LMICs) may come from global collaboration initiatives toward a less fragmented approach to scaling and integrating digital health [61].

5.4.3   Opportunities and Future Prospects of eHealth in Developing Countries

Indeed, the use of digital technology in healthcare presents exciting opportunities for the future. It has the potential to revolutionize traditional healthcare by enabling patient-centric and data-driven approaches. New eHealth technology solutions are constantly being developed, offering promising avenues for improving healthcare delivery in both developed and developing countries. In developing countries, there are numerous opportunities and solutions to embrace digital healthcare. These include leveraging mobile technologies for telemedicine and remote patient monitoring, using electronic health records (EHRs) to enhance care coordination and continuity, adopting health information exchange platforms to facilitate data sharing, and implementing digital tools for health education and behavior change. However, despite the potential benefits, there are inherent barriers that need to be addressed to successfully put innovative digital health solutions into practice.

The ultimate objective of eHealth is indeed to shift the focus of healthcare services from a physician and hospital-centered model to one that empowers individuals and prioritizes their well-being. This transformation is made possible through the use of digital technology and encompasses various aspects of healthcare delivery. One aspect of eHealth is the implementation of ePrescriptions, which enables patients to access prescribed medications more conveniently and with greater mobility. Instead of relying on physical prescriptions, electronic prescriptions can be transmitted directly from healthcare providers to pharmacies, allowing patients to pick up their medications from any participating pharmacy, saving time and effort.

Integrating patient data into a single electronic health record (EHR) is a crucial aspect of eHealth. Healthcare professionals can obtain a more thorough and current understanding of a patient's medical history by combining health information from several sources, including clinics, hospitals, and laboratories, into one all-inclusive digital record. Patient safety is increased, test and procedure duplication is decreased, and greater care coordination is made possible. Apart from integrating data, eHealth utilizes contemporary technology such as artificial intelligence (AI) and big data tools to examine vast amounts of data and detect trends, deviations, or possible hazards. By applying advanced analytics to health data, eHealth solutions can help identify early signs of diseases, predict disease outbreaks, and provide personalized recommendations or interventions for patients. This data-driven approach has the potential to enhance preventive efforts and improve health outcomes on both individual and population levels.

Future developments in digital health technology have the potential to bring medical treatment closer to the patient, including in scenarios where triage is necessary. Triage is a process used in emergency rooms to prioritize patients based on the urgency of their condition. With the use of modern technologies, this process can be simplified and made more accessible. Digital interfaces, such as smartphone applications or web-based platforms, can allow patients to input their symptoms and relevant information. These interfaces can utilize well-established symptom-tracking techniques and algorithms to digitally assess the severity and urgency of the symptoms. This can help in assigning different levels of priority or severity to patients, enabling more efficient triage processes.

Moreover, sophisticated telemedicine technologies can enable healthcare professionals to remotely evaluate patients' conditions and provide appropriate guidance or interventions. Through video consultations, remote monitoring devices, and secure communication platforms, healthcare providers can assess and treat patients virtually, bringing healthcare competencies closer to the patient's home. This approach has several potential benefits, including increased accessibility to healthcare services, reduced need for unnecessary hospital visits or emergency room visits, and improved efficiency in the delivery of care. It can be particularly advantageous in situations where physical access to healthcare facilities is limited, or where patients prefer the convenience and comfort of receiving care from their own homes. It is important to note that while digital health technologies have the potential to enhance the delivery of healthcare, there are considerations to address, such as ensuring the privacy and security of patient data, addressing potential disparities in access to technology, and

maintaining the human touch and empathy that is integral to healthcare.

In the future, it is indeed plausible that the objective of digital health technology could be to facilitate patient access to healthcare services through innovative approaches. One such approach could involve the setup of medical kiosks or similar decentralized units that enable individuals to remotely communicate with healthcare professionals and receive medical advice and prescriptions.

These medical kiosks could serve as a convenient alternative to traditional doctor's office visits, particularly for non-emergency cases or routine healthcare needs. By leveraging telecommunication technologies, individuals would be able to connect with healthcare providers remotely, discuss their symptoms or concerns, and receive appropriate guidance and prescriptions, if necessary.

However, even if such decentralized units were to serve as the primary access points for digital health services, they would still rely on key areas of strength. These areas could include:

- Centralized digital trust: In order to guarantee patient data security and privacy, a centralized digital trust system would be necessary. The implementation of this system would guarantee the secure transmission and storage of patient data by establishing and upholding standards for data security, authentication, and encryption.
- Provider network and collaboration: The success of decentralized units would depend on a network of healthcare providers who are available to provide remote consultations and care. Collaboration among healthcare professionals, including specialists, would be crucial to ensure comprehensive and coordinated care for patients.
- Infrastructure and technical support: Medical kiosks and other similar devices would require a strong infrastructure to support their operation. This infrastructure would need to include safe data storage, dependable internet access, and sufficient technical assistance. This infrastructure would guarantee the smooth opera-

tion of digital health services and allow patients and healthcare providers to communicate with each other.

- Regulatory frameworks and policies: Clear regulatory frameworks and policies would be necessary to govern the operation of medical kiosks and ensure compliance with healthcare standards, patient safety, and privacy regulations. These frameworks would help establish guidelines for the use of digital health technologies and protect patient rights.

While the concept of decentralized units for remote healthcare delivery is promising, it is important to address potential challenges, such as ensuring equitable access to these services, maintaining continuity of care, and addressing any limitations in physical examinations or diagnostic capabilities that may arise from remote consultations.

Applications for digital health are essential to improving healthcare because they give a number of advantages, such as decision support, better patient-provider communication, patient care management, and higher-quality treatment overall. However, a number of difficulties must be resolved in order to guarantee the long-term viability and success of digital health apps in low- and middle-income nations:

- Regional integration: Achieving regional integration is crucial for seamless data exchange and collaboration among healthcare systems and providers. Developing interoperable systems and standardized protocols can facilitate the secure sharing of health information across different regions and improve continuity of care.
- Privacy and security concerns: Building public confidence and acceptance of digital health applications requires addressing concerns about security and privacy. To allay worries, it's imperative to put strong data protection measures into place, adhere to privacy laws, and guarantee safe infrastructure and data storage.
- Interoperability challenges: Developed and developing nations alike confront the diffi-

culty of achieving interoperability, or the capacity of disparate systems to share and utilize information. Encouraging data sharing agreements, establishing common data standards, and implementing interoperability frameworks can help ensure smooth system integration and information transmission.

- Workforce training and development: Building a trained workforce capable of effectively utilizing and managing digital health applications is crucial. Training programs, capacity building initiatives, and continuous professional development opportunities can enhance the skills and knowledge of healthcare professionals in utilizing digital health tools.
- Infrastructure limitations: Poor infrastructure, such as restricted power supplies and internet connectivity, is a common problem in developing nations. Innovative strategies including utilizing mobile technology, putting offline functionality in place, and customizing solutions for low-resource environments are needed to overcome these obstacles.
- Funding and technical assistance: For digital health applications to be successfully deployed and sustained in resource-constrained areas, there must be sufficient financing and technical support. The provision of funding, materials, and technical know-how to facilitate the execution and expansion of digital health projects can be greatly aided by governments, international organizations, and development partners.

Through the resolution of these concerns, nations can surmount obstacles and fully utilize digital health applications to enhance healthcare provision and results in lower- and middle-class environments.

References

1. Sheikh A, Anderson M, Albala S, Casadei B, Franklin BD, Richards M, et al. Health information technology and digital innovation for national learning health and care systems. Lancet Digit Health. 2021;3(6):e383–96.
2. Cline GB, Luiz JM. Information technology systems in public sector health facilities in developing coun-

tries: the case of South Africa. BMC Med Inform Decis Mak. 2013;13(1):13.

3. Ndlovu K, Scott RE, Mars M. Interoperability opportunities and challenges in linking mhealth applications and eRecord systems: Botswana as an exemplar. BMC Med Inform Decis Mak. 2021;21(1):1–12.

4. Patel D, Msosa YJ, Wang T, Mustafa OG, Gee S, Williams J, et al. An implementation framework and a feasibility evaluation of a clinical decision support system for diabetes management in secondary mental healthcare using CogStack. BMC Med Inform Decis Mak. 2022;22(1):1–11.

5. Chen H, Hailey D, Wang N, Yu P. A review of data quality assessment methods for public health information systems. Int J Environ Res Public Health. 2014;11:5170–207.

6. Reeder B, Hills RA, Demiris G, Revere D, Pina J. Reusable design: a proposed approach to Public Health Informatics system design. BMC Public Health. 2011;11:116.

7. WHO. Global strategy on digital health 2020–2025. Geneva: World Health Organization; 2021.

8. Mathur A. Designs of healthcare trade: role of information technology. Econ Polit Wkly. 2004;39(20):2036–47.

9. Omotosho A, Emuoyibofarhe J. ICT in Health care delivery system: a framework for developing nations. Ota: Covenant University and Bells University of Technology; 2011.

10. WHO. Framework and standards for country health information systems. 2nd ed. Geneva: World Health Organization; 2008.

11. Herman H, Grobbelaar SS, Pistorius C. The design and development of technology platforms in a developing country healthcare context from an ecosystem perspective. BMC Med Inform Decis Mak. 2020;20(1):1–24.

12. Chambers DA, Glasgow RE, Stange KC. The dynamic sustainability framework: addressing the paradox of sustainment amid ongoing change. Implement Sci. 2013;8(1):1–11.

13. Tabak RG, Khoong EC, Chambers DA, Brownson RC. Bridging research and practice: models for dissemination and implementation research. Am J Prev Med. 2012;43(3):337–50.

14. Proctor E, Silmere H, Raghavan R, Hovmand P, Aarons G, Bunger A, et al. Outcomes for implementation research: conceptual distinctions, measurement challenges, and research agenda. Adm Policy Ment Health Ment Health Serv Res. 2011;38(2):65–76.

15. Davis FD. User acceptance of information: system characteristics, user perceptions and behavioral impacts. Int J Man Mach Stud. 1993;38:475–87.

16. Rabin BA, Brownson RC, Haire-Joshu D, Kreuter MW, Weaver NL. A glossary for dissemination and implementation research in health. J Public Health Manage Pract. 2008;14(2):117–23.

17. Rye CB, Kimberly JR. The adoption of innovations by provider organizations in health care. Med Care Res Rev. 2007;64(3):235–78.

18. Henggeler SW, Letourneau EJ, Chapman JE, Borduin CM, Schewe PA, McCart MR. Mediators of change for multisystemic therapy with juvenile sexual offenders. J Consult Clin Psychol. 2009;77(3):451–62.

19. Dusenbury L, Brannigan R, Falco M, Hansen WB. A review of research on fidelity of implementation: implications for drug abuse prevention in school settings. Health Educ Res. 2003;18(2):237–56.

20. Carroll C, Patterson M, Wood S, Booth A, Rick J, Balain S. A conceptual framework for implementation fidelity. Implement Sci. 2007;2(1):1–9.

21. Glasgow RE, Vogt TM, Boles SM. Evaluating the public health impact of health promotion interventions: the RE-AIM framework. Am J Public Health. 1999;89(9):1322–7.

22. Moullin JC, Sabater-Hernández D, Fernandez-Llimos F, Benrimoj SI. A systematic review of implementation frameworks of innovations in healthcare and resulting generic implementation framework. Health Res Policy Syst. 2015;13:16.

23. Nilsen P. Making sense of implementation theories, models and frameworks. Implement Sci. 2015;10(1):1–13.

24. Glasgow RE, Harden SM, Gaglio B, Rabin B, Smith ML, Porter GC, et al. RE-AIM planning and evaluation framework: adapting to new science and practice with a 20-year review. Front Public Health. 2019;7:64.

25. Damschroder LJ, Aron DC, Keith RE, Kirsh SR, Alexander JA, Lowery JC. Fostering implementation of health services research findings into practice: a consolidated framework for advancing implementation science. Implement Sci. 2009;4(1):1–15.

26. Feldstein AC, Glasgow RE. A practical, robust implementation and sustainability model (PRISM) for integrating research findings into practice. Jt Comm J Qual Patient Saf. 2008;34(4):228–43.

27. Suhanic W, Crandall I, Pennefather P. An informatics model for guiding assembly of telemicrobiology workstations for malaria collaborative diagnostics using commodity products and open-source software. Malar J. 2009;8(1):1–11.

28. Alam S, Elwyn G, Percac-Lima S, Grande S, Durand MA. Assessing the acceptability and feasibility of encounter decision AIDS for early stage breast cancer targeted at underserved patients. BMC Med Inform Decis Mak. 2016;16(1):1–13.

29. Pagalday-Olivares P, Sjöqvist BA, Adjordor-Van De Beek J, Abudey S, Silberberg AR, Buendia R. Exploring the feasibility of eHealth solutions to decrease delays in maternal healthcare in remote communities of Ghana. BMC Med Inform Decis Mak. 2017;17(1):1–13.

30. Tracy CS, Dantas GC, Upshur REG. Feasibility of a patient decision aid regarding disclosure of personal health information: qualitative evaluation of the Health Care Information Directive. BMC Med Inform Decis Mak. 2004;4:1–7.

31. Hage E, Roo JP, Van Offenbeek MAG, Boonstra A. Implementation factors and their effect on. BMC Health Serv Res. 2013;13:19.

32. Gururajan R, Hafeez-baig A. An empirical study to determine factors that motivate and limit the implementation of ICT in healthcare environment. Med Inform Decis Mak. 2014;14:98.

33. Sambasivan M, Esmaeilzadeh P, Kumar N, Nezakati H. Intention to adopt clinical decision support systems in a developing country: effect of Physician's perceived professional autonomy, involvement and belief: a cross-sectional study. BMC Med Inform Decis Mak. 2012;12(1):1–8.

34. Yusof MM, Kuljis J, Papazafeiropoulou A, Stergioulas LK. An evaluation framework for health information systems: human, organization and technology-fit factors (HOT-fit). Int J Med Inform. 2008;77(6):386–98.

35. Yusof MM, Stergioulas L, Zugic J. Health information systems adoption: findings from a systematic review. Stud Health Technol Inform. 2007;129:262–6.

36. Zanaboni P, Wootton R. Adoption of telemedicine: from pilot stage to routine delivery. BMC Med Inform Decis Mak. 2014;12(1):1–9.

37. Jimma BL, Enyew DB. Barriers to the acceptance of electronic medical records from the perspective of physicians and nurses: a scoping review. Inform Med Unlocked. 2022;31:100991.

38. Tong WT, Lee YK, Ng CJ, Lee PY. Factors influencing implementation of a patient decision aid in a developing country: an exploratory study. Implement Sci. 2017;12(1):1–12.

39. Matthews SD, Proctor MD. Public health informatics, human factors and the end-users. Health Serv Res Manag Epidemiol. 2021;8:1–3.

40. Boyle LD, Husebo BS, Vislapuu M. Promotors and barriers to the implementation and adoption of assistive technology and telecare for people with dementia and their caregivers: a systematic review of the literature. BMC Health Serv Res. 2022;22(1):1–19.

41. O'Connor S, O'Donoghue J, Gallagher J, Kawonga T. Unique challenges experienced during the process of implementing mobile health information technology in developing countries. BMC Health Serv Res. 2014;14(S2):6963.

42. Le PTD, Eschliman EL, Grivel MM, Tang J, Cho YG, Yang X, et al. Barriers and facilitators to implementation of evidence-based task-sharing mental health interventions in low- and middle-income countries: a systematic review using implementation science frameworks. Implement Sci. 2022;17(1):1–25.

43. Ishijima H, Mapunda M, Mndeme M, Sukums F, Mlay VS. Challenges and opportunities for effective adoption of HRH information systems in developing countries: National Rollout of HRHIS and TIIS in Tanzania. Hum Resour Health. 2015;13(1):1–14.

44. Detmer DE. Capacity building in e health and health informatics: a review of the global vision and informatics educational initiatives of the American Medical Informatics Association. Yearb Med Inform. 2010;19:101–5.

45. Luna D, Almerares A, Mayan JC, de Quirós FGB, Otero C. Health informatics in developing countries: going beyond pilot practices to sustainable implemen-

tations: a review of the current challenges. Healthc Inform Res. 2014;20(1):3–10.

46. Mosa M, Yoo I, Sheets L. A systematic review of healthcare applications for smartphones. BMC Med Inform Decis Mak. 2012;12(67):1–31.

47. Salleh MIM, Abdullah R, Zakaria N. Evaluating the effects of electronic health records system adoption on the performance of Malaysian health care providers. BMC Med Inform Decis Mak. 2021;21(1):1–13.

48. Idoga PE, Toycan M, Nadiri H, Çelebi E. Assessing factors militating against the acceptance and successful implementation of a cloud based health center from the healthcare professionals' perspective: a survey of hospitals in Benue State, Northcentral Nigeria. BMC Med Inform Decis Mak. 2019;19(1):1–18.

49. Colicchio TK, Facelli JC, Del Fiol G, Scammon DL, Bowes WA, Narus SP. Health information technology adoption: understanding research protocols and outcome measurements for IT interventions in health care. J Biomed Inform. 2016;63:33–44.

50. Alzghaibi HA, Hutchings HA. Exploring facilitators of the implementation of electronic health records in Saudi Arabia. BMC Med Inform Decis Mak. 2022;22(1):1–13.

51. Bentley CL, Otesile O, Bacigalupo R, Elliott J, Noble H, Hawley MS, et al. Feasibility study of portable technology for weight loss and HbA1c control in type 2 diabetes. BMC Med Inform Decis Mak. 2016;16(1):92.

52. Tumuhimbise W, Atwine D, Kaggwa F, Musiimenta A. Acceptability and feasibility of a mobile health application for enhancing public private mix for TB care among healthcare workers in Southwestern Uganda. BMC Digit Health. 2023;1:9.

53. Hébert RJ. Economics of health informatics in developing countries. Stud Health Technol Inform. 2011;164:162–7.

54. Luna D, Otero C, Marcelo A. Health informatics in developing countries: systematic review of reviews. Contribution of the IMIA Working Group Health Informatics for Development. Yearb Med Inform. 2013;8:28–33.

55. Jawhari B, Ludwick D, Keenan L, Zakus D, Hayward R. Benefits and challenges of EMR implementations in low resource settings: a state-of-the-art review. BMC Med Inform Decis Mak. 2016;16(1):1–12.

56. Ibeneme S, Ukor N, Ongom M, Dasa T, Muneene D, Okeibunor J. Strengthening capacities among digital health leaders for the development and implementation of national digital health programs in Nigeria. BMC Proc. 2020;14(Suppl 10):1–12.

57. Lang A. Government capacities and stakeholders: what facilitates ehealth legislation? Glob Health. 2014;10(1):1–14.

58. Bashiri A, Shirdeli M, Niknam F, Naderi S, Zare S. Evaluating the success of Iran Electronic Health Record System (SEPAS) based on the DeLone and McLean model: a cross-sectional descriptive study. BMC Med Inform Decis Mak. 2023;23(1):10.

59. Wozney L, Newton AS, Gehring ND, Bennett K, Huguet A, Hartling L, et al. Implementation of eMental Health care: viewpoints from key informants from organizations and agencies with eHealth mandates. BMC Med Inform Decis Mak. 2017;17(1):1–15.
60. Saigí-Rubió F, Torrent-Sellens J, Jiménez-Zarco A. Drivers of telemedicine use: comparative evidence from samples of Spanish, Colombian and Bolivian physicians. Implementn Sci. 2014;9(1):128.
61. Labrique AB, Wadhwani C, Williams KA, Lamptey P, Hesp C, Luk R, et al. Best practices in scaling digital health in low and middle income countries. Glob Health. 2018;14(1):1–8.

Leadership and Governance of Public Health Informatics

6

Zeleke Abebaw Mekonnen
and Moges Asressie Chanyalew

Abstract

Public health informatics is implemented within a governmental environment, wherein it is crucial to address to the legislative, regulatory, and public occurrences in a transparent and accountable way. Along this, establishing a robust governance structure is important to define the specific roles and responsibilities of all stakeholders within the digital health ecosystem. This ensures adherence to laws, regulations, and standards, and promotes efficient coordination and decision-making processes for the optimal utilization of health information systems.

Health information exchange (HIE) refers to the electronic exchange of health information among various healthcare organizations. When engaging in the exchange of health information, it is vital to prioritize the security, confidentiality, and privacy of the data. The capability of health information systems to collaborate within and between organizational boundaries is commonly referred to as interoperability. In developing countries, the absence of interoperability and integration among different health systems presents a significant barrier to realizing the potential advantages of digital health.

Health information standards play a critical role in various aspects of healthcare, including data storage and analysis, data security and confidentiality, data exchange, and utilizing data for informed decision-making. In this ever-evolving landscape, healthcare information systems managers need to closely monitor legal advancements and be ready to adapt policies and procedures accordingly. This is especially important when it comes to complying with changing national and international standards of care, particularly concerning health information standards.

In the realm of public health informatics, health program managers frequently employ monitoring and evaluation to enhance the effectiveness of their plans, initiatives, and other endeavors. Besides, to facilitate evaluation, it is essential to have a reliable monitoring system in place. The focus of the public health community on illness and injury surveillance, communities rather than individuals, prevention, and longitudinal analysis

Z. A. Mekonnen (✉)
Policy, Strategy and Research Lead Executive Office, Federal Ministry of Health, Addis Ababa, Ethiopia

SMART Health, Research and Publication Department, Bahir Dar, Ethiopia
e-mail: Zeleke.abebaw@moh.gov.et

M. A. Chanyalew
SMART Health, Research and Publication Department, Bahir Dar, Ethiopia

Planning, Monitoring, and Evaluation Directorate, Amhara National Regional State Health Bureau, Bahir Dar, Ethiopia

© The Author(s), under exclusive license to Springer Nature Switzerland AG 2024
K. D. Gashu et al. (eds.), *Public Health Informatics*, Sustainable Development Goals Series,
https://doi.org/10.1007/978-3-031-71118-3_6

create special opportunities for research, assessment, and best practices. Through research in public health informatics, new ideas undergo thorough examination prior to implementation, and it aids in establishing priorities for the efficient allocation of resources, particularly in developing countries.

Keywords

Public health informatics · Health information · Interoperability · Standard

6.1 Policies Supporting Public Health Informatics

Public health informatics is employed in a governmental context, where it is essential for the responses to public events, laws, and regulations to be transparent and accountable. In order to effectively harness technology and data in the healthcare field, it is imperative for all stakeholders, including governments, legislators, providers, administrators, and the general public, to undergo a process of social change, leadership, and cultural transformation. This management of decisions and their execution concerning the Health Information System (HIS) is referred to as HIS governance [1, 2].

Nowadays, the health systems in developing nations are information-poor and data-rich characterized by having limited access to health information while possessing a wealth of data. As technology becomes increasingly prevalent and information exchange becomes more seamless through consolidation and shared information sources, healthcare services are expected to become less fragmented.

The absence of effective governance structures, policies, procedures, and uniform standards in the global health sector poses significant threats to the integrity of health services and the equitable provision of healthcare. Inefficiencies, wastage, fraud, and errors are perpetuated by inadequate governance, leading to compromised health services. This issue is particularly severe in Low and Middle-Income Countries (LMICs),

where public health informatics encounters similar challenges [3, 4].

Generating high-quality data in emerging nations is becoming increasingly challenging for health information systems. The absence of reliable health-related information hampers the development of effective health policies. According to a study, the performance of health information systems in underdeveloped countries will always be at risk without a national health information management plan. Hence, the production of high-quality data poses growing difficulties for health information systems in resource limited settings [5].

On the other hand, the efficient utilization of digital interventions in health systems necessitates the coordinated implementation of scalable, sustainable, and integrated digital solutions [6, 7]. Policies regarding digital health in developing countries must swiftly establish mechanisms for collaboration in order to avoid repeated and fragmented vertical implementations. It is crucial to manage solutions at scale and put an end to the recurring challenges of implementation.

When properly integrated, digital health solutions enable different healthcare provider systems to communicate, share data, and exchange information among themselves and with other technology and software programs [8]. This interoperability enhances the continuity of care. However, achieving interoperability requires effective policy implementation and oversight in the field of digital health. In addition to transforming the current care-focused model of healthcare delivery into a health-focused one, effective governance of digital health systems improves their performance and supports broader health objectives. The guiding values of good digital health governance include accountability, adherence to the rule of law, responsiveness, equity, efficiency, and confidentiality.

Following the introduction of various digital health solutions, such as electronic medical records, many countries have encountered challenges in executing well-informed investment decisions due to inadequate governance. It falls upon governments to promote digital transformation by enacting laws and policies that facilitate a conducive environment for its implementation. Creating an enabling environment involves factors like demonstrating high-level political commitment, establishing stable and predictable policy frameworks, implementing investment-friendly policies for the private sector, adopting best practices in regulation, and fostering increased demand for digital solutions.

Creating a conducive environment that promotes digital transformation across key pillars is of utmost importance. Regulators and policymakers need to remain abreast of technological advancements, address evolving regulatory landscapes, and establish the necessary foundations for digital transformation to reach its maximum potential. Being prepared for the advent of digital transformation and emerging technologies such as 5G, artificial intelligence (AI), and the Internet of Things (IoT) is crucial. To enable digital transformation across industries and nations, it is essential to establish modern, flexible, incentive-based, and market-driven legal, regulatory, and public policy frameworks [9].

Developing countries face various challenges related to resources and infrastructure when implementing long-term health information systems and digital health initiatives. The necessary infrastructure to support such implementations is often unevenly distributed and limited in quantity. Developing nations often experience structural deficiencies in their physical networks due to factors like high costs, geographical dispersion, and a large rural population. These issues are particularly pronounced in rural areas [10].

To ensure the success of any public health informatics implementation, it is crucial to anticipate and address potential obstacles. This is particularly vital in LMICs where instability and uncertainty are common. The issues that should be recognized and tackled includes the imperative to establish national agendas for digital health to attain sustainable implementations, strategies to address public concerns regarding privacy and security, the shared challenges of achieving interoperability faced by both developed and developing nations, and the importance of a skilled workforce in health informatics along with ongoing initiatives for its development.

Along with this, global health organizations like the World Health Organization (WHO) and their affiliated entities have been advocating for the development and adoption of sustainable and scalable health information technology (IT) solutions in healthcare settings with limited resources [11, 12]. The maturity of the ecosystem, encompassing information and communication technology (ICT) infrastructure and supporting components, plays a pivotal role in determining the suitability and impact of recommended digital health solutions. As outlined in Table 6.1 below, this encompasses workforce capabilities, standards and interoperability, leadership, governance mechanisms, regulatory and policy frameworks, strategic and financial investments, and sociocultural considerations,

Table 6.1 Aspects of the digital health policy landscape

Components	Description
Leadership and governance	It entails establishing national coordinating systems, garnering political support, aligning with health objectives, and involving relevant stakeholders
Strategy and investment	It includes guaranteeing funds to meet the strategy's goals and coordinating finance with health priorities
Services and applications	It includes the essential components and mechanisms required to facilitate the accessibility, utilization and distribution of health information to relevant stakeholders
Infrastructure	It encompasses the required physical infrastructure that underpin a country's digital health ecosystem
Standards and interoperability	It pertains to the guidelines that guarantee the uniform and precise gathering and exchange of data or information within diverse systems and providers
Health workforce	It includes the educational and training opportunities in the field of digital health

all of which are relevant to digital health initiatives [13].

6.2 Why Leadership and Governance in Digital Health?

Although many proven, accessible, and adaptable digital health solutions are already available to all countries, there is still an early stage of development for a global framework that brings together resources, knowledge, and strategies to fully leverage the impact of eHealth. While guidelines, procedures and resources to assist developing countries are being established, policymakers face challenges in integrating technology into their own health systems [14].

To establish a global digital health framework, low- and middle-income nations need to collaborate with international partners to build essential infrastructure. This includes developing national plans, enhancing skills, improving information and communication technology (ICT) infrastructure, and implementing governance mechanisms that strike a balance between innovation and data security.

To facilitate the effective utilization of technological interventions in the health sector and optimize healthcare service delivery, it is essential to have robust digital health governance and leadership. This mechanism oversees and enhances decision-making concerning digital health planning, funding, implementation, and monitoring by employing appropriate digital health policies, legislation, compliance, and standards. It is crucial to employ strategic policy frameworks alongside efficient coalition building, oversight, regulation, system design, and accountability considerations [15, 16]. Strong and enduring leadership and governance facilitate the integration of digital health investments with national health priorities, provide guidance, and ensure adherence to organizational standards and norms.

According to a study, developing nations, including those in Africa, require efficient health systems to achieve the SDGs health related goals and UHC [17, 18]. Nevertheless, most investments in these countries are focused on specific programs, driven by vertical partnerships, and thus have limited impact on the overall healthcare system. Due to a lack of capacity, these systems are unable to effectively gather comprehensive information among multiple programs, resulting in inadequate linkages among them.

Moreover, there is a deficiency in leadership capabilities to effectively implement technological health interventions that are tailored to meet local requirements.

Additionally, there is a lack of management and governance capability to implement digital health solutions that are responsive to local needs. Therefore, governance plays a crucial role in bringing together the diverse stakeholders required to support the widespread development and implementation of digital health systems at both national and international levels.

6.2.1 Factors for Successful Leadership and Governance in Digital Health

To achieve digital transformation in developing countries, it is imperative to have political commitment at the highest level, alignment of policies and sector regulations, and a significant increase in investment and allocation of resources towards the foundational pillars and critical sectors of digital transformation. Many countries are implementing digital health solutions, such as electronic medical records, digital disease surveillance systems, and social health insurance payment procedures. However, a comprehensive and holistic approach to digital health is often lacking, highlighting the need for effective governance to ensure successful adoption and long-term sustainability across the healthcare system.

This implies that good digital health governance serves as the cornerstone for bringing together stakeholders and policies that support efficient ICT within a robust health system. To accomplish this, the approaches employed to implement the digital health global strategy will differ based on the countries context, the priorities of countries health and well-being, and the specific needs and capacities of each country's digital infrastructure.

Countries and stakeholders were further encouraged to develop an action plan to realize this vision and align the eHealth vision with national health priorities and available resources [19]. The global strategy framework is guided by three principles, aimed at ensuring appropriateness and sustainability:

1. Recognize the importance of an integrated approach to maximize the effectiveness of digital health projects.
2. Promote the responsible application of digital health technology.
3. Address the key challenges faced by less developed nations in implementing digital health technologies and acknowledging their pressing need for resolution.

6.2.2 Domestic Digital Health Governance

Policymakers play a vital role in ensuring that domestic regulations on data governance enable the smooth exchange and transfer of health data across national borders. It is important for policymakers to prioritize policies that not only enable access to and sharing of health information but also promote data sharing. Presently, most regulations pertaining to health data prioritize the ability to disclose personal information for the common good, with limited emphasis on empowering individuals to restrict the use of their health data.

To ensure robust data protection within a country, policymakers should adopt an accountability-based approach. However, the adoption of best practices and standards for health data exchange is currently limited in many countries. According to the WHO's 2015 Atlas of eHealth Country Profiles, only 34% of the surveyed countries have established a framework to regulate the sharing of electronic health records (EHRs) among healthcare providers within the same country. Furthermore, only 22% have such a framework in place to regulate the sharing of EHRs between countries. Policies that facilitate data sharing for research purposes are even less common, with only 39% of nations having a framework to govern the exchange of personal and health information between research entities [20].

Hence, there is a need to establish a national interoperable digital health ecosystem that enables the sharing of health data between health information technology infrastructures across different countries, while ensuring compatibility and accommodating variations in national laws and policies. The essential components of digital health legislation, policy, and compliance necessary to facilitate the creation and operation of the national digital health ecosystem are outlined in Table 6.2.

6.2.3 Digital Health Governance Mechanisms

For a health information system to function effectively, it necessitates various policy administrative, organizational and financial prerequisites. Supportive laws and regulations are essential to ensure data privacy, security, ownership, sharing, and retention. Leadership and

Table 6.2 Components related to digital health legislation, policy and compliance

Components	Description
Legislation and policy	The legal, policy, and regulatory frameworks that govern the sharing, storage, and access of health information within and across countries are crucial. To foster the development of a national digital health ecosystem, comprehensive public health informatics policies are required to provide a more enabling environment
Digital health specific policy	Policies that specifically focus on safeguarding the privacy of health-related data stored in digital format play a critical role in shaping digital health services
Compliance	There are key elements that are necessary to enable the development of digital health products which are compatible to the nation's digital ecosystem

expertise at the national and subnational levels are also vital in overseeing data utilization and ensuring data quality. Additionally, infrastructure and policies must be established to facilitate the seamless exchange of information between producers and users within and beyond the healthcare system [21].

The healthcare systems face significant challenges that hinder the realization of the full potential of digital technologies. These obstacles encompass a range of issues, such as inadequate infrastructure investments, limited funding, insufficient human resources, high costs associated with scaling up, and coordination issues within the healthcare systems. Furthermore, the lack of systems thinking and design has contributed to the fragmentation and incompatibility of various applications, further impeding progress in this domain.

Improving workforce and public capacity, as well as strengthening governance and management of digital health, can contribute to enhancing information sharing, privacy, and security. In LMICs, it is crucial to prioritize initiatives such as establishing regulations for privacy and security, understanding existing security conditions and solutions, and selecting appropriate standards for patient identification and authentication. These measures are essential to ensure robust information security and protect the privacy of individuals in the digital health context [22, 23].

To successfully implement the HIS and digital health solutions across the healthcare system, several factors are crucial. These include engaging end users, developing a digital health strategy and strategic plan aligned with national health priorities, strengthening governance, and providing guidance and monitoring for HIS and digital health advancements. By addressing these factors, the deployment of HIS and digital health can be effectively carried out, ensuring their acceptance and utility within the healthcare system.

The decisions made by funders and policymakers, as well as the structures, roles and practices of the health sector, significantly influence the effectiveness of the information system.

Therefore, it is essential to establish a governance mechanism for health information systems (HIS) and digital health that fulfills the following objectives:

- Generate intelligence to inform policies, strategic plans, and decision-making processes.
- Develop policies and strategic plans to guide the operations and reforms of HIS.
- Implement tools to support the execution of policies and strategic plans, such as coordination mechanisms, concrete roadmaps and indicators for measuring progress.
- Ensure accountability by implementing transparent and controllable processes and procedures.

By adhering to these principles, the governance mechanism can enhance the effectiveness and efficiency of HIS and digital health initiatives, promoting better coordination and facilitating informed decision-making within the health sector of developing countries.

6.3 Health Information Exchange

6.3.1 Why Health Information Exchange?

In the healthcare domain, numerous interactions occur that involve healthcare professionals, patients, and other stakeholders, making it a highly transaction-intensive field. To ensure continuity of care, it is essential to foster efficient teamwork and enable the exchange of critical information among all parties involved. This exchange of health information among healthcare organizations is commonly referred to as health information exchange (HIE). By reducing redundant services and providing comprehensive information at the point of care, HIE has the potential to improve healthcare quality while simultaneously lowering costs.

The collection of data, clinical management, administrative procedures, and the care process are all hindered by the widespread dispersion and fragmentation of information across multiple sources, often operating in isolated silos. This challenge is prevalent in both developed and developing nations, and no country is exempt from its impact [21, 24].

As digital health technologies become increasingly prevalent in healthcare settings worldwide, Health Information Exchange (HIE) is gaining significant attention. HIE facilitates the sharing of data between healthcare institutions, particularly during pandemics, and contributes to improved patient safety, effectiveness and affordability of health care.

The development of policies and standards for Health Information Exchange (HIE) is vital in order to facilitate a seamless shift from independent technological applications to interconnected national digital health ecosystems. HIE strategies establish guidelines for the implementation of HIE within digital health systems. These policy and standards elements play a vital role in promoting seamless and effective data exchange within healthcare systems.

Effective client care management stems from well-coordinated communication between patients and healthcare providers. Patients have the right to control the disclosure of their health information, determining when and how it is shared. However, there is increasing concern regarding the security of electronically stored patient health information. Both healthcare workers and legislators anticipate that organizations will electronically share pertinent information, while also digitizing the data that healthcare workers rely on to provide optimal care to their clients [25].

The importance of fundamental requirements, such as interoperable data standards, is frequently overlooked, leading to limitations in data sharing and impeding the flow of information across multiple sites.

To achieve interoperability, all applications must adhere to established standards. Well-structured processes for acquiring, exchanging, assessing, and utilizing health-related data in decision-making are vital elements of a robust health information system. Strengthening coun-

tries health system structure necessitates the adoption and adaptation of global health information standards that align with broader initiatives aimed at improving the accessibility and quality of health information.

6.3.2   Privacy, Confidentiality and Security

When exchanging health information, it is essential to prioritize the security, confidentiality, and privacy of data. The concerns related to privacy, security, and confidentiality should encompass aspects such as data integrity, the potential misuse of illegally accessed client information, and compliance with laws and regulations that safeguard the public. It is worth noting that terms like security, confidentiality, and privacy may have varying interpretations. To provide clarity, the distinctions between these concepts are explained below.

6.3.2.1   Privacy

Within healthcare settings, privacy pertains to an individual's entitlement to control access to their personal data. It encompasses the freedom individuals possess to maintain the confidentiality and concealment of their personal information. Under this definition, private information is not shared with any third party without explicit consent. Individuals retain the authority to determine what information they disclose, to whom, and in what manner. Privacy is a foundational principle within the client-health professional relationship, playing a vital role in facilitating the effective delivery of healthcare services.

Threats to client privacy and information security can be classified into two main categories. Firstly, there are organizational threats that arise from improper access to client data. These threats can occur when internal individuals abuse their privileges or external agents exploit vulnerabilities in information systems. Secondly, there are systemic threats that occur when an agent within the information flow chain misuses the disclosed data for purposes other than the intended ones.

The intersection of privacy policies and public health raises a fundamental conflict between the right to privacy and the need for accessible information by public health organizations to enable population tracking and monitoring. With the increasing availability of electronic data about individuals, the public is becoming more aware of privacy concerns and more capable of engaging in public health initiatives. Addressing these challenges on a daily basis necessitates transparency, as public health workers must maintain the trust of the communities they serve to effectively carry out their duties.

6.3.2.2 Confidentiality

Confidentiality ensures that personally identifiable information is not shared without consent (unless mandated by law), as its disclosure would infringe upon the right to privacy. Within this framework, "identifying information" encompasses any data, whether demographic or not, that can identify individual clients or papers. In the context of healthcare, it refers to the obligation placed on professionals with access to patient information to maintain its privacy.

Confidentiality can also be understood as privileged communication between two individuals in a professional relationship, such as a client and a healthcare provider. The level of confidentiality of an institution's data largely depends on the technical, administrative, and physical safeguards it has implemented to safeguard its systems.

Public health organizations regularly handle sensitive data that is legally mandated to be protected, making confidentiality a significant concern for them. The regulations should encompass electronic information systems, necessitating confidentiality standards that restrict the disclosure of data. These standards are necessary to prevent inadvertent identification of individuals during the data release process.

6.3.2.3 Security

Security encompasses various measures and mechanisms that prevent unauthorized access to or alteration of health information and health information systems. With the increasing use of electronic health record systems, the need for specific regulations regarding electronic health information has become more apparent. The objective is to safeguard personally identifiable information stored electronically while ensuring healthcare providers have appropriate access to data and flexibility in utilizing technology, while considering administrative and technical safeguards.

System security includes safeguards related to hardware, software, personnel, and institutional regulations. Data security focuses on protecting data and computer programs from unwanted events and exposures. It involves implementing confidentiality policies in computer systems, such as access control, data integrity, and system availability. A comprehensive security solution should encompass administrative measures (such as limiting employee access rights and providing support for security policies), technical measures (such as firewalls, encryption, and digital certificates), and physical measures (such as locked doors and security patrols). Establishing comprehensive confidentiality policies lays the foundation for developing an effective security system to uphold them.

6.3.3 Information Sharing in Public Health Information

The value of information lies in its utilization, sharing, and documentation. To facilitate this, nations can promote sharing of information by establishing and implementing organizational structures, standards for information and robust security measures. By doing so, they create a framework that promotes effective and secure information exchange [23].

In order to effectively address public health concerns, it is necessary to have access to highly sensitive, personally identifiable information. However, the acquisition of this information requires a careful balance between societal needs and individual liberties. Public health practices have a commendable track record of upholding the privacy of information collected from indi-

Table 6.3 Safeguards to protect privacy, security and integrity of health information

Physical safeguards	The measures include device isolation, which involves limiting direct physical access to authorized health workers, as well as data backup and copying.
Technical safeguards	It consists of firewalls and safe communication channels such virtual private networks and encryption methods.
Administrative safeguards	It includes organizational security policies accompanied by training for personnel to ensure their understanding and adherence to these policies. Enforcing policies that govern the storage and retention of electronic data and system backups is crucial. Additionally, it is important to clearly document accountability measures for any violations of policies and procedures.

viduals, with very few exceptions. This ensures that individuals will continue to be willing to provide public health professionals with sensitive information and helps to maintain community trust. In developing nations, preventing the unintentional identification of specific individuals through the use of aggregated health data remains a challenge.

Hence, public health institutions need to establish and effect confidentiality regulations that address the management and dissemination of health related information, while adhering to the principles of fair information practices. Developing and implementing these standards with clear definitions of privacy, confidentiality, and security is essential to prevent the unauthorized disclosure of protected health information. Additionally, ensuring public trust in integrated information systems relies on thoughtful consideration of privacy and confidentiality protections, which ultimately contribute to the advancement of public health.

Preserving the privacy of electronically stored patient data is widely recognized as the foremost ethical concern in public health informatics. However, the profession also grapples with a range of additional ethical dilemmas, including the appropriate utilization and application of informatics technologies in clinical settings [26]. Moreover, public health informatics gives rise to significant legal and regulatory considerations. To ensure the confidentiality, security, and accuracy of recorded health information, health care workers are granted appropriate access for client care and management. This is accomplished through the implementation of physical, technical, and administrative measures, as shown in Table 6.3.

6.4 Health Information Systems Interoperability

Interoperability refers to the ability of various information systems, devices, and applications to integrate and use data or information in an organized approach. This collaboration occurs within and among regional or national boundaries to enhance individual and community health and facilitate the efficient delivery of healthcare services.

Interoperability involves the capacity of multiple information systems to effectively exchange and utilize information according to established standards. This enables the smooth and timely transfer of information, maximizing health outcomes worldwide.

Interoperability entails the ability of two or more information systems or components to utilize and exchange information based on established standards. This enables the seamless and timely portability of information, optimizing the health outcomes of individuals and populations globally. Through interoperability, different health information systems can collaborate within and beyond organizational boundaries to enhance health of the community and improve the efficiency of healthcare provision. Health data exchange frameworks, application interfaces, and standards enable the accurate and secure access and sharing of data across the entire spectrum of care, in various contexts and with relevant stakeholders, including individuals [27, 28].

When multiple organizations merge, it is crucial for all systems and technologies to effectively share data in various formats and structures. This transparent sharing and exchange of information present complex challenges related to compatibility and interoperability. The architecture must enable the integration of work across multiple disciplines, allowing integrated teams to provide comprehensive care to a single client, even when they are geographically dispersed and belong to different organizations.

Data interoperability plays a vital role in ensuring the secure, reliable, and consistent transfer of data between devices, applications, and platforms. It is essential for maximizing the efficient use of health information [29]. Interoperability is primarily characterized by the ability of systems to communicate with each other through a shared channel, indicating compatibility between them. In the context of a specific task, two applications are considered interoperable when one application can receive data from the other, including service requests, and successfully and satisfactorily complete the task without requiring additional intervention from an operator, as determined by the user of the receiving system.

The interoperability stack comprises three layers:

1. The communication and transport layer, which focuses on the mechanisms and protocols for exchanging information between systems.
2. The document layer, which addresses the format of messages and documents exchanged, as well as the coding systems utilized.
3. The business process layer, which involves the interaction choreography. In this layer,

two applications must agree on interfaces in order to achieve interoperability.

Please refer to Fig. 6.1 below for a visual representation (Fig. 6.1).

6.4.1   Why Interoperability?

The lack of interoperability is widely recognized as a significant barrier to the adoption and effective implementation of digital health technologies and the broader digital transformation of healthcare. This challenge is particularly evident in low and middle-income countries, where the diversity of health information systems hampers the adoption of health interoperability standards.

Large healthcare organizations cannot rely on a single health information system to fulfill their clinical and administrative information technology requirements. Therefore, achieving interoperability becomes crucial in such fragmented environments, necessitating the establishment of interoperability standards.

In regions like Africa, the lack of integration and interoperability among diverse health systems presents a major obstacle to realizing the potential benefits of digital health. Incompatibility between health information systems leads to wasted resources and compromised quality of client management. Consequently, there is an urgent need to develop integration methods that

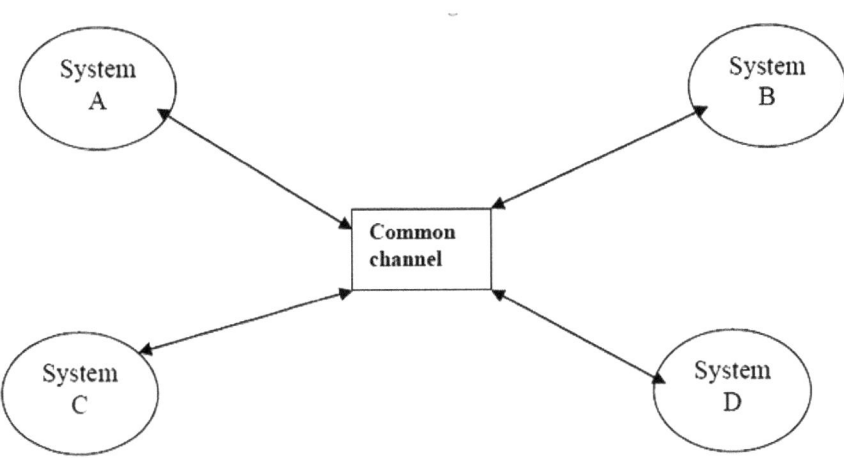

Fig. 6.1 Interoperability between systems

bridge the gap between various health information systems [30, 31].

Interoperability in digital health does not rely on a single standard. Instead, numerous standards, specifications, and profiles have emerged from different organizations and initiatives, addressing specific interoperability requirements. In comparison to sectors like banking, mobile communications and commerce, healthcare has lagged behind in achieving concrete examples of interoperable data flows while maintaining competition. The lack of interoperability poses a significant obstacle to the digital transformation of healthcare.

It is widely recognized that unlocking the potential of digitalization in the healthcare industry requires breaking down data silos and enabling improved sharing and flow of data. Concrete examples of this potential include:

- Advanced clinical decision support, where easily accessible patient-centric information can enhance diagnosis and treatment.
- Data sharing in standardized formats that all stakeholders can understand, leading to improved care coordination.
- Empowering clients with access to their own medical records, enabling them to actively manage their conditions and strive for a healthy lifestyle.
- Streamlining workflows and facilitating outcomes-driven improvement cycles through operational data.

The lack of interoperability in health information systems leads to inconsistent data collection, increased susceptibility to misunderstandings and challenges or impossibility in effective communication. To address these issues, it is crucial to establish an organization or leadership group dedicated to ensuring interoperability from a governance standpoint. Interoperability plays a vital role in delivering better care at a reduced cost, leading to improved patient outcomes and career support. Achieving these objectives requires the widespread interpretation and free accessibility of relevant data.

The importance of interoperable digital health systems cannot be overstated in today's healthcare landscape. Without the ability of health information systems (HISs) to exchange information, the full benefits of investments in digital health become harder to realize. Interoperability enables fast access to client information whenever and wherever it is needed. Additionally, it reduces the need for redundant data capture in each system and mitigates the challenges associated with entering the same data multiple times, minimizing data capture issues.

The importance of implementing interoperability standards in the healthcare industry is widely recognized, as the compatibility between health information systems is essential for the success of digital health projects and ICT benefits in general. There are several significant advantages associated with the use of interoperability standards. Firstly, standards play a crucial role in facilitating and supporting the delivery of improved health services. They enable seamless data exchange and interoperability between different systems, leading to enhanced coordination and continuity of care. Secondly, interoperability standards yield financial gains by streamlining processes, reducing duplication of efforts and promoting efficiency in healthcare operations. By enabling the seamless flow of information, standards contribute to cost savings and resource optimization.

The implementation of interoperability standards in the healthcare industry brings numerous advantages, including improved health services, financial gains, enhanced safety and collaboration facilitation [30]. Most importantly, interoperability standards enhance the safety of front-line service delivery, benefiting individuals as a whole. It ensures that accurate and relevant information is available when needed, supporting informed decision-making and reducing the risk of errors or miscommunication. Standards also serve as a common ground for collaboration when multiple software systems need to work together. For example, if two systems utilize comparable terminology for recording information, they can exchange valuable data despite having distinct user interfaces, thus promoting interoperability and data sharing.

Interoperability in healthcare offers significant benefits to all stakeholders involved in the delivery and receipt of healthcare, as described below:

- **Individuals:** People can experience improved treatment quality and safety, with healthcare available when and where it is needed. Interoperability enables the creation of integrated care plans by healthcare providers from multiple organizations, ensuring comprehensive and well-coordinated healthcare.
- **Healthcare practitioners:** By strengthening coordination across various care delivery sites, healthcare practitioners have the opportunity to enhance the quality and safety of the care they provide. Interoperability allows practitioners to access comprehensive patient information, enabling informed decision-making and ultimately improving the overall quality of care.
- **Efficiency:** Interoperability reduces redundant data entry, such as entering the same demographic information multiple times. This streamlines processes and enhances efficiency for both individuals and healthcare professionals, freeing up time for more focused patient care.
- **Cost reductions:** Interoperability has the potential to yield cost reductions through various means. These include minimizing unnecessary tests and procedures, facilitating early disease detection, and reducing expenses associated with adverse events. Improved client outcomes contribute to long-term cost savings in the healthcare system.
- **Access to care:** Interoperability enables quicker access to care, diagnosis, and treatment of illnesses. The efficiency benefits resulting from the adoption of healthcare interoperability standards benefit both providers and clients, leading to reduced costs and improved healthcare access.

In summary, interoperability in healthcare brings significant advantages, including improved treatment quality and safety for individuals, enhanced coordination and care quality for practitioners, increased efficiency through reduced redundant data entry, potential cost reductions, and improved access to care for both health care pro-viders and clients. These benefits contribute to better healthcare outcomes and cost-effectiveness in the healthcare system.

6.4.2   Types of Interoperability

To facilitate the interoperability and meaningful exchange of data between systems, health information standards need to address both the structure (syntax) and meaning (semantics) of the exchanged data. In the field of public health informatics, interoperability standards can be categorized into three main types: semantic interoperability, syntactic interoperability, and foundational/technical interoperability. These standards, when combined, enable secure, efficient, and timely data exchange across nations, organizations, institutions, and individuals. The following section describes the various types of interoperability in more detail [22].

6.4.2.1 Semantic Interoperability

Semantic interoperability, also known as knowledge level interoperability, refers to the ability of different information systems, components, applications, and services to communicate information based on agreed-upon definitions of terms and expressions. It allows multiple systems or elements to share and utilize information effectively.

Semantic interoperability utilizes both the language and structure of data exchange to ensure that receiving information technology systems can understand the data. This level of interoperability facilitates the electronic sharing of client summary data, client-provided wellness data, and health-related financial data among authorized parties and caregivers. It enables the integration of potentially incompatible mobile technologies, medical equipment, electronic health record (EHR) systems, and other systems to enhance wellness and improve the availability, affordability, safety, and quality of healthcare services.

Furthermore, semantic compatibility ensures that users can receive and interpret the communicated information. Semantic interoperability plays a crucial role in the healthcare industry through semantic mediation, which involves translating healthcare messages defined in one standard format into another. By utilizing pre-established shared meanings for concepts, semantic interoperability allows different systems to interpret transferred data in a consistent manner. The publication, maintenance, and retrieval of semantic services within a repository are important for achieving this level of interoperability.

Semantic interoperability goes beyond simple data transfer and encompasses the interpretation of data. According to the HL7 group, semantic interoperability is the process of communicating data in a way that both the originating and receiving information systems understand it in the same manner. This type of interoperability focuses on standardizing data representation to ensure comprehension across different information systems.

Unlike human-centric aspects, semantic interoperability primarily addresses the interactions between information systems, including programming, information transmission, and information utilization. It plays a vital role in healthcare interoperability by enabling disparate information systems to understand shared data at the application level. This promotes more efficient, secure, confidential, and higher-quality healthcare delivery [29, 32, 33].

6.4.2.2 Syntactic Interoperability

Syntactic interoperability is achieved when two or more systems agree to communicate and exchange data using agreed-upon formats. However, it does not guarantee that the recipient will receive and interpret the message accurately. Syntactic interoperability relies on predefined data formats, communication protocols, and similar elements to ensure communication and data exchange. While the shared information can be processed by the respective systems, there is no guarantee of consistent interpretation. Semantic interoperability is employed to ensure the interoperability of message content as received by the end-user.

The challenges associated with syntactic interoperability include:

1. Identifying Elements in Various Systems: One challenge is identifying all the elements present in different systems that need to communicate with each other.
2. Establishing Rules for Element Structuring: Defining rules for how these elements should be structured to enable effective communication and data exchange is another challenge.
3. Mapping and Bridging Equivalent Elements: Creating mappings, bridges, and crosswalks between equivalent elements using schemas is crucial to ensure compatibility between different systems.
4. Agreeing on Equivalent Rules: Agreeing on equivalent rules to bridge different cataloguing and registry systems is necessary to facilitate interoperability.

6.4.2.3 Technical Interoperability

Technical interoperability facilitates data sharing between different systems, but it does not guarantee that the receiving system can effectively utilize the shared data in a meaningful manner. It focuses on the transfer of data between systems without the systems having an understanding of the significance of the data being exchanged.

The primary objective of technical interoperability is to enable the transmission of data rather than its interpretation. It emphasizes the tools and processes involved in data transfer, with a primary focus on hardware-related characteristics such as interfaces and protocols. By leveraging underlying networks, protocols, and a well-established communication architecture, technical interoperability enables the exchange of data across various information systems.

For example, information systems allow a healthcare worker to request a client's medical record from another health worker, regardless of their geographical distance. This communication capability is made possible by technical compatibility. Even when two experts are physically separated, there is a means of communication and sharing of health data. Technical interoperability thus helps overcome the impact of distance and facilitates the interchange of healthcare data through the utilization of networks, hardware, software, and various other technological instru-

Table 6.4 Levels of interoperability

Levels of interoperability	Description
Semantic interoperability	Ensure that the phrases and idioms used in data exchange have agreed-upon and consistent interpretations
Syntactic interoperability	Change information using a pre-established data structure and format
Technical interoperability	Enable technical end-to-end data interchange between systems

ments. Levels of interoperability are summarized in Table 6.4 below.

Achieving interoperability relies on the following components:

1. **Adoption and optimization:** The implementation and optimization of Health Information Exchange (HIE) services and Electronic Health Records (EHRs) are crucial for attaining interoperability. In many low-middle income countries, healthcare workers and organizations traditionally kept client medical records on paper, limiting access to one person at a time in a specific location. The adoption of electronic files allows for secure and simultaneous information flow among authorized users in different locations, enabling better care coordination.

2. **Privacy and security:** Clients must have confidence that their health information will be protected and secured, especially when it is shared across different care sites. All stakeholders involved in healthcare delivery, including the government, developers, health plans, providers, and clients, share the responsibility of ensuring privacy and security.

3. **Rules of engagement:** A framework is needed to establish and implement trusted national exchange practices that promote good governance within and across communities. This framework encompasses four categories of principles:

   - **Trust principles:** Educate health information exchange governance entities on data management, meaningful choice and client privacy.
   - **Business principles:** Focus on prudent financial and operational policies to safeguard the best interests of clients, empha-

sizing transparency and the sharing of health information.
   - **Technical principles:** Prioritize the application of standards to enhance interoperability implementation while upholding trust and business principles.
   - **Organizational principles:** Develop broadly applicable approaches for effective self-governance.

6.5   Health Information Standards

Standards are a set of guidelines established by international organizations such as Health Level Seven (HL7), Integrating the Healthcare Enterprise (IHE), World Health Organization (WHO), and the International Organization for Standardization (ISO). These standards enable uniform and consistent sharing and processing of data. By providing common naming conventions and data models, these standards prevent isolated and non-scalable implementations, making it easier to share information across the digital health ecosystem. Notable examples include the International Classification of Diseases (ICD) by the WHO.

ISO defines standards as documents created through consensus and authorized by official organizations. They offer norms, guidelines, or specifications for actions or their outcomes, aiming to achieve the highest level of order in a specific situation. These specifications are intended for consistent and repeated use.

A widely accepted and reliable mechanism for capturing and sharing health information is the healthcare data interchange standard. In the context of healthcare, data standards refer to procedures, terminologies, and guidelines that govern the capture and exchange of various healthcare applications such as medical records, prescription drugs and organizational procedures.

Standardizing healthcare data encompasses several aspects, including:

- **Definition of data elements:** Clearly defining the specific data elements that are relevant to healthcare information exchange.
- **Data interchange formats:** Establishing standardized formats for the exchange of healthcare data, ensuring compatibility and interoperability between different systems.
- **Terminologies:** Employing standardized terminology systems to ensure consistent and accurate representation of medical concepts and terms.
- **Knowledge representation:** Utilizing standardized methods to represent medical knowledge, enabling effective sharing and interpretation of healthcare information.

In summary, healthcare data standardization involves defining data elements, determining data interchange formats, implementing standardized terminologies, and employing knowledge representation techniques. These measures promote consistency and enhance the exchange and utilization of healthcare information [34].

Data interoperability is a crucial component of modern health information technology. In order to exchange essential data and leverage the vast amounts of collected data for research, trend analysis, safety improvements, and cost reduction, healthcare information systems must be interoperable. Accessible data standards play a vital role in facilitating interoperability [35]. Standards are essential for various aspects of digital health systems, including interoperability, data interchange, data analysis and storage, data security and privacy, and data-driven decision-making. Guidelines covering different mediums, content, and transit formats should be followed when exchanging health data.

To enable consistent communication among health information systems across regional and national boundaries, healthcare interoperability standards have been established. Without standardized formats for reporting electronic data,

the correct acceptance, analysis, and aggregation of such data by public health systems would be costly and unfeasible. By adopting global standards, countries can save significant resources and make substantial progress more efficiently.

Standardizing digital health, in particular, is an inherently complex field. It involves linking various stakeholders, including hospitals, pharmacies, healthcare providers, clients in their homes, and administrative organizations such as insurance companies or government agencies. Each of these entities possesses a wide range of installed technologies, information systems, and medical devices, often built to proprietary specifications.

One of the major challenges in achieving technical standardization is the electronic integration of these diverse entities. The sensitive nature of health data requires robust privacy safeguards, quality assurance measures, and stringent security protocols, further complicating the standardization landscape in digital health. Isolated or non-communicative public health systems can be attributed to several key factors:

1. **Functional requirements:** Variations in design can arise from the specific functions served by different systems, such as case management versus population surveillance.
2. **System architecture:** Failure to consider the importance of system integration and architecture when constructing new systems can result in isolated and non-integrated systems. Standardization plays a critical role in facilitating system integration.
3. **Variations among exchange partners:** In public health, there is a diverse range of exchange partners, making it challenging to achieve consensus and integrate a single norm. These partners include hospitals, laboratories, public health groups, the general public, individuals with personal health records, and other institutions generating data.

In summary, the complexity of standardizing digital health arises from the diverse stakeholders involved, the need for robust privacy and security measures, and challenges related to functional requirements, system architecture, variations among exchange partners, and policy requirements. Overcoming these barriers is crucial for achieving effective interoperability and advancing digital health initiatives.

6.5.1 Why Standards in Health Care?

The lack of standardized data standards and the incompatibility of healthcare information systems have been persistent challenges in the field of health informatics. Healthcare interoperability issues arise from gaps in data standards, the presence of multiple overlapping standards, diverse groups developing data standards, and the absence of a centralized system overseeing their creation and application.

Recognizing the need for standardized terminology and data standards in the healthcare industry has been long-standing. The urgency for initiatives like electronic health record sharing and health information exchanges is growing, further emphasizing the importance of these standards.

Public health informatics standards continue to evolve due to several reasons:

1. **Growth in the field of public health**: As new tools for diagnosis and treatment are developed, new ideas emerge alongside existing ones. This gradual progression leads to the expansion of semantic code sets and the development of format or syntax standards, incorporating new disciplines as necessary.
2. **Changing healthcare organization and delivery:** The way healthcare is organized and delivered is constantly evolving. Various stakeholders, including healthcare organizations, public authorities, insurers, citizens and clients, shape and maximize their resources and procedures based on their roles, responsibilities, decision-making authority, liabilities, and mutual dependencies. This process gives rise to new procedures and care delivery methods, necessitating the creation of new workflow or domain standards. For example, the increasing importance of tele-monitoring services for remote patient monitoring.
3. **Evolving laws and regulations:** New or evolving laws impose organizational and technical constraints on healthcare delivery, often requiring new interoperability criteria. Rapid changes may introduce new areas that require standards or necessitate the development of standards to address unique functional aspects like data privacy and patient consent. Public authorities are increasingly providing top-down incentives and direction to promote greater interoperability.
4. **Rapid advancements in ICT standards and technologies:** Information and communication technology (ICT) standards and technologies are constantly evolving at a fast pace. Public health informatics standards need to adapt and take advantage of these advancements.

In summary, public health informatics standards evolve due to the growth of the field, changes in healthcare organization and delivery, evolving laws and regulations, and advancements in ICT standards and technologies. Adapting and updating these standards is crucial to keep pace with progress and facilitate interoperability in public health information systems. The establishment and adherence to data standards are crucial for expediting interoperability. Data standards and interoperability play pivotal roles in leveraging healthcare information technology for positive healthcare reforms.

Standardization is a fundamental requirement for achieving interoperability. The current landscape of diverse and competing standards poses significant challenges to the standardization of digital health. Many standards overlap, compete, and even contradict each other. Consequently, standardization provides a valuable framework for effective communication and the realization of interoperability. Various standards development organizations (SDOs) contribute to facilitating complex levels of interoperability.

The adoption and promotion of standards, as well as active participation in their development, are more urgent than ever due to the expanding use of electronic data interchange in public health. To overcome the significant obstacles hindering standards adoption, the field of public health and its numerous stakeholders need to reach consensus on the selection and value of standards. Joint agreement on standards is essential to advance interoperability efforts.

6.5.2   Type of Standards

In general, standards can be categorized into two main types: proprietary and open. Proprietary standards are developed by profit-driven industry groups for their specific purposes. These standards are typically kept confidential and protected by copyright laws. On the other hand, open standards can be created by both profit and non-profit organizations. They are available for use by anyone interested, with the required documents and specifications accessible to the public. In the realm of public health informatics, standards can be further subdivided into process or data standards.

Process standards encompass procedures and policies, covering aspects such as architecture, workflow, security rules, data use agreements, and metadata standards. These standards often overlap with data standards. Data or content standards, on the other hand, focus on common terms and methods that enhance data sharing between systems. They consist of vocabulary and format components.

To achieve interoperability in health information exchange, adherence to standards for healthcare data interchange is crucial. Public healthcare standards can often fall into one or more of the following categories based on their functionality:

1. **Terminology standards:** These standards provide guidelines, coding systems, terminology and accepted language for data transfer between computer systems. They serve as a dictionary of sorts for the healthcare domain.
2. **Messaging standards:** Messaging standards define common structures for exchanging clinical data, financial information, and medical images among different institutions and service providers.
3. **Document standards:** Document standards establish a common format for sharing and documenting medical and patient demographic data, including information like prescriptions and illness details.
4. **Application standards:** Application standards outline standardized methods for integrating and operating various healthcare applications seamlessly.
5. **Legal standards:** Legal standards describe the rules, legislation, and guidelines related to patient confidentiality.

Interoperability and digital health standards enable the consistent and accurate gathering and exchange of health information across geographic and health sector boundaries. Without these elements, it would be challenging or even impossible to exchange health information due to data structure and terminology incompatibilities, inconsistent data collection practices and the potential for misinterpretation. The examples of common digital health standards are described below in Table 6.5.

Table 6.5 Examples of common digital health standards and interoperability components

Component	Description
Data structure standards	To ensure the proper handling and interpretation of health datasets, these standards define guidelines for presenting the information within software applications and maintaining it using standardized data structures.
Common terminologies	These standards facilitate the adoption of a unified language for electronic information communication, enabling consistent descriptions of symptoms, diagnoses and treatments.
Secure messaging standards	To ensure secure communication and accurate delivery of information to the intended recipient, these standards pertain to secure transmission and delivery of messages, as well as the proper identification of message recipients.
Software accreditation standards	These standards establish the criteria that digital health software products and services must meet in order to obtain certification, enabling them to seamlessly exchange health information within the country's digital health ecosystem.

6.6 Regulatory Operations

The laws and regulations that pertain to healthcare organizations handling personal information generally extend to the collection, use, and dissemination of public health information. While certain regulations may exempt specific public health functions, it is crucial to carefully consider these exemptions to fully understand their implications and limitations. Healthcare information systems administrators need to stay vigilant about legal developments in this dynamic environment and be ready to adapt policies and procedures in line with evolving national and international laws and healthcare standards.

The healthcare industry has generated vast amounts of complex and diverse data due to record-keeping, regulatory compliance, and client care. However, if health informatics and the data it generates are not effectively managed and utilized, clients will not benefit from the valuable information it holds. Currently, there is a growing trend towards rapid digitization of these extensive data sets, as evidenced by the recent computerization of healthcare facilities worldwide, particularly in underdeveloped countries [35].

To ensure the sustainability, quality, safety, and security of advanced health technologies and digital health products used in the healthcare industry, it is necessary to establish policies, regulations, and standards. Both healthcare providers and clients need to have confidence in the confidentiality and security of a client's health information in order to fully harness the potential of digital health information for improving health outcomes, making informed budget decisions, and promoting overall well-being [36, 37].

In an interoperable digital health ecosystem, all clients, health service providers, and other stakeholders are subject to a rigorous and reliable process of digital identification, authentication, and authorization. This process ensures trust in the secure sharing of health data and complies with nationally appropriate methods. These measures are implemented both from an organizational and legal perspective to uphold the integrity of the ecosystem [19].

Clients within healthcare systems rely on their trust in the individuals responsible for safeguarding their private data. While these concerns are present globally, they can have particularly severe consequences in underdeveloped nations where legal systems may offer less support for digital initiatives. Moreover, security concerns and legal responsibilities can pose significant challenges during the implementation process.

The establishment of legal and regulatory frameworks surrounding the creation and utilization of health information is crucial. These frameworks enable the development of systems that ensure data accessibility, interchange, quality, and sharing. Particularly regarding a health information system's ability to access data from non-health and public health sectors, as well as both, legislation and regulation play a paramount role. A legal framework can also define ethical guidelines for data collection and dissemination.

Health information policies should outline key stakeholders and their coordination mechanisms, ensure program oversight, and establish accountability procedures. Institutional policies within health organizations should outline distinct functions to protect data integrity and promote accountability.

Government regulatory agencies contribute to the development of regulations that facilitate the adoption of electronic health records. To ensure that clients and healthcare professionals have timely access to high-quality, safe, and effective digital health products and services, regulations must strike a balance between fostering innovation and expedited technology access while upholding ethical standards and data protection considerations. Regulation plays a crucial role in instilling public and user confidence regarding the reliability of the system and the use of data, software, and devices in healthcare delivery [38].

Public health organizations have essential responsibilities in gathering, analyzing, and disseminating information about illnesses and health conditions. This information can be obtained from various sources, including clinical records from healthcare providers, statistics from health plans, and research conducted by agencies. In developing nations, provider records are particularly valuable in generating information. Such data can be shared through different processes and systems or consolidated in disease registries, providing valuable insights into disease prevention and promoting good health.

Limited financial resources may jeopardize patient privacy in developing nations, making it challenging to adopt advanced health information security tools or make significant investments in educating medical staff about the ethical standards associated with the use of new communication and digital technologies in the field [15, 39].

To enhance the use of eHealth, it is crucial to leverage existing frameworks and, where necessary, develop robust and sustainable regulatory frameworks. Standardization is also essential at both national and international levels to establish an interoperable digital health ecosystem.

Developing modern and integrated health information systems is vital to facilitate service delivery and informed decision-making in healthcare. These systems generate reliable data for relevant users and stakeholders. Key components of this foundation include data transformation, integration, archiving, management, and analytics. This involves identifying relevant data sources, extracting and harmonizing data for analysis, establishing and maintaining secure data repositories, enforcing data governance guidelines, improving data exchange standards, and utilizing powerful data analytics tools.

Many healthcare systems will need to make political and legislative adjustments to fully leverage digital health in achieving universal healthcare goals and integrating it seamlessly into daily healthcare services. Additionally, to unlock the full potential of digital health, the legal framework surrounding healthcare provision must be modified. Therefore, a comprehensive legal framework for digital health is necessary to govern the sharing and application of data between healthcare professionals and clients.

An effective legal framework must also encompass data quality and integrity, serving as the basis for clinical and patient decision-making. It should provide provisions for modi-

fying professional liability regulations to accommodate digitally or remotely delivered care. It is essential to ensure that legislation addresses the procurement of digital health tools, such as electronic health records (EHRs), telemedicine systems, and monitoring systems, and that medical devices have provisions for ensuring system interoperability. In addition to conventional legal considerations such as privacy and liability, these aspects are crucial to be covered by the legal framework [39].

While legislative frameworks have made progress in incorporating essential digital health tools like electronic health records, many countries still need to establish robust governance to facilitate the integration of mHealth and telehealth technologies into healthcare delivery systems. This is particularly evident in developing nations, where there is a lack of consistency in meeting the legislative requirements for full integration into healthcare systems. This undermines the potential return on investment and the ability of digital health to accelerate the achievement of universal health coverage targets.

6.6.1   Enforcement of Policies and Regulations

Evidence indicates that progress has been made in the development and enforcement of policies and regulations in public health informatics. According to the WHO Global Health Observatory Report, only 33% of member countries have legislative policies for eHealth services. This suggests that general regulations for eHealth are evolving slowly but steadily. However, 47% of states have laws in place to support the security, quality, and standards of health-related data.

Regarding the enactment of laws concerning the privacy of health data, 78% of member nations have laws protecting the privacy of personal data, and 55% have laws protecting the privacy of electronically stored patient data. However, laws facilitating the global exchange of electronic health record data for patient treatment are being adopted slowly. Only 22% of member states have laws addressing the exchange of health-related patient data globally, compared to 34% who reported that their laws cover sharing such data among healthcare practitioners within their own country.

The development of patient rights concerning electronically stored health data is progressing steadily. Approximately 29% of countries have enacted laws to ensure patients' access to electronic health records (EHRs), while a similar 28% reported that laws grant authority clients to specify who can retrieve their records. In terms of data accuracy, 32% of respondents stated that patients can request corrections to inaccuracies in their EHRs, but only 18% allow for the removal of specific entries.

6.6.2 Key Regulatory Issues

Many countries, including those in developing nations, now have national policies or strategies on digital health. Therefore, it is crucial for developing nations to establish regulatory standards and guidelines that address the key regulatory issues associated with the use of health applications, in addition to their national policies and strategies on digital health. Studies have indicated that standards, privacy, confidentiality, and security should be the primary regulatory objectives for digital health [40].

The utilization of big data analytics in health informatics holds great potential for transforming how healthcare professionals leverage advanced technology to extract knowledge from their clinical and data repositories, enabling informed decision-making. The future adoption of big data analytics in healthcare organizations and the sector as a whole is expected to be rapid and widespread. However, several key issues need to be addressed (as shown in Table 6.6) to ensure privacy, security, establish standards and governance, and continuously advance the tools and technology associated with big data analytics.

While health information technology has the potential to enhance patient safety and improve the quality of care, it also introduces new risks and hazards. Regulators are increasingly identifying the potential negative consequences of health information technology, even though positive uses of technology and digital maturity are strongly correlated with overall organizational quality. Commonly recognized factors that negatively impact quality and safety include inadequate technology usability, challenges in accessing systems and data, and improper use of health information technology.

To effectively guide future practices and legislation, it is imperative to have a comprehensive understanding of the risks and benefits of health information technology from the perspectives of all stakeholders, including patients, end-users, providers, and regulators. This holistic approach ensures that the diverse needs and concerns of all parties are taken into account [41]. Key regulatory issues relevant for public health informatics are summarized below.

Key regulatory issues pertinent to public health informatics in resource-limited settings include:

Table 6.6 Security measures in health information system and digital health

Security measure	Description
Administrative Safeguards	Administrative safeguards refer to the set of rules, practices, and activities implemented to prevent, detect, mitigate, and respond to security breaches. These safeguards encompass the entire process of selecting, developing, implementing, and maintaining security procedures aimed at protecting health information.
Physical Safeguards	These precautions encompass physical barriers, regulations, and guidelines that ensure the safety of associated structures, equipment, and electronic information systems from external threats, as well as natural and human-induced risks. These protective measures involve the use of technology, alongside guidelines and protocols that govern the management of access to health information and the associated infrastructure.
Policies and Procedures	To meet the requirements of the security rule, it is necessary to implement appropriate and sufficient policies and processes.

- Data Access and Ownership: Ensuring appropriate access to and ownership of data, defining who has rights to access and control the data.
- Privacy and Confidentiality: Establishing safeguards to protect the privacy and confidentiality of patient information in digital health systems.
- Informed Consent for Data Use: Defining procedures and requirements for obtaining informed consent from patients for the use of their data in digital health initiatives.
- Access Rights to Patient Data: Establishing guidelines for access rights to patient data, ensuring appropriate and authorized access by healthcare providers.
- Data Integrity: Ensuring the accuracy, completeness, and reliability of data in digital health systems.
- Patient Safety and Secure Data Transmission: Addressing the secure transmission of patient data to protect patient safety and prevent unauthorized access.
- Electronic and Physical Security: Implementing measures to secure electronic systems and physical infrastructure supporting digital health initiatives.
- Sustainability of Electronic Patient Medical Records: Ensuring the long-term integrity and accuracy of EMRs.
- Quality of Care Using eHealth Processes: Evaluating and monitoring the quality of care delivered through digital health processes.
- Efficient and Effective Communication Systems: Establishing efficient and effective communication systems for the secure transfer of patient data.

6.6.3   Establishing Legal and Regulatory Framework for Data Security

The capacity of digital health tools to collect, analyze, and generate precise data that can be shared with clients, healthcare providers, and researchers is a fundamental aspect of their effectiveness. Whether utilized for direct client care via electronic health records, telehealth,

mobile health, or big data applications, this data plays a crucial role. Moreover, legal frameworks that establish access control, medical liability, and ensure the integrity of health data movement and storage are vital for enabling the advancement and utilization of digital health [42].

Prior to deploying a health system that is interoperable, it is of utmost importance to develop a strong framework that safeguards and regulates the integrity and confidentiality of health information, while also ensuring the availability of the system. This framework should be built upon widely accepted show cases within the healthcare sector.

A suitable legal framework should encompass people's rights to transparent information, accountability and a robust mechanisms for auditing and control. To prevent unauthorized access to information, appropriate actions must be taken in accordance with national or local data protection regulations.

Enforcing regulations to guarantee the confidentiality and integrity of medical records is of utmost importance. When clients have confidence in the health system and health information technology to protect their health information, they can make better decisions and have a comprehensive view of their overall health. However, breaches in health information can have significant repercussions on the finances and reputation of healthcare organizations.

Healthcare providers rely on people, data, technology, and facilities to fulfill their primary objective of delivering care to clients or the community. It is essential to safeguard these resources. The security rule includes various requirements and precautions that must be adhered to, as outlined in Table 6.6 below.

In response to the rapid expansion of electronic health records, countries have implemented policy and regulatory frameworks to guide and oversee the implementation of laws and procedures aimed at protecting patient health information. While striving for improved access, healthcare institutions also have the responsibility to ensure the preservation of confidentiality and privacy. Striking a balance between maintaining patient privacy and facilitating authorized access to the data is essential, as patient information is sensitive and confidential. Safeguarding the security and integrity of patient information has become a legal requirement for healthcare organizations. However, resource limitations pose a significant challenge in achieving this goal.

In developing nations, it is crucial to establish appropriate governance and legal frameworks, data ownership and usage agreements, as well as security and privacy guidelines for health data. These elements serve as the foundation for establishing comprehensive and interoperable technical standards [22].

6.7   Monitoring and Evaluation

Monitoring and evaluation play a crucial role in facilitating goal attainment and performance improvement. The primary objective of monitoring and evaluation is to track and assess performance, allowing for more effective management of outputs and outcomes, commonly referred to as development results. Performance is defined as the progress made towards and the achievement of goals.

In the past, monitoring and evaluation primarily focused on examining implementation methods and inputs. However, in present times, the emphasis has shifted towards assessing various factors such as outputs, collaborations, policy advice and discussions, advocacy, and coordination, all contributing to a specific development outcome. Program managers are actively utilizing information-based monitoring and evaluation to enhance strategies, programs, and other activities, aiming for continuous improvement [43].

6.7.1   Why Monitoring and Evaluation

Results-oriented monitoring and evaluation have several key objectives, which include enhancing organizational and development learning, making informed decisions, promoting substantive accountability, and building national capacity for monitoring and evaluation as well as general functioning. These objectives are interconnected and form a continuous process, as illustrated in Fig. 6.2.

Learning from the past enables better decision-making in the future. Improved decision-making increases stakeholder accountability. Enhanced decision-making leads to increased outputs, allowing for ongoing alignment of initiatives. Maintaining strong connections with key stakeholders throughout this process facilitates the exchange of information and knowledge, supports the transfer of expertise, and strengthens the planning, monitoring, and evaluation capabilities of national offices and projects. These stakeholders also provide valuable feedback that can be utilized to enhance learning and performance.

By consistently reinforcing good practices at the core of monitoring and evaluation, the overall effectiveness of development initiatives is enhanced. This interconnected process fosters continuous improvement and contributes to the overall success of development efforts.

Monitoring and evaluation share the objective of deriving insights from actions and methods, with a focus on efficiency, effectiveness and

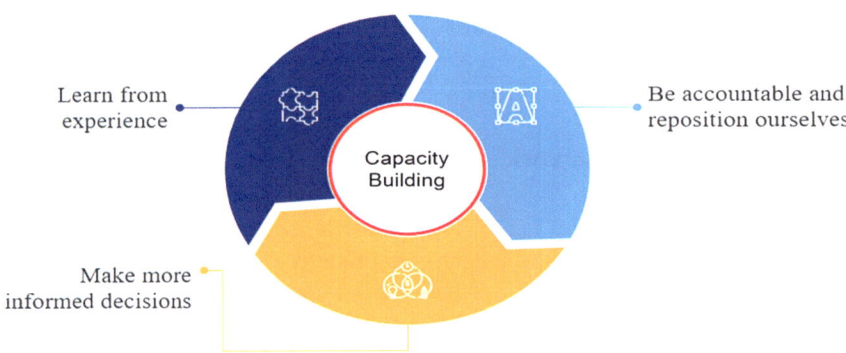

Fig. 6.2 Objectives of monitoring and evaluation

impact. Efficiency pertains to ensuring that the resources invested in the program or project yielded appropriate results. This encompasses contributions such as financial resources, labor, personnel, and other resources. When managing a project and considering its scalability or replicability, it is crucial to ensure efficiency is optimized. The effectiveness of a development program or project is also determined by its ability to achieve specific goals.

Impact refers to the extent to which the targeted situation has improved as a result of the actions taken. It is important to ensure that the actions being taken align with the desired impact before deciding to scale up or replicate the initiative elsewhere.

In summary, monitoring and assessment are aimed at learning from actions and methods, with a focus on evaluating efficiency, effectiveness and impact. It is essential to consider these factors to ensure that the project's objectives are met and that the intended impact is realized before considering expansion or replication.

6.7.2 Definition of Monitoring and Evaluation

Monitoring involves the continuous collection and analysis of program-related data, comparing actual outcomes with expected outcomes, and making assessments regarding the effective implementation of an intervention. It involves comparing individuals, types of programs, and geographical regions using data provided by the program itself, such as participant characteristics, enrollment and attendance, beneficiaries' post-program situations, and program expenses.

A reliable monitoring system is a prerequisite for conducting evaluations. Monitoring is an internal function within any project or organization. Monitoring involves several key steps, including establishing metrics to measure impact, efficacy, and efficiency, implementing mechanisms to collect data on these indicators, gathering and recording the data, analyzing the data, and utilizing the insights gained from the data to inform daily managerial decisions [43, 44].

Evaluation is a purposeful undertaking that systematically and impartially assesses the achievement of a goal and the steps taken to reach it. It involves a comprehensive examination of a program's overall value and relevance by impartially evaluating its various components, such as design, implementation, and achieved results. The objective is to provide decision-makers with reliable information that enables them to identify strategies for achieving more of the intended outcomes.

Evaluation is a process that encompasses multiple evaluations of varying depth and scope, conducted at different times in response to evolving demands for evaluative insights and learning throughout the pursuit of a goal. It is not a one-time occurrence. Evaluations of any kind, including project evaluations that assess performance, relevance, and other factors, should be linked to outcomes rather than solely focusing on implementation or immediate results [43, 45].

Evaluation entails:
- Conducting an evaluation to assess the progress made towards the intended impact and desired outcomes. What was the desired outcome or impact that the initiative or organization aimed to achieve?
- Analyzing the strategy of the project or organization. Was there a well-defined plan in place? Was the implementation of the plan successful? If not, what were the reasons for the lack of success?
- Examining the operational aspects of the project or organization. Were the resources utilized effectively? What were the opportunity costs associated with the chosen operational approach?
- Assessing the sustainability of the project or organization's operational model. How does the working style of the organization impact different stakeholders?

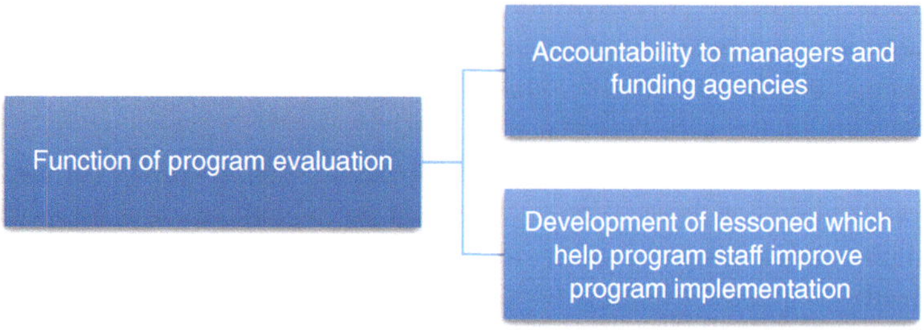

Fig. 6.3 Functions of program evaluation

6.7.3 Function of Monitoring and Evaluation

Program evaluations should fulfill two essential purposes, as depicted in Fig. 6.3. Firstly, they should enable program managers and funding organizations to gain insights from the assessment outcomes regarding resource utilization, program goal attainment, and the execution of planned activities. Secondly, evaluations should generate lessons that program personnel can utilize to improve future program implementation. While many evaluations generate data for accountability purposes, they often fall short in producing actionable lessons for the future [46].

There are different approaches to conducting program evaluations, and program managers need to choose the strategy that aligns with their specific needs. Selecting the most suitable evaluation technique involves considering several crucial factors, such as: who will be responsible for conducting the evaluation? Should it focus on process evaluation or outcome evaluation? Should the emphasis be on deriving lessons for the future or identifying areas of weakness?

6.7.4 Engaging Stakeholders

Most evaluators concur that it is essential to engage in collaboration with stakeholders, and evaluations that prioritize utilization should primarily focus on maximizing the intended usage by the intended users [47]. This section focuses on the techniques and involvement of stakehold-

ers. These techniques include: (1) identifying the key stakeholders, especially those who will use the evaluation information; (2) clarifying the purposes and goals of the evaluation; and (3) determining which stakeholders to engage with, how to engage with them, and at what stages of the evaluation process, in order to maximize the likelihood of the evaluation fulfilling its intended purpose for its intended users.

6.7.4.1 Knowing What Constitutes a Stakeholder, Particularly a Key Stakeholder

Taking into account stakeholders from both practical and ethical perspectives has emerged as a widely recognized strategy in the field of evaluation. Empirical evidence indicates that considering and involving key stakeholders improves the design and implementation of evaluations, as well as the utilization of evaluation findings in decision-making processes [47]. According to Wholley et al., stakeholders refer to individuals, organizations, or groups who have the potential to influence or be affected by an assessment process or its outcomes. The term is deliberately broad to encompass all possible stakeholders. Within this larger group, there exists a subset of significant stakeholders; however, identifying the key players is always subject to debate and judgment [48]. The guiding ideas are:

Develop Facilitation Skills
Effective engagement with stakeholders in evaluation necessitates evaluators to possess interpersonal communication skills, the ability to build relationships, conflict management capabilities, political awareness, and the skills to navigate

group dynamics. Merely having technical proficiency and expertise in social science is inadequate for ensuring that evaluation results are utilized. People skills are essential. Despite the emphasis on rational decision-making in modern organizations, real-world outcomes are influenced by interpersonal and political factors. If evaluators lack the political astuteness and interpersonal acumen, their work is likely to be disregarded or, even worse, misused.

Find and Train Evaluation Information Users

During the evaluation process, it is crucial to identify individuals who are not only interested in acquiring knowledge but also willing to utilize the information obtained from the assessment. This identification is important to establish collaboration with key intended users and to achieve the intended purposes of the evaluation. The number of individuals identified may vary, ranging from a single primary user to a substantial group that includes representatives from diverse constituencies. For instance, this could involve forming a task force comprising community members, donors, program personnel, administrators, board members and legislators.

Find Tipping Point Connectors

Authority and formal positions alone are insufficient indicators of key users in the evaluation process. Evaluators must instead identify individuals who hold influential positions and possess traits such as dependability, knowledge, and extensive networks. These individuals, known as tipping point connectors, are the ones to whom others turn for information. Creating a stakeholder influence diagram that includes the main intended users can serve as a useful foundation for this process. By determining who has influence over important decision-makers and understanding the connections between stakeholders, evaluators can gain valuable insights into key individuals within the evaluation context.

Facilitate High-Quality Interactions

The quality of interactions with targeted users is important, but so are the number and timeliness of those interactions. Excessive interactions without substantive content can diminish stakeholder interest. When requesting time and participation from busy individuals, evaluators must approach them with tact and kindness. It is essential to ensure that conversations are held with the appropriate individuals, addressing relevant concerns. Simply increasing contact without a focused approach is unlikely to have a significant impact, and engaging with individuals who are not invested in the evaluation may not be beneficial.

What truly matters is the type and standard of communication between decision-makers and evaluators. Establishing clear guidelines for what constitutes high-quality interactions with these individuals is crucial to enable meaningful engagement. Additionally, jointly assessing the progress of the evaluation process against these standards is important to ensure its effectiveness.

Nurture Interest in Evaluation

Evaluators often need to invest effort in generating and sustaining enthusiasm for the utilization of evaluations. It requires a combination of nurturing and selection to identify and collaborate with desired users. Some potential users may have negative perceptions or limited interest in assessments due to past negative experiences or simply not having paid much attention to the benefits of evaluation. To foster an interest in evaluation, it is important to understand what matters to the individuals involved in the evaluation process and the intended application of assessment results. By aligning the evaluation with their concerns, evaluators can engage and collaborate with these individuals and organizations, placing their evaluation efforts at the center of addressing these specific issues.

Ensuring Cultural Integrity

Ensuring cultural integrity is a fundamental element in establishing the credibility of assessments, particularly when dealing with individuals from diverse backgrounds. It is important to actively seek input from individuals regarding their top concerns and any cultural sensitivity issues that may arise. Avoid restricting your actions based on personal biases or preconceptions. Instead, consult competent individuals and those directly affected to gather their perspectives and insights on these concerns. Obtain and apply feedback to improve the evaluation process and outcomes.

Anticipate Turnover of Intended Users

High reliance on interpersonal relationships in evaluation can lead to challenges with turnover. Unless evaluators proactively anticipate and prepare for turnover among major intended users, it can become a critical flaw in the evaluation process. In order to gain the support of new team members and foster their sense of ownership over the evaluation, it may be necessary to make adjustments to the design at a later stage, if feasible. When selecting the initial group of intended users, it is advisable to include backup individuals and potential replacements. Regularly checking in with stakeholders involved throughout the evaluation process helps to monitor any changes in their circumstances.

6.7.4.2 Dealing with Power Differentials

While an evaluation may involve a single primary intended user or a small group of known collaborators, power differentials become more relevant in larger, more intricate evaluations where multiple stakeholder constituencies have competing or opposing interests, as depicted in Fig. 6.4. Using a power versus interest grid, the position of individuals on the grid guides the approach to be taken with them:

- **High-power, interested individuals:** These are the stakeholders who hold significant influence and are highly interested in the evaluation. It is crucial to actively engage with them and make concerted efforts to satisfy their needs and expectations.
- **High-power, less interested individuals:** While these stakeholders possess considerable power, they may have limited interest in the evaluation. It is important to engage them with enough effort to maintain their interest, without overwhelming them with excessive information.
- **Low power, interested individuals:** These stakeholders may have limited power but are genuinely interested in the evaluation. It is essential to ensure they are well-informed and engaged to prevent any potential issues. They can often provide valuable assistance regarding specific aspects of the evaluation.
- **Low power, less interested individuals:** Although these stakeholders have lower power and may demonstrate limited interest, it is still important to monitor their involvement. However, it is advisable to avoid inundating them with excessive communication that may be perceived as bothersome.

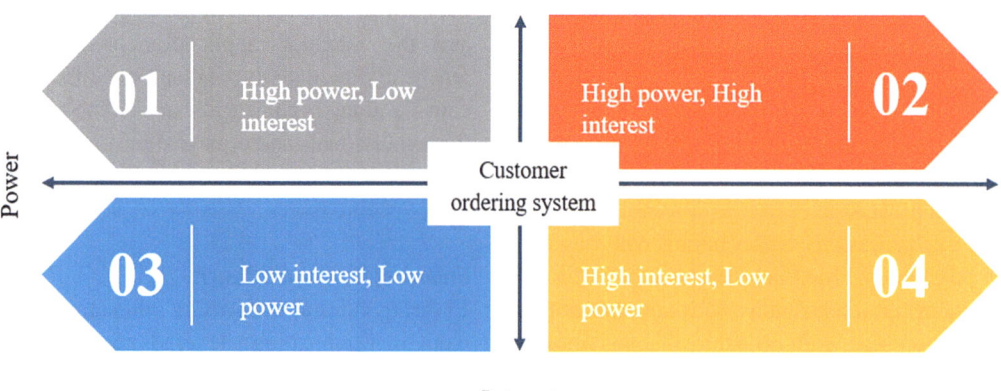

Fig. 6.4 Power/interest grid

6.7.5   Approaches of Program Evaluation

6.7.5.1 The Approach Driven by Experts

This approach involves the assignment of one or more external evaluators to undertake the entire evaluation process. This encompasses establishing the evaluation goals, crafting the methods, gathering and scrutinizing data, and drawing independent conclusion and recommendation.

There is a common misconception that hiring external evaluators ensures a more "objective" assessment. However, when external "specialists" are solely responsible for program evaluation, it often creates a top-down dynamic.

Traditional assessment methods sometimes discourage program staff from participating in the evaluation of their own programs. When evaluation specialists are given full authority to determine the direction of the assessment, program personnel may feel marginalized. Consequently, they may reject or disregard the findings and recommendations of the evaluators, leading to a sense of alienation.

6.7.5.2 Participatory Approach

Implementing a participatory approach for program evaluation entails a designated evaluation coordinator, often external to the program or organization and engages in collaborative efforts with program stakeholders at every stage of the evaluation process.

With this context, stakeholders are people who vested interest in the outcomes of the evaluation and will utilize the assessment data to make informed decisions. The specific composition of program stakeholders may vary depending on the context and nature of the evaluation. Evaluation planners must determine the relevant stakeholders in each case and the appropriate level of their involvement. It is not always necessary or beneficial to include a large number of stakeholders.

In the participatory approach, stakeholders fulfill the following roles: sharing their program-related experiences, actively participating in gathering information about implementation of the program, collaborating with the team to ana-lyze collected data and reported experiences, and contributing to the drawing of conclusions regarding program outcomes. By incorporating the subjective perspectives of program implementers alongside the impartial viewpoint of an external evaluator, the participatory approach aims to generate evaluation findings of good quality.

The underlying premise of participatory evaluation is that involving stakeholders ensures that relevant topics are addressed and that stakeholders own the findings generated through the evaluation process. Additionally, the implementation of the participatory approach provides an opportunity to all involved stakeholders. This strengthens the capacity to evaluate programs and enhances their understanding of the strengths and weaknesses of their program design. Furthermore, the interaction itself has the potential of improving communication among different stakeholders operating at various stages of program implementation, which is an additional benefit of participatory assessment.

6.7.6   Theory of Change

During the planning process, organizations and stakeholders outline their long-term objectives and identify the necessary conditions for achieving those goals. This robust and inclusive approach is commonly referred to as the theory of change. In a causal framework, these conditions are visually depicted as desired outcomes. An outcomes framework, on the other hand, maps out the outcomes using interventions, which can be a single program or a coordinated effort, as described in the theory of change.

The causal framework establishes connections between actions and outcomes, revealing the complex web of interconnected activities required to bring about change. This framework provides a working model for evaluating theories and assumptions regarding the most effective course of action to achieve the desired results depicted in the model [49]. It is a means of redefining planning and evaluating development such that the main emphasis is on improvements for our target groups rather than on our intended course of action.

Program staff have the flexibility to make adjustments and revisions to their change model as they gain more insights into what strategies are effective and what are not. By adhering to the theory of change method, the implementation and evaluation processes remain transparent, ensuring that everyone involved understands the actions being taken and the reasons behind them. It is important that each outcome in the theory is clearly defined, and success indicators are established for each outcome. As implementation progresses, organizations collect and analyze data on these key indicators to monitor progress towards achieving the theory of change.

A theory of change utilizes rationales to describe the relationships between outcomes and the underlying reasons why achieving one result is dependent on achieving another. These rationales are based on assumptions and are often supported by research, which enhances the credibility of the theory and increases the likelihood of achieving its intended objectives. In addition to the visual representation, the theory of change includes a textual narrative that provides contextual explanations and reasoning behind the framework. The theory of change (ToC) can be used for tracking and evaluating changes, as well as planning and issue formulation.

Various processes such as goal-setting procedures, visioning papers, strategic plans, and yearly plans rely on the theory of change to articulate long-term outcomes, preconditions, and actions. The theory of change serves as an assessment tool, precisely defining the program's goals and linking them to specific interventions. Once the objectives are established, data can be collected to assess the effectiveness of the interventions in working towards achieving the desired outcomes.

The theory of change (ToC) outlines your initiative in a step-by-step manner. It starts by defining the long-term objectives and the underlying assumptions. Next, it traces a backward path from the long-term objective to identify the prerequisites or requirements necessary to achieve that objective, providing justifications for each step.

The ToC also expresses your assumptions about the elements of the system that your theory relies on and explains why certain outcomes are necessary preconditions for other outcomes. Additionally, the ToC involves evaluating and selecting the most effective interventions to bring about the desired change. It includes the creation of metrics to track progress towards the desired outcomes and finally, it evaluates the overall effectiveness of your initiative.

6.7.6.1 When Is ToC Appropriate?

A theory of change is a crucial component of impact evaluations and should be incorporated in some form in every evaluation program. When preparing for an impact evaluation and creating the terms of reference, it is important to evaluate any existing theory of change associated with the program or policy. This evaluation should assess its appropriateness, thoroughness, and accuracy to make necessary modifications accordingly. The theory of change should be revised to match any modifications made to the intervention itself or any new insights gained regarding its functioning or intended operation during the evaluation [50].

According to Serrat et al., a theory of change should answer six overlapping questions depicted below in Fig. 6.5 [51]:

(i) What concern, its underlying causes, and consequences, does one and others wish to ameliorate in the long term (external context)?
(ii) Who does one seek to benefit or influence (beneficiaries)?
(iii) What benefits does one aim to deliver (results)?
(iv) When will the benefits be realized (time span)?
(v) How will one and others make that happen (interventions)?
(vi) Why, and based on what evidence, does one believe the theory of change will bear out (assumptions)?

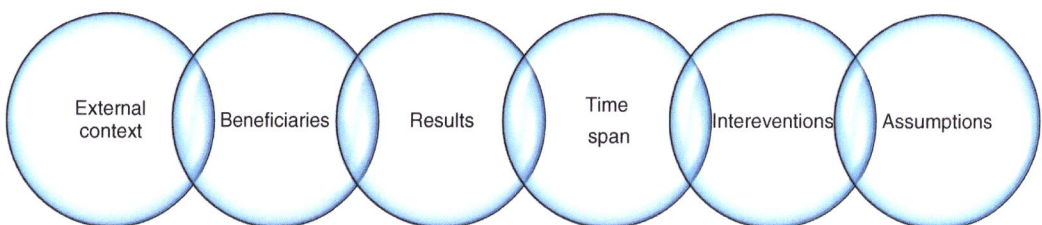

Fig. 6.5 Focusing and scoping a theory of change. Reproduced with permissions from Serrat, O. (2017). Theories of Change. In: Knowledge Solutions. Springer, Singapore. https://doi.org/10.1007/978-981-10-0983-9_24.   Creative Commons Attribution-Non Commercial 3.0 IGO license (http://creativecommons.org/licenses/by-nc/3.0/igo/)

6.7.7   Frameworks in Monitoring and Evaluation

6.7.7.1 Logic Model

Bickman et al. define a logic model as a rational and reliable depiction of how a program will function within a specific context to tackle identified problems. It forms the basis for a compelling storyline that elucidates the program's expected achievements, communicating to stakeholders and other concerned individuals the problem the program aims to address and its suitability for doing so. The logic model comprises resources, actions, outputs, as well as short-term, intermediate, and long-term outcomes [48, 52].

For over two decades, program administrators and evaluators have employed the logic model approach as a means to depict the efficacy of their programs. This model elucidates the logical links between resources, activities, target audiences, outputs, and the short, intermediate, and long-term outcomes of a program, all within the context of a specific issue or situation. By utilizing the logic model, it becomes possible to identify crucial performance indicators for assessing program effectiveness [53]. Logic models provide you an idea of how your program is supposed to operate, which might help you with evaluation.

Logic models outline the fundamental components of a program and elucidate their interrelationships. These models encompass both process and result components. They serve as narrative or visual representations of real-world processes, illuminating the underlying assumptions that connect actions to anticipated outcomes. By presenting a series of cause-and-effect connections, logic models offer a systems-based approach to communicate the necessary steps for achieving a goal [47, 53, 54].

Logic models serve multiple purposes in program development and evaluation. They contribute to comprehension and clarity by outlining the necessary resources, sequencing activities, and establishing a foundation for program assessment. When determining what aspects of the program to evaluate and prioritize, logic models are valuable for refining the scope of the evaluation process. They can be constructed as nested logic models, focusing on specific actions or components or as global logic models, providing an overview of the entire program's functioning. Furthermore, logic models aid program implementers and evaluators by offering a visual representation of the intended functionality of the program. They identify the key elements of the software and explain how they should seamlessly integrate.

Descriptions of the Elements of the Logic Model

Resources: To support the program, partnerships are essential along with other critical inputs such as financial and human resources. Among these resources, one of the most vital is the availability of information regarding the nature and extent of the issue being addressed.

Activities: The crucial actions that must be taken in order to generate program outcomes.

Outputs: The supplies, commodities, and services provided to program participants or direct clients are considered as outputs. In many evaluation cases, actions and outputs are not clearly distinguished. However, we prefer to separate the two as it simplifies the evaluation of program implementation. Activities typically refer to the actions performed by the program, while outputs represent the tangible or intangible results produced by the program.

Outcomes: The expected changes or benefits that are anticipated to occur as a result of engaging in program activities and achieving program outcomes can be described as outcomes. Programs typically have a sequence of outcomes that collectively form the program's outcome structure. The first type of outcomes are short-term outcomes, which are the immediate modifications or benefits directly linked to or caused by the program's outputs. These anticipated short-term outcomes are expected to lead to intermediate objectives, which come next in the sequence. Program impacts or long-term consequences, are anticipated to arise from the benefits derived from the intermediate results.

In the logic model, important contextual elements that are beyond the program's control and can influence its success are considered essential components. These contextual elements can have both positive and negative impacts. There are two categories of circumstances that affect how the program is designed and delivered: antecedental factors and mediating factors. Antecedent elements at the program's inception include factors such as client characteristics, location-specific variables, and economic conditions [55].

Mediating factors refer to the variables that arise during the program's implementation, including factors like personnel turnover, changes in regulations, economic fluctuations and the emergence of other competing priorities. Therefore, evaluators of the program should consider these factors when developing and assessing the program. Additionally, it is essential to recognize the potential influence of specific client characteristics on the program's outcomes. Taking into account these client characteristics is crucial for understanding and evaluating the program's effectiveness.

How to Use a Logic Model

Elucidating the Theory behind the Program

1. **Statement of problem:** Provide a concise explanation of the issues or problems that the program aims to solve.
2. **Community Resources:** Identify the assets or requirements present in your community that have inspired your organization to create a program aimed at resolving the recognized problem.
3. **Desired achievements:** Define the desired achievements and future visualization by outlining both short-term and long-term goals.
4. **Influential Factors:** Compile a list of factors that may impact the transformation of the community.
5. **Strategies:** Present a list of effective "best practices" or tactics that have proven successful in similar communities in achieving the desired outcomes promised by the program.
6. **Assumptions:** Describe the underlying assumptions that guide why and how the change management techniques will be successful in the specific public domain.

Implementation of program- Illustrating the Advancement of Your Program:

1. **Outputs:** Identify the intended outcomes (service delivery/implementation objectives) for each program activity.
2. **Outcomes:** Enumerate the immediate and long-term results that aim to achieve for each task.
3. **Impact:** Articulate the anticipated effects that each program activity will have on the community over the next 7 to 10 years.
4. **Activities:** Provide a concise description of each planned activity of the program that will be undertaken during implementation.
5. **Assets:** Enumerate the resources or crucial elements accessible to bolster the program's functioning.

Indicator and questions for the program, evaluation:

1. **Priority areas:** Compile a list of the key components that constitute the most significant

aspects of the program, utilizing the logic model derived from the program theory.

2. **Target Audience:** Determine the primary recipients for each focus area. Further, identify the individuals or groups with a vested interest in the program.

3. **Questions:** Generate a list of potential questions that the target audience may have regarding the program for each specific area of focus.

4. **Information use:** Determine the ways to utilize the evaluation data to address the needs of each audience and address the identified questions.

5. **Indicators:** Describe the data that can be collected for each question to provide insight into the current state of the program and its participants.

6. **Technical assistance:** Demonstrate the level of experience the organization possesses in conducting evaluations and managing data to gather and analyze relevant information for these indicators.

6.7.7.2 Log-Frame

The logical framework, commonly known as the logframe, is a widely used planning tool. It has garnered both popularity and criticism. Initially designed for simple, time-limited projects, it is now used for interventions of various scales, ranging from small initiatives to major organizational funding. The logical framework serves as a foundation for monitoring and evaluation activities, providing a framework for assessing project progress and outcomes [56].

The development of the logframe was a response to various common weaknesses found in projects, such as a lack of consensus among partners regarding project scope, poorly defined objectives, insufficient identification and management of risks and assumptions, inadequate exploration of cause-and-effect relationships between different levels of objectives, inadequate alignment of activities and outputs with higher-level objectives, and a lack of systematic monitoring and evaluation.

The versatility of the logical framework may explain its widespread popularity, as it can serve multiple purposes depending on the context. Originally designed as a planning tool to assist in the management of scheduled procedures, the logframe can also function as a program management tool, provide a foundation for monitoring and evaluation (M&E) within a project or program, serve as an accountability mechanism, offer a concise description of work, provide insights into the operations of an organization or complex program, present a linear theory of change, or even serve as a mechanism for securing funding, depending on the specific circumstances.

Components of a Log-Frame

The logframe comprises several components. To ensure a comprehensive understanding and effective utilization, each component is explained in detail in the following subsections.

1. **Overall goal:** This represents the desired impact of the project, often at a program or sector level. It serves as the overarching objective that aligns with other initiatives within a portfolio. It can also be referred to as the "main objective" or "aim."

2. **Project purposes:** The project's purposes define the reasons for its implementation and outline the intended results. Ideally, a project should have a single goal to provide clear direction for actions and outputs. Projects with multiple goals and a wide range of outcomes may suffer from a lack of guidance. The terms "objective" or "goal" can also be used to refer to project purposes.

3. **Outputs:** Outputs are the tangible deliverables that the project aims to produce. A mutual issue is that program deliverables may not be all-inclusive enough, as they often focus on specific deliverables without considering important institutional or managerial aspects necessary for success.

4. **Activities:** Activities outline how the project or program will be executed, the steps required to achieve the desired results and the necessary inputs. Activities may include standard project management procedures such as scheduling periodic meetings, conducting

event monitoring and carrying out assessments.

5. **Verifiable indicators:** Verifiable indicators are metrics used to measure project progress and success. When developing indicators, three factors should be prioritized: quantity, quality and timeliness. These indicators should be feasible and provide a financially sustainable basis for evaluating and tracking the project's performance.

6. **Assumptions:** Assumptions in the logframe represent necessary conditions or events that are beyond the project's control. They are factors that are assumed to be in place for the project to succeed, such as timely budget releases or stable security conditions. The strength of a project's design increases as the level of risk or uncertainty associated with assumptions decreases.

6.7.8   Types of Monitoring and Evaluation

6.7.8.1 Process Evaluation

Process evaluation, in contrast to outcome evaluation, focuses on the execution of a program and entails an examination of the methods employed, as well as suggestions for enhancing its implementation. It delves into the manner in which various tasks were accomplished and addresses challenges encountered. While a process evaluation can involve quantitative measurement of task completion, the acquisition of qualitative data is deemed more crucial.

6.7.8.2 Outcome Evaluation

The initial drive for program assessment originated from funding agencies demands for accountability from implementers of the program. Primary emphasis has been on quantifying the achievements of a program, particularly in terms of completed tasks. However, both funding agencies and program administrators are increasingly recognizing that simply knowing the quantity of activities is insufficient. There is an increasing recognition that assessments should also capture, qualitatively, both the achievements and difficulties encountered during the implementation process, aligning with a perspective that prioritizes learning and enhancement.

6.7.8.3 Formative Evaluation

Formative evaluation involves gathering and analyzing user feedback during the development or implementation of a project, program or product. It identifies the strengths, weaknesses, and areas for potential improvement, enabling adjustments to be made to enhance the quality and effectiveness of the final outcome. Formative assessment is crucial because it provides valuable data that can inform and improve the development or implementation process. By identifying areas requiring adjustments early on, it can ultimately save resources, time and money. Moreover, it ensures that the end product or program meets the needs of the target audience, leading to increased satisfaction and success [57–59].

In addition, formative assessment can foster a culture of continuous learning and improvement within an organization. By consistently gathering feedback and making necessary adjustments, businesses can progressively enhance their processes and outcomes. This iterative approach can lead to increased effectiveness, efficiency and creativity.

Purpose of Formative Evaluation

1. **Offer feedback:** Formative evaluation aims to provide feedback to program stakeholders, including program creators, staff, and funders, in order to guide further program growth and improvement.

2. **Identify issues:** Formative assessment is employed to identify problems and areas for improvement in program design, implementation, and delivery, allowing for timely and effective interventions.

3. **Monitor progress:** Formative evaluation is utilized throughout the development and implementation of a program to monitor progress and outcomes, ensuring that the program is on track to achieve its desired objectives.

Aim of Formative Evaluation

Formative assessment aims to improve program design by identifying both strengths and weaknesses in program components, including content, delivery and staffing. It plays a crucial role in enhancing program implementation by pinpointing areas where program personnel may require additional training or support, or where adjustments in program delivery may be necessary. Furthermore, formative assessment is utilized to maximize program outcomes by identifying opportunities to enhance program effectiveness, such as through modifications to program components or delivery methods.

6.7.8.4 Summative Evaluation

It is an evaluation conducted upon the conclusion of a project or program, aiming to evaluate its complete effectiveness. The main objective of this type of evaluation is to ascertain whether the project or program successfully accomplished its objectives or not.

These evaluations serve as an accountability mechanism to determine how well a standards are met during implementation. Therefore, it is crucial for these evaluations to be reliable and credible [60, 61]. Summative evaluations provide various types of information, including data that identify the strengths and weaknesses in performance.

6.7.9   Monitoring and Evaluation Focus Areas

Monitoring primarily focuses on documenting inputs (activities) and outputs, with some consid-eration given to intermediate results. On the other hand, evaluation takes place at specific intervals and allows for a more comprehensive assessment of a program's progress. Evaluation tracks changes and places greater emphasis on the outcomes and degree of impact.

The relationship between the chain of inputs, outputs, outcomes and impacts throughout the planning cycle is illustrated in the accompanying diagram, highlighting these distinctions. Output measurement assesses how tasks are executed, while outcome measurement gauges the extent to which specific goals and expected outcomes are achieved. Impact evaluation, as depicted in Fig. 6.6, evaluates the extent to which the program ultimately fulfills its overarching purpose.

Effective monitoring and evaluation (M&E) necessitate a clear definition of goals, objectives, and activities during the design phase. This entails developing quantifiable indicators that allow for objective verification at a reasonable cost. These indicators should be specific, measurable, achievable, agreed upon, relevant and time-bound [62].

6.7.9.1 Performance Indicators

Performance indicators refer to the measures used to assess inputs, processes, outputs, outcomes, and impacts of strategies, programs, or development initiatives. By employing reliable methods for data collection, such as formal surveys, analysis, and reporting, managers can monitor progress, present findings, and implement corrective actions to improve service delivery based on these indicators. It is important to involve key stakeholders in the definition of indi-

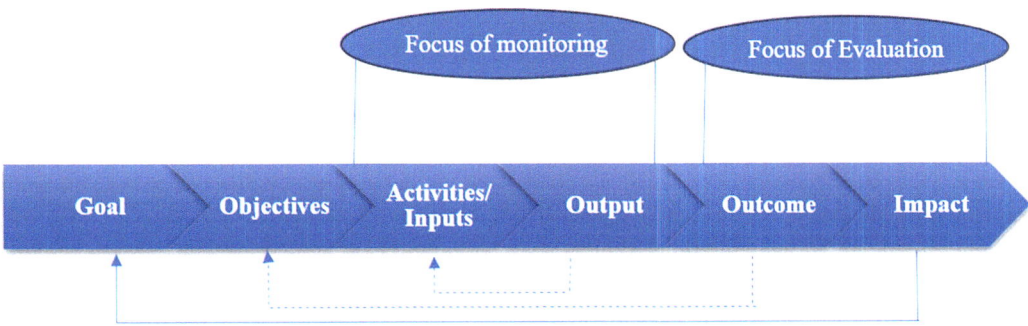

Fig. 6.6 Focus area of monitoring and evaluation

cators, as this increases the likelihood that they will understand and apply them to decision-making processes [63].

6.7.9.2 Selecting Indicators

The selection of indicators should be based on a comprehensive examination of goals, desired changes, and the availability of financial, technological and human resources. A good indicator should closely align with the target it is meant to monitor and should consider potential threats. Two types of indicators are necessary:

1. Outcome/Impact indicators, which assess systemic changes resulting from strategic action plans.
2. Output/Process indicators, which measure the amount of work being done, such as the quantity of stakeholder developed strategic action plans.

To ensure that multiple individuals can measure the indicator reliably and obtain equally trustworthy findings, it should be precise and clear. Each indicator should focus on a single type of data. While qualitative data dependent on personal opinions may sometimes be the only available option, it still holds significance. However, quantitative measures or numerical data are generally more beneficial. It is easier to select indicators for explicit goals or activities compared to goals that involve behavioral shifts, such as improved community empowerment or increased awareness.

6.7.9.3 Criteria for Selecting Indicators

The process of selecting appropriate indicators can be challenging. It is important to involve multiple stakeholders in an effective accountability system, including those responsible for data collection, utilization, and those with technical expertise in evaluating different measures. The following questions can help guide the selection of indicators:

- Does the indicator provide direct evidence of the expected result or condition? Indicators should, to the extent possible, offer the most direct information about the phenomena or results they are monitoring.

- Is the indicator consistently defined over time? Consistency in indicator definition is crucial for making consistent decisions over time. Decision-makers need confidence that the data they are evaluating measure the same phenomenon (referred to as dependability). For example, when evaluating successful employment, the indicator should be consistently measured against the same success benchmark, such as 3 months in a full-time position. Similarly, when working with percentages, the denominator must be recognized and applied consistently.

- Will data be available for the indicator? The frequency of data collection should be sufficient for decision-makers to use the indicators effectively. Result data is often available on an annual basis, while data on inputs, processes, and outputs are more commonly collected regularly.

- Is data currently being collected for the indicator? Accountability demands are increasing, but resources for monitoring and evaluation are decreasing. In some cases, data may already be collected, especially for input and output indicators and certain common outcome indicators. When data is not being collected, the cost of additional data collection efforts must be weighed against the potential benefits.

- Is the indicator important to a wide range of stakeholders? Publicly shared indicators need to be highly credible, providing sufficient information about a condition or outcome to persuade both supporters and critics. The information they convey should be understandable and acceptable to key stakeholders. However, certain indicators may require more explanation or be highly technical (such as indices), and they may be necessary for those more directly involved in the programs.

- Is the indicator quantitative? Numerical indicators are often used to provide decision-makers with relevant and easily comprehensible data. However, in some cases, qualitative data may be needed to better understand the event being measured.

6.7.9.4 Implementing M&E

The terms of reference (TOR) should clearly outline the monitoring and evaluation (M&E)

tasks, as day-to-day management concerns can often overshadow the importance of monitoring activities. Sufficient time should be allocated for analysis and interpretation of data. It is crucial to oversee the implementation of the responsibilities outlined in the M&E strategy and make necessary adjustments when needed. Separate plans may be required for different components, but all significant sectoral components should be included in the overall M&E strategy. The most effective monitoring occurs when it is conducted by the relevant parties themselves or in close collaboration with their full cooperation.

6.7.9.5 Performance Monitoring Plan (PMP)

Performance monitoring plans play a crucial role in ensuring the proper implementation of monitoring and evaluation activities. Within the project management cycle, monitoring and evaluation serve distinct purposes. While they are intended to complement each other, they should be conducted independently to provide an unbiased assessment of program and project implementation. Due to differences in frequency, strategy, technique, and scope, it is necessary to handle them as separate components in the project management plan (PMP).

6.8 Supporting Innovations and Research Development of Public Health Informatics

Health informatics, which involves the integration of data, communication, information systems, and medical treatment, is currently driving transformative changes in the healthcare sector. Technological advancements have fostered innovation across various disciplines within the medical field. Technology is playing a leading role in the ongoing evolution of the healthcare system, with developments such as 3D bioprinting and artificial intelligence. Here are some ways in which technology and health informatics will shape the future of healthcare.

6.8.1 Innovations in Health Informatics

The field of health informatics is currently experiencing a period of great advancement. Substantial investments in health information technology (IT) have aligned with a notable rise in eHealth, particularly in the use of client information. While the history of information technology has seen its share of ups and downs, the core objectives and motivations, along with the ongoing introduction of new technologies, have remained consistent since the year 2000, even though they may not have prioritized patient-centric approaches to a sufficient extent [64].

6.8.1.1 mHealth

The integration of mobile technology in healthcare, known as "mHealth," is simplifying medical treatment and enhancing the patient experience. With a growing array of smartphone applications, patients now have the ability to conveniently schedule appointments, communicate with healthcare professionals, efficiently monitor their health, and access relevant health information. Additionally, technology is assisting physicians in enhancing patient compliance by enabling remote monitoring of specific medical conditions and equipment. This technological advancement is improving patient engagement and contributing to more effective healthcare management.

6.8.1.2 Telemedicine

Similar to mobile health, telemedicine utilizes virtual connections between health care providers and patients. Through telemedicine, patients can receive medical consultations and treatment without the need to physically visit the health facility. This is particularly advantageous for individuals residing in rural areas, lacking transportation options, or facing mobility limitations, as it provides them with access to healthcare services. Telemedicine experienced a significant surge in usage following the COVID-19 pandemic in 2020. By leveraging telemedicine, healthcare providers can help prevent infections and ensure the uninterrupted delivery of care for both COVID-19 and non-COVID-19 patients.

6.8.1.3 Electronic Health Records

By ensuring that clinicians have access to a comprehensive view of patients' past and current health, electronic health records (EHRs) contribute to improved continuity of care and better patient outcomes. EHRs not only reduce healthcare disparities and streamline processes like telehealth and electronic prescriptions, but they also enhance coordination of care among healthcare providers.

In our digitally connected world, EHRs help health care providers organize patient care and ensure accuracy, while also empowering patients to advocate for themselves. Through patient portals offered by many health facilities, patients have immediate access to their health history, test results, medical information, and the ability to connect with their health care workers. The widespread adoption of EHRs brings several benefits, including enhanced patient care, improved diagnoses, increased practice efficiency and cost savings.

6.8.1.4 Health Information Technology Systems Interoperability

Interoperability refers capability of secure systems which enables authorized stakeholders, regardless of their location, to access and share information instantly. Interoperability facilitates the smooth and timely transfer of information, thereby improving population and individual health services globally.

Before the implementation of interoperable health IT systems, patients had to gather and provide all their medical records to health workers, rely on the hope that their medical network shared the necessary information, or simply verbally communicate their prior care to clinicians. However, with the presence of health IT systems, healthcare practitioners can access a patient's complete medical information and history, even if it is stored in different computer systems across various locations. This access ensures that medical caregivers at any healthcare facility have a comprehensive understanding of a patient's medical history, which is vital for maintaining continuity of treatment.

6.8.1.5 Wearables

In addition to electronic health records, wearables offer an additional means of gathering information, promoting prevention and improving user outcomes. The availability and capabilities of wearables have significantly expanded in recent years. One valuable feature of wearables is their ability to notify users and health workers about sudden medical concerns. Wearables collect real-time data, which is then aggregated and analyzed by a system to alert health workers of potential issues with their patients. This proactive approach enables medical professionals to reach out to patients who may not even be aware that they require urgent care.

6.8.1.6 The Cloud and Data Analytics

The proliferation of data from wearables, electronic health records (EHRs), and other sources has made the cloud and data analytics emerging and reliable methods for storing and exchanging large volumes of data. These technologies enable the healthcare industry to operate and advance more rapidly and efficiently than ever before. Through data analytics initiatives and cloud computing services, healthcare organizations can leverage insights derived from real-world data to evaluate numerous possibilities and determine the optimal course of action. This accelerated availability of information and decision-making speed holds significant importance in the field of healthcare.

6.8.1.7 3D Bioprinting

While still in its nascent stages, this state-of-the-art medical advancement holds immense potential for the production of medications, prosthetic limbs, and even human tissue and organs. A noteworthy milestone in 3D printing occurred in 2018 when researchers successfully created human ears and successfully attached them to the skin of mice. Another remarkable breakthrough took place in Australia, where a 3D printed spine was successfully implanted into a human patient suffering from chordoma cancer. Additionally, 3D orthopedic implants are revolutionizing joint and bone replacement procedures by providing better-fitting, longer-lasting, and more functional implants. These advancements in 3D printing technology hold great promise for the future of medical interventions.

6.8.1.8 Artificial Intelligence

The new capabilities of artificial intelligence (AI) have facilitated significant advancements in medical settings. Healthcare and health informatics are leveraging AI and machine learning to aid health workers in more accurate patient diagnoses and predict high-risk cases. Additionally, AI is contributing to personalized therapy by providing clinicians with enhanced insights into symptom patterns and effective treatment plans. These applications of AI are enhancing medical practices and improving patient care outcomes.

6.8.1.9 Robotics

The utilization of robotics is on the rise in the fields of care administration and facility maintenance, thanks to the advancements in AI and machine learning. Robots with advanced artificial intelligence capabilities are being employed to assist in tasks such as delivery, transportation, and even serving as surgical assistants. These intelligent robotics are enhancing efficiency and effectiveness in various aspects of healthcare and facility management.

6.8.1.10 Blockchain

Blockchain technology is revolutionizing data security across various sectors, including healthcare. Acting as an immutable shared ledger, blockchain simplifies asset tracking and transaction recording within a corporate network. Tangible assets as well as intangible assets like intellectual property, patents, copyrights, and branding, can be efficiently tracked and traded on a blockchain network. This technology reduces costs and mitigates risks for all involved stakeholders. The fundamental concept behind blockchain is that once data is entered, it becomes unalterable, ensuring exceptional security while remaining accessible.

6.8.2 Research Development in Health Informatics

Health informatics is currently experiencing a period of significant growth and advancement. Although information technology has been marked by ups and downs over the years, the core objectives and motivations, along with the ongoing introduction of new technologies, have remained consistent since 2000, even if they may not have prioritized patient needs to the fullest extent [64].

While clinical and bioinformatics share similarities with Public Health Informatics (PHI), the latter presents distinct prospects for research and the establishment of best practices. PHI places emphasis on prevention, community-based approaches, disease and injury monitoring, and longitudinal analysis. Conducting research in this field ensures thorough evaluation of innovative concepts before implementation and aids in setting resource priorities.

To address both short- and long-term needs, a research agenda must be developed, prioritizing regional, state wide and national initiatives. When feasible and appropriate, it is important to review and leverage existing knowledge and techniques from health informatics. The involvement of interdisciplinary research teams enhances the likelihood of productive and relevant outcomes that benefit public health.

In summary, a comprehensive research agenda is essential in public health informatics, addressing short and long-term needs. The research should concentrate on areas that hold promise and relevance to public health concerns. Leveraging existing medical informatics knowledge and techniques when suitable will further enhance the research efforts. The involvement of multidisciplinary research teams improves the chances of productivity and relevance to public health.

References

1. Magnuson JA, Fu PC Jr. Public health informatics and information systems. Springer; 2014.
2. World Health Organization. Guidance for health information system governance. WHO; 2021.

3. HISA. Leadership in clinical informatics. HISA; 2018.
4. Holeman I, Cookson TP, Pagliari C. Digital technology for health sector governance in low and middle income countries: a scoping review. J Glob Health. 2016;6(2):020408.
5. Koumamba AP, Bisvigou UJ, Ngoungou EB, Diallo G. Health information systems in developing countries: case of African countries. BMC Med Inform Decis Mak. 2021;21(1):232.
6. Elina Laukka TP, Kanste O. Leadership in the context of digital health services: a concept analysis. J Nurs Manag. 2022;30(7):2763–80.
7. Karamagi HC, Muneene D, Droti B, Jepchumba V, Okeibunor JC, et al. eHealth or e-Chaos: the use of digital health interventions for health systems strengthening in sub-Saharan Africa over the last 10 years: a scoping review. J Glob Health. 2022;12:04090.
8. Marcelo A, Medeiros D, Ramesh K, Roth S, Wyatt P. Transforming health systems through good digital health governance. Asian Development Bank; 2018.
9. African Union. The digital transformation strategy for Africa (2020–2030). African Union; 2020.
10. Luna D, Almerares A, Mayan JC 3rd, González Bernaldo de Quirós F, Otero C. Health informatics in developing countries: going beyond pilot practices to sustainable implementations: a review of the current challenges. Healthc Inform Res. 2014;20(1):3–10.
11. Harding K, Biks GA, Adefris M, Loehr J, Gashaye KT, Tilahun B, et al. A mobile health model supporting Ethiopia's eHealth strategy. Digit Med. 2018;4(2):54–65.
12. World Health Organization. WHO guideline: recommendations on digital interventions for health system strengthening. WHO; 2019.
13. World Health Organization. National eHealth strategy toolkit. Geneva: World Health Organization and International Telecommunication Union; 2012.
14. Nigel Cory and Philip Stevens. Building a global framework for digital health services in the era of COVID-19. Nigel Cory and Philip Stevens; 2020.
15. Ministry of Health. Digital health blueprint. Ministry of Health; 2021.
16. Health Information Technology Directorate. Federal Ministry of Health. National Digital Health Strategy, 2020–2029. HITD; 2021.
17. Ibeneme S, Karamagi H, Muneene D, Goswami K, Chisaka N, Okeibunor J. Strengthening health systems using innovative digital health technologies in Africa. Front Digit Health. 2022;4:854339.
18. Yasnoff WA, Overhage JM, Humphreys BL, LaVenture M. A national agenda for public health informatics: summarized recommendations from the 2001 AMIA Spring Congress. J Am Med Inform Assoc. 2001;8(6):535–45.
19. WHO. Global strategy on digital health 2020–2025. WHO; 2021.
20. World Health Organization. Atlas of eHealth country profiles.The use of eHealth in support of universal health coverage. Based on the findings of the third global survey on eHealth 2015. Global Observatory for eHealth. WHO; 2016.
21. World Health Organization. Framework and standards for country health information systems. 2nd ed. WHO; 2012.
22. Mamuye AL, Yilma TM, Abdulwahab A, Broomhead S, Zondo P, Kyeng M, Maeda J, Abdulaziz M, et al. Health information exchange policy and standards for digital health systems in Africa: a systematic review. PLoS Digit Health. 2022;1(10):e0000118.
23. World Health Organization. Regional action agenda on harnessing e-health for improved health service delivery in the Western Pacific. 2019;
24. Desai S. Health information exchange, interoperability, and network effects. 2015; University of Pennsylvania. Publicly Accessible Penn Dissertations. 1040. http://repository.upenn.edu/edissertations/1040.
25. Walker J, Pan E, Johnston D, Adler-Milstein J, Bates DW, Middleton B. The value of health care information exchange and interoperability. Health Aff. 2013;Suppl Web Exclusives:W5-10-W5-18.
26. Goodman RC, Miller RA. Ethics in biomedical and health informatics: users, standards, and outcomes. In: Biomedical informatics. Springer; 2014. p. 391–423.
27. Global Digital Health Partnership. Advancing interoperability together globally. GDHP; 2021.
28. MedTech Europe. Interoperability standards in digital health. MedTech Europe; 2021.
29. GSMA. Digital healthcare interoperability. GSMA; 2016.
30. Health Information and Quality Authority. Overview of healthcare interoperability standards. HIQA; 2013.
31. Torab-Miandoab A, Samad-Soltani T, Jodati A, Rezaei-Hachesu P. Interoperability of heterogeneous health information systems: a systematic literature review. BMC Med Inform Decis Mak. 2023;23:18.
32. Garlapati R. Interoperability in healthcare—a focus on the social interoperability. LAP LAMBERT Academic Publishing; 2011.
33. Benson T. Training material on principles of healthcare interoperability HL7 and SNOMED. Springer; 2009.
34. Aspden P, Corrigan JM, Wolcott J, Erickson SM. Patient safety: achieving a new standard for care. National Acadamics Press; 2004.
35. Miraj SSA. Challenges and perspectives of health informatics and its management in developing Asian countries. Biosci Biotech Res Comm. 2017;10(4):597–600.
36. Kira B, Phillips T, Dolan J, Natih P, Tartakowsky A. Digital technology governance: developing countries' priorities and concerns. Digital Pathways at Oxford; 2020.
37. The Office of the National Coordinator for Health Information Technology. Guide to privacy and security of electronic health information. The Office of the National Coordinator for Health Information Technology; 2015.
38. Bell K. Public policy and health informatics. Semin Oncol Nurs. 2018;34(2):184–7.

39. World Health Organization. Global diffusion of eHealth: making universal health coverage achievable. Report of the third global survey on eHealth. WHO; 2016.
40. World Health Organization. Global strategy on digital health 2020–2025. WHO; 2021.
41. Martin G, et al. A regulatory perspective on the influence of health information technology on organisational quality and safety in England. Health Informatics J. 2020;26:897–910.
42. World Health Organization. mHealth New horizons for health through mobile technologies. Based on the findings of the second global survey on eHealth, Global Observatory for eHealth series, vol. 3. WHO; 2011.
43. UNDP. Handbook on monitoring and evaluating for results. International Federation of Red Cross and Red Crescent Societies; 2002.
44. International Labour Organization. Basic principles of monitoring and evaluation. ILO; 2017.
45. Kusek JZ, Rist RC. Ten steps to a result-based monitoring and evaluation systems. World Bank Publications; 2004.
46. Aubel J. Participatory program evaluation manual: involving program stakeholders in the evaluation process. Catholic Relief Service; 1999.
47. Patton MQ. Utilization focused evaluation the new century text. 3rd ed. Sage; 1997.
48. Wholey JS, Hatry HP, Newcomer KE. Handbook of practical program evaluation. Nonprofit Volunt Sec Q. 2010;41:1269–72.
49. Taplin DH, Clark H. Theory of change basics: a primer on theory of change. ActKnowledge; 2012.
50. Gangloff D. Theory of change. Am For. 2014;113(2):3.
51. Serrat O. Theories of change. In: Knowledge solutions. Singapore: Springer; 2017. https://doi.org/10.1007/978-981-10-0983-9_24.
52. Bickman L. The function of program theory. Wiley; 1987.
53. Mccawley PF. The logic model-for program planning and evaluation. University of Idaho Extension; 2015.
54. Kusek JZ, Rist RC. Ten steps to a results-based monitoring and evaluation system. World Bank Publications; 2004.
55. Harrell FE Jr, Lee KL, Mark DB. Multivariable prognostic models: issues in developing models, evaluating assumptions and adequacy, and measuring and reducing errors. N Engl J Med. 1996;15:361–87.
56. Pfenning F. Tools for development: a handbook for those involved in development activity. Department for International Development of the United Kingdom; 2002.
57. Stetler CB, Legro MW, Wallace CM, Bowman C, Guihan M, Hagedorn H, et al. The role of formative evaluation in implementation research and the QUERI experience. J Gen Intern Med. 2006;21(Suppl. 2):1–8.
58. Donaldson S, Scriven M. Evaluating social programs and problems: visions for the new millennium. Taylor & Francis; 2008.
59. Rossi PH, Freeman HE, Lipsey MW. Evaluation a systematic approach. Sage; 1990.
60. Education V. Formative and summative assessment: trends and practices in basic education. J Educ Pract. 2019;10(27):39–45.
61. Panchal AC. Formative and summative evaluation: challenges and remedy. Int J Res All Subj Multi Lang. 2020;8(3):15–20.
62. Taylor-Powell E, Henert E. Developing a logic model: teaching and training guide. Madison: University of Wisconsin-Madison Division of Extension, Program Development and Evaluation; 2008.
63. Lamhauge N, Lanzi E, Agrawala S. The use of indicators for monitoring and evaluation of adaptation: lessons from development cooperation agencies. Clim Dev. 2013;5(3):229–41.
64. Bond CS. Innovation in health informatics: much is underpinned by eHealth and better information for patients. J Innov Health Inform. 2015;22(4):374–6.

Ethics in Public Health Informatics

Kassahun Dessie Gashu
and Habtamu Alganeh Guadie

Abstract

According to UN's Universal Declaration, human right recognizes individual's intrinsic freedom, pride and equality. Human right serves as the foundational requirements for civic, political, and legal freedoms that uphold human dignity. Ethical complexities can diminish organization's and individual's rights. Therefore, it is vital to address ethical dilemmas during the development as well as deployment of new technologies. The misuse or excessive reliance on technology can lead to detrimental consequences. The use of e-Health systems often presents ethical dilemmas, including concerns about privacy, confidentiality, dignity, security, and safety of personal information. During the development and implementation of e-Health technologies, it is vital to uphold ethical values such as respect for life, the intention of doing good, the avoidance of harm, and the pursuit of justice. The code of ethics should adhere to the fundamental ethical principles. Ensuring ethical considerations is particularly challenging in resource-limited settings. In this chapter, we discussed the fundamental ethical principles, ethical dilemmas related to public health informatics, and strategies to improve privacy, access, security, accountability, and integrity in the area of public health informatics.

Keywords

Ethics · Public health informatics · Privacy
Access · Security · Equity · Accountability
Integrity

K. D. Gashu (✉)
Department of Health Informatics, Institute of Public Health, College of Medicine and Health Sciences, University of Gondar, Gondar, Ethiopia

SMART Health, Research and Publication Department, Bahir Dar, Ethiopia
e-mail: kassahun.dessie@uog.edu.et

H. A. Guadie
SMART Health, Research and Publication Department, Bahir Dar, Ethiopia

Department of Health System Management and Health Economics, School of Public Health, College of Medicine and Health Sciences, Bahir Dar University, Bahir Dar, Ethiopia
e-mail: Habtamu.Alganeh@bdu.edu.et

7.1 Fundamentals of Ethics

7.1.1 Overview

According to UN's Universal Declaration of Human right [1], "all human beings are born free and equal in dignity and rights". It emphasizes the universal entitlement of every individual to dignity and human rights. The proclamation was declared in 1948. It was a globally recognized framework of human rights that holds legal significance. When individuals are treated in a manner that disregards their humanity, their rights are violated. Human rights serve as the fundamental prerequisites for civic, political, and legal freedoms that uphold and safeguard human dignity.

The Declaration establishes the principles that underpin the laws governing the respect for rights, pride, and autonomies. Its purpose is addressing the ethical complexities that can violate human rights. By incorporating bioethics within the framework of international human rights, the declaration recognizes the intrinsic connection between ethical conduct and human rights. Furthermore, it ensures the preservation and reverence for human life.

UNESCO has played a significant role in shaping the basics ideologies in the bio-ethics fields of study. Notably, the organization contributed to the development of the "Universal Declaration on the Human Genome and Human Rights," which was unanimously adopted by the General Conference in 1997 and subsequently endorsed by the United Nations General Assembly in 1998. Additionally, UNESCO was involved in the formulation of the "International Declaration on Human Genetic Data," which received unanimous approval from the General Conference on October 16, 2003 [2].

The lessons learned from failure of ethical misconducts in research projects conducted in the past has laid a huge benchmark on how we engage with people now. Some of the historic research misconducts include the Tuskegee Syphilis study, Nazi war crimes during second World War, the Willow brook's study, among others.

7.1.1.1 The Tuskegee Syphilis Study (1932–1972)

The U.S Public Health Service (PHS) initiated a study to investigate the natural history of Syphilis disease among black-male Afro-Americans live in rural areas. Their study involved approximately 400 participants with syphilis and 200 uninfected individuals serving as a control group. Unfortunately, informed consent was not obtained from the participants. When penicillin became widely available as a standard treatment for syphilis by 1947, the subjects involved in the study were intentionally denied to get access to this effective therapy.

This study has become a symbol of racism in the fields of medicine and science, ethical misconduct in research, and exploitation of vulnerable populations by the government. In 1997, President Clinton formally apologized on behalf of the U.S. government for the injustices inflicted by the study. The Tuskegee study gained public attention following the release of the Belmont Report in 1972. As a result, the National Commission for the Protection of Human Subjects of Biomedical and Behavioral Research was established in 1974 [3].

After conducting its investigations, the commission presented a report titled "The Belmont Report: Ethical Principles and Guidelines for the Protection of Human Subjects of Research." This report established the core ethical principles that form the basis for conducting research involving human participants in an acceptable manner. These principles encompass autonomy, beneficences, and fairness.

7.1.1.2 Nazi War Crimes During Second World War (1940s)

During the time of the Nazi regime, physicians and scientists carried out experiments on prisoners in concentration camps without their consent. The horrific lessons learned from these unethical experiments led to the development of the Nuremberg Code, which established guiding principle that helps to conduct researches that involve humans as a study participants. The absolute necessity of obtaining voluntary consent from the human subjects is the commonest guiding principle [4].

7.1.1.3 The Willow Brook Study (1963–1966)

Deliberate infection with a hepatitis virus was inflicted upon mentally disabled children. The study involved more than 700 children, including those in both experimental and control groups [5].

7.1.2 What Is Ethics?

Some authors interchangeably use the terms "morals" and "ethics," both of which encompasses "good and bad", and "right and wrong" within the social order. Some authors draw a distinction between these two concepts, considering morality as a personal conduct and ethics as a societal norm. Others describe morality as a practical application while ethics deals with hypothetical basis. The ethical questions often lack definitive right or wrong answers. However, specific contexts require adherence to established ethical frameworks [6]. It is generally agreeable that philosophy had opened the door and played a facilitation role in the groundwork of ethics.

7.1.3 Basic Ethical Philosophies

Philosophy has played a crucial role shaping our understanding of ethics in guiding our moral judgments. The philosophy's key role was addressing fundamental questions about morality. The ancient Greek philosophers Socrates, Plato, and Aristotle laid the foundation for ethical investigation. Ethics is closely linked to metaphysics and epistemology, as beliefs about reality and knowledge influence ethical theories. Through philosophical exploration, various ethical theories like consequentialism, deontological ethics, and virtue ethics have emerged. Philosophy aids in comprehending ethical dilemmas and encourages critical thinking. It prompts individuals to reflect on their ethical beliefs, promotes open dialogue, and fosters the examination of diverse perspectives [7, 8].

The field of ethics is fundamentally based on three major ethical philosophies that can steadily define which act is right or wrong [7–10]. The three major ethical philosophies are explained below.

7.1.3.1 Deontology
Deontology is known as the Kantian approach, places emphasis on honesty, accountability, and the belief that moral principles serve as the foundation for all ethical actions. It directs attention towards the action itself rather than its consequences or outcomes. According to this perspective, actions are evaluated as morally right or wrong, just or unjust, independent of their results. Consequently, the end result can never justify the

means, in contrast to the utilitarian viewpoint. Kant's ethical system aims to establish a universally acceptable code of conduct applicable to all individuals. It is closely tied to the concepts of duty and obligation towards others. However, critics argue that this approach is overly individualistic and limited in its universal applicability across diverse cultures and belief systems [7, 9].

7.1.3.2 Consequentialism
The utilitarian perspective involves selecting actions that yield the most favorable overall outcomes while minimizing harm. However, due to the presence of numerous uncontrollable factors, utilitarianism has inherent limitations in its ability to predict events accurately. This method often favor for benefiting the majority while potentially neglecting the interests of minority groups, leading to their marginalization. Additionally, it may justify immoral tactics under the guise of pursuing the greater good [10].

7.1.3.3 The Virtue Model of Ethics
According to Hursthouse [8], virtue model is "agent-centered" rather than "act-centered" and emphasizes virtues and moral character in comparison to rules or duties (deontology) or consequences (utilitarianism). The virtue model is not concerned with consequences or ethical actions but, rather, with subjective nonrationality impulses (instincts) that influence how people act when clear rules are not present.

Ethics can further be sub-divided into three different categories [9]:

- *Meta-ethics:* It describe ethical theories
- *Normative ethics:* It focus on the process of reaching moral conclusions
- *Applied ethics:* concerned with their practical application in certain contexts

Ethical issues and dilemmas are present in various professional pursuits. Numerous academic disciplines, particularly those in the health sciences, are deeply concerned with ethics. While the establishment of institutional ethical committees has contributed to a more standardized approach to research ethics and professional conduct, the interpretation of ethical implications in specific research methodologies and practices can vary across fields and cultural contexts. Bioethics, a broader term encompassing clinical medical ethics, is a normative ethics branch applied in biology, medicine, health care decision-making, and public policy. It also addresses ethical concerns linked to fundamental scientific inquiry. As a relatively emerging and expansive area of exploration, bioethical science is flourishing in response to the advancements of the biological revolution, which have presented new capabilities, options, and challenges [11].

7.1.4 Ethical Principles

Ethical principles form an integral part of normative theories that provide justification and defense for moral rules and judgments. They are not contingent upon individual subjective perspectives. Fundamental ethical principles and basic professional codes of ethics apply to all social interactions.

7.1.4.1 Fundamental Ethical Principles

According to Beauchamp and Childress [12], For a code of ethics to be considered comprehensive, it should align with the four core-principles of ethics such as, beneficences, non-maleficence, autonomy, and justice.

The Principle of Respect for Autonomy

It entails showing respect for individuals and acknowledging their personal rights. Every person possesses a fundamental entitlement to self-determination [13]. The application of the principle of respect for autonomy gives rise to the following moral principles or obligations [14].

- Tell the truth
- Respect other people's privacy
- Safeguard sensitive data
- Ask for consent before intervening with patients

The Principle of Beneficence

It is promoting good and acting in the best interest of others. Every individual has an obligation to promote the well-being of others, provided that the nature of this well-being aligns with the fundamental and ethically justifiable values of the parties involved. This concept can be traced back to the Hippocratic oath (fourth century BC), which primarily focused on the doctor-patient relationship and emphasized the physician's code of conduct. It stated, "I will use treatment to help the sick according to my ability and judgment." In contemporary terms, this obligation extends to various aspects, such as a physician's duty to refer patients to other healthcare professionals when necessary and to continuously stay informed about the latest advancements and discoveries in medical science, among other responsibilities [15]. The principle of beneficence supports the moral principles or obligations listed below [14].

- Protect and defend the rights of others
- Prevent injury to others
- Remove conditions that will cause harm
- Assist people with disabilities
- Rescue people in danger

The Principle of Non-maleficence

It is to mean "not doing harm". Every individual has the responsibility to prevent harm to others to the extent that it is feasible without causing undue harm to themselves. This principle can be traced back to the Hippocratic Oath (fourth century BC), which pertains to the doctor-patient relationship and emphasizes the physician's code of conduct. The oath states, "I will use treatment to help the sick according to my ability and judgment, but I will never use it to injure or wrong them." [16]. The following guidelines are supported by the principle of non-maleficence [14].

- Avoid killing
- Avoid causing suffering or agony
- Do not render helpless
- Avoid offending others

The Principle of Equality and Justice

In the realm of public health, justice entails the equitable allocation of the threats, expenses and related-benefits in the society. Every individual, regardless of their status, possesses an inherent right to be treated with equality and impartiality. Fairness specifically pertains towards impartial allocation of paybacks, risks, costs, and resources. The principles advocate equitable distribution to each individuals based on [14]:

- Equal allocation
- Individual need
- Personal effort
- Individual contribution
- Merit-based considerations

7.1.4.2 Basic Professional Code of Ethics

Most professional societies or organizations have established fundamental codes of ethics for their members, in addition to upholding the four core ethical principles [14]:

(a) Respect for human dignity
(b) Maintenance of confidentiality

(c) Protection of privacy
(d) Safeguarding patient rights

7.1.5   Ethics in Public Health

It is evident that the bioethical concepts cannot be used in public health practice in the same manner [17]. Within public health, there exist additional fundamental principles such as equality, utility, and stewardship, as illustrated in Fig. 7.1. These fundamental ethical principles should be integrated with these basic public health principles.

Reaching a consensus among all stakeholders in public health regarding the moral dilemmas arising from certain initiatives is often challenging and not straightforward. However, there are various tools available, such as codes of ethics for public health that can facilitate progress and provide safeguards against potential abuses. Codes of ethics encompass a collection of ideals and principles that should be considered in any conflict, although they are not designed to provide straightforward solutions to intricate ethical

Fig. 7.1 The basic principles of public health

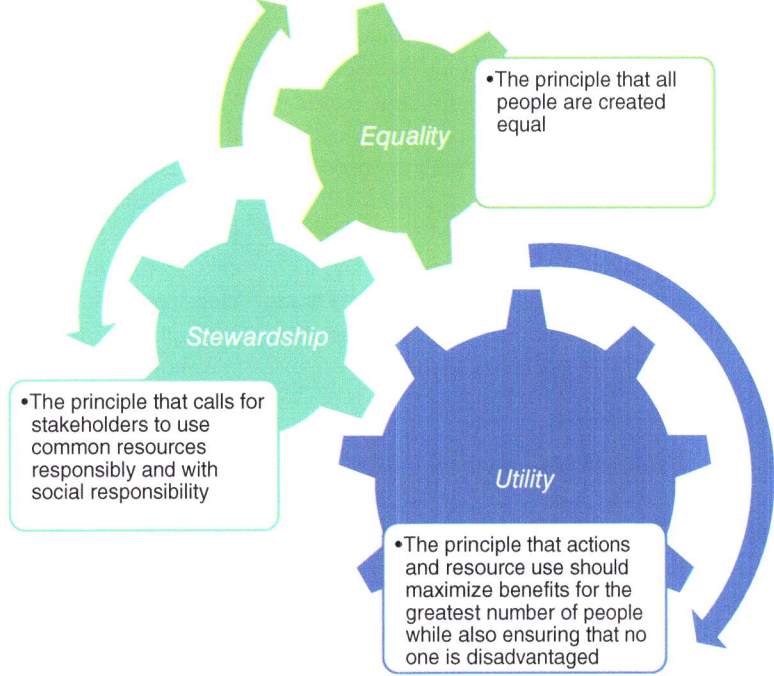

- The principle that all people are created equal

Equality

Stewardship

- The principle that calls for stakeholders to use common resources responsibly and with social responsibility

Utility

- The principle that actions and resource use should maximize benefits for the greatest number of people while also ensuring that no one is disadvantaged problems [17]. Accordingly, the code of ethics specifies the following public health principles.

- Primarily focus on addressing the underlying source of illnesses and preventing health and health-related problems.
- Expected to respect community's rights.
- Prioritize, initiate, and involve procedures that allow for community input during their design and evaluation.
- Targeted to ensure accessibility to essential healthcare services including empowerment of marginalized community members.
- Strives for demanding best available data and evidences to formulate policy, programs and to inform routine activities.
- Offer the required data to make informed decisions and seeking community approval before implementation.
- Obligated to take prompt action based on the available resource and directives set forth.
- Integrate diverse strategies that respect community's norms.
- Enhance the physical and social environment integrated into public health initiatives and policies.
- Ensure data security, if disclosed, could jeopardize the well-being of an individual or community. Exceptions should only be made when there is a chance to have substantial harms in the community.
- Have sufficient manpower with the necessary competence and expertise
- Create collaborations and partnerships between public health organizations and their staff members should be conducted in a manner that enhances the effectiveness of the institution and promotes public trust.

7.1.6   Ethics in Informatics

Historically, the field of information and communication technology, including software development, did not prioritize the practice of ethics. Software development progressed gradually and did not always have a direct impact on everyday

life. However, in today's interconnected world, software is ubiquitous, and advancements in big data and data analytics have significant implications for each individual.

In general, software design and development, and specifically in the context of public health, adhere to eight guiding principles of code of ethics. The items listed under each guiding principle serve as a means to evaluate whether the software development process aligns with the code of ethics. Each item provides a range of response categories, including strongly favor, favor, uncertain, oppose, and strongly oppose [18]. Hence, the following are the guiding principles of ethics in software development.

7.1.6.1 Software Products with Satisfactory Quality

The software design and development process should ensure that the end product is free of errors, delivered within the set timeframe, and of satisfactory quality for the general public, employers, clients, and users. The process begins by comprehending the requirements and expectations of all stakeholders and formulating a thorough project plan. During the design phase, the emphasis is on establishing a strong foundation that adheres to the defined requirements. The quality assurance and testing play a vital role in early detection and resolution of errors. Continuous and effective collaboration and communication among team members and stakeholders ensure congruence and satisfaction. Continuous improvement allows for learning from errors and refining the development process. In return, the software design and development process can result in error-free and high-quality products that fulfills the needs of all stakeholders.

7.1.6.2 Independent and Scientific Judgments

Although ethical codes are not laws, they do provide policy makers with information and practical guidance on matters that concern professionals and their clients. Software engineers must safeguard both their professional judgment's independence and its reputations.

7.1.6.3 Products for Public Wellbeing

Software engineers must always act in a way that promotes the general welfare, health, and safety of the public. It requires to follow the laws, regulations, and ethical guidelines that govern software development to ensure public safety. Prioritizing user-centric design, conducting risk assessments, and implementing security measures are essential for this purpose. Collaborating with experts and continuously learning contribute to the creation of secure software solutions. Transparency, effective communication, and responsiveness to feedback are vital for maintaining public trust and addressing any concerns that may arise.

7.1.6.4 Continuous Self-Development

Developers should constantly work to improve their skills so they can perform their work as it should be performed.

7.1.6.5 Loyal Developer-Client Relationship

Software developers are required to consistently work within their professional roles, behaving as dutiful representatives. They should consider the well-being and security of the general public while performing their duties.

7.1.6.6 Effective Leadership

When acting in a managerial or leadership role, a software engineer must act ethically and support and motivate individuals they are responsible for in fulfilling their individual and group commitments.

7.1.6.7 Professional Integrity

Software engineers are obligated to maintain the integrity and standing of their profession, ensuring that their actions do not compromise the well-being of the community. In order to achieve this, it is essential for healthcare software engineers to adhere to professional codes of conduct and continually enhance their knowledge and skills through ongoing education and training. They should employ ethical decision-making frameworks to assess the impact of their actions, while also promoting accountability and creating an environment that encourages the reporting of unethical behavior. Collaboration, peer review, and open discussions centered on ethical challenges play a vital role in identifying and resolving potential issues. Additionally, advocating for industry standards and regulations, as well as leading by example and providing mentorship, further contribute to upholding professional integrity. By implementing these strategies, software engineers for healthcare can ensure that their actions align with the well-being of the community and uphold the esteemed reputation of their profession.

7.1.6.8 Promoting Fairness in Teamwork

Software developers must treat everyone equally with whom they interact and actively promote teamwork that would create a positive and productive working environments. Promoting the culture of fairness in any teamwork needs a continuing efforts and commitments.

7.2 Ethics in Public Health Informatics

As e-Health services and their users continue to advance, ethical conflicts arise that have the potential to affect fundamental human rights. These dilemmas arise from the combination of the e-Health solutions used to provide the healthcare services and how the data they contain is utilized. The ethical hurdles that emerge can undermine individual's and organization's rights. Some of the major ethical concerns include trustfulness, confidentiality, data security, proprietorship, dignity, and fairness are key aspects where technology and data overlap that demands careful planning. Furthermore, when developing and implementing e-Health technology, it is essential to consider overarching ethical principles such as respect for life, the pursuit of beneficence, the avoidance of harm, and the promotion of justice [19].

7.2.1 Why Ethics in Public Health Informatics?

As a result of the rapid and worldwide revolution in information technology, there is a discernible shift towards a new paradigm of communication and service provision. Information technology possesses a dual nature, capable of both positively and negatively impacting the well-being of individuals, organizations, and countries. When utilized appropriately, information technology enables countries to make significant strides in their social and economic development. However, misuse and excessive reliance on technology can lead to detrimental consequences.

Similarly, when engaging with technology, especially in the context of e-Health systems, ethical dilemmas arise, encompassing concerns such as privacy, confidentiality, dignity, security, and safety in relation to personal information [20]. Consequently, ethical principles are essential for effectively addressing the practical ethical dilemmas that arise in the field. When developing and implementing e-Health technology, it is vital to uphold the overarching ethical values of respect for life, the pursuit of beneficence, the avoidance of harm, and the promotion of justice. Moreover, specific ethical principles must be established and applied to safeguard the rights of individuals and organizations.

7.2.2 Ethical Principles in Public Health Informatics

The fundamental ethical principles are also essential ethical components public health informatics. Taking that in to account, the ethical principles in health informatics including PHI consists of [19]:

7.2.2.1 Privacy

Citizens possess the autonomy to determine which personal details they wish to disclose. This encompasses the following concepts:

- Safeguarding the privacy, anonymity, and confidentiality of individuals and ensuring their voluntary consent when sharing personal information in e-Health.
- Ensuring that health data is regarded as the property of the patient.
- Implementing measures to secure data from unauthorized access by third parties.

- Obtaining explicit consent from individuals before sharing their health information.

7.2.2.2 Beneficence

Beneficence stands as a core ethical principle, particularly in the realm of e-Health initiatives. Within this framework, it entails promoting the well-being of individuals. Beneficence in e-Health encompasses the following aspects:

- Maximizing the benefits for individuals by harnessing the potential of IT in improving data quality and facilitating data-informed decision-making.
- Leveraging the capabilities of cybersecurity functions to safeguard against unauthorized access to data by third parties.

7.2.2.3 Non-maleficence

The principle of non-maleficence entails preventing the potential harm that affect individuals or communities welfare. The process of eliminating the potential harms, starts early at the designing stage and continues to the developing, and implementing phases of an e-Health projects. This principle encompasses the following elements:

- Avoiding the use of data that may lead to erroneous clinical decisions by healthcare providers, which could potentially harm patients.
- Preventing the misuse of personal information that could result in social exclusion, stigma, discrimination, or job rejection.

7.2.2.4 Justice

Equality and equity are integral to the concept of justice in e-Health. This entails ensuring that everyone has equal opportunities to access similar e-Health services. The pursuit of justice involves addressing and preventing inequities. For example, certain groups such as the elderly, individuals with limited education, those without employment, and those residing in rural areas may not have equal access to e-Health services. It is observed that individuals with lower levels of education tend to utilize digital services less frequently compared to those with higher levels of education.

7.2.2.5 Trust

It is crucial to instill public confidence by ensuring correct data processing, up-to-date and high-quality information, and adequate consideration of security threats. The successful development of e-Health systems can positively influence end-users' trust in adopting the new system. This encompasses various concepts, including:

- Competence of the personnel involved in e-Health initiatives.
- Maintaining accuracy, consistency, legitimacy, integrity, and confidentiality of e-Health data.
- Ensuring the security and safety of data.

7.2.3   Ethical Guiding Principles

According to the e-Health Ethics Summit in 2000 [21, 22], the guiding principles of e-Health code of ethics has been set by the Internet Healthcare Coalition in collaboration with WHO as mentioned below.

- *Disclose details that, if known by consumers, would probably alter how they perceive or utilize the product:* Individuals who rely on the Internet for health-related purposes should have the autonomy to assess the reliability and trustworthiness of the websites and services they utilize.
- *Be truthful (being honest) and not deceptive:* Internet users seeking health information should have confidence that the information they acquire is both accurate and presented in a transparent and non-misleading manner.
- *Provide current, accurate, and understandable health information:* Ensure the provision of up-to-date, precise, and comprehensible health information. It is essential for individuals to have the right and reasonable expectation that websites will offer reliable,

well-substantiated information, along with high-quality goods and services. This enables them to make informed decisions regarding their healthcare.

- *Request and accept users' right to choose (Informed Consent):* Acknowledge and respect users' autonomy in determining the gathering, utilization, and sharing of their personal information. Individuals accessing health-related information should be informed about the potential collection of their personal data and be empowered to make decisions regarding their consent for the collection, use, and sharing of such information. Furthermore, individuals possess the right to choose when and how they actively participate in a business partnership, and their consent should be obtained accordingly.
- *Respecting basic ethical obligations (Professionalism):* Respecting fundamental ethical obligations is paramount. Healthcare professionals must uphold ethical norms when providing specialized and confidential medical advice or care through online platforms.
- *Make sure the organizations and websites they affiliate with are reliable (Responsible partnering):* Ensure that healthcare professionals establish affiliations with reliable organizations and websites. This involves forming partnerships with trustworthy individuals or entities that can be relied upon for providing accurate and ethical information and services.

Ensure that users have relevant opportunities to provide the website with feedback (Accountability): It is crucial for individuals to have confidence that businesses and individuals operating websites providing health-related information, goods, or services on the internet prioritize users' concerns and uphold ethical business practices. The e-Health tools should incorporate user-friendly features that allow users to provide feedback and enable prompt response to complaints.

7.2.4   Ethical Dimensions in Public Health Informatics

There are various dimensions of public health informatics and yet on the way of advancement. This book included some well-articulated ethical perspectives in public health informatics such as:

- Information privacy and disposition
- Data access
- Data security
- Data equity
- Data accountability
- Data integrity

This book further illustrates in the proceeding chapters focusing on the list of ethical dimensions in public health informatics.

7.3   Privacy and Disposition of Health Data

7.3.1   What's Privacy?

Several scholars from various disciplines have attempted to define privacy due to its uncertainty. According to Nissenbaum [23], Privacy can be conceptualized as "contextual integrity," wherein the flow of information aligns with expectations and norms regarding information disclosure. In line with the theory of contextual integrity, privacy is considered a characteristic of sociotechnical systems that individuals navigate and comprehend based on their personal expectations and societal standards.

According to Fried [24], Privacy refers to the individual's entitlement to maintain the confidentiality of personal information and exercise control over its dissemination. It can also be defined as the assertion of individuals, groups, or institutions to independently determine the timing, manner, and extent of the communication of information about themselves to others [25]. In general, the concept of privacy recognizes that every individual possesses a fundamental right to privacy. This right entails having control over various aspects such as the collection, storage, access, use, communication, manipulation, and disposal of personal data.

7.3.2   Types of Privacy

It is of utmost importance to protect consumer privacy in the modern era, where organizations extensively collect, store, and process personal data. When it comes to the health industries, data privacy becomes a priority and critical agenda. To ensure responsible handling of data, legal frameworks, industry standards, and technological measures are implemented to safeguard consumer privacy and promote secure data practices.

Generally, consumer privacy can be broadly categorized into three types [25–27], namely: information privacy, communication privacy, and individual privacy. They are interconnected and often intersect with each other. The three types of privacy are discussed below.

7.3.2.1   Information Privacy
Information privacy pertains to the consumer's entitlement to exercise control over the access, use, and dissemination of their personal data. It grants individuals the freedom to make decisions regarding when, how, and to what extent others can access their information. When submitting personal information online for medical purposes, it is ensured that the information will be treated as private. This is particularly crucial for sensitive health-related information, as improper disclosure can lead to significant consequences.

7.3.2.2   Communication Privacy
It entails safeguarding private communications or interactions to prevent unauthorized listening, searching, or interception. The objective is to maintain the privacy of conversations and ensure they remain free from external surveillance.

7.3.2.3   Individual Privacy
The protection and preservation of individual privacy are prioritized. Threats to individual privacy can arise from invasions of personal space, emotional manipulation, physical interference, and similar factors.

7.3.3   Privacy Legislations and Policies

Some of the relevant legislations stated to protect data and personal health information (PHI) are as follows:

- The Privacy Act in Australia, 1988
- The Data Protection Directive by European Union in 1995
- The HIPAA in the USA in 1996
- The COPPA in the USA in 1998
- The Gramm-Leach-Bliley in the USA in 1999
- The Data PIPEDA in Canada, 2000
- The Act09–08 in Morocco, 2009
- The GDPR by European Union in 2015
- The Consumer Privacy Act (CCPA) in California, enacted in June 2018
- The General Data Protection Law (LGPD) in Brazil passed in 2018
- The Consumer Data Protection Act (CDPA) in Virginia enacted on March 2, 2021.

In addition, the International Standard ISO/IEC 29100 defines 11 privacy principles as listed in the Fig. 7.2.

A "privacy policy" is a document that outlines an institution's approach to handling individuals' data. However, it may not always align with the preferences of the individuals involved. The primary objective of a privacy policy is to safeguard individuals' privacy when it comes to the disclosure of personal information. There are four common goals that a privacy policy aims to achieve:

- Empowering patients/individuals with complete control over their electronic health records
- Determining authorized individuals who can access and track the information
- Ensuring secure transfer of information
- Reducing the possibility of illegal data access

7.3.4   Why Privacy in Public Health Informatics?

As everyone is entitled to equal rights under the law, so that all the laws that oppose or undermine this equality are morally unjust. One of these rights is the right to privacy. Privacy can be defined as the ability to overcome or be free from

Fig. 7.2 List of data privacy principles

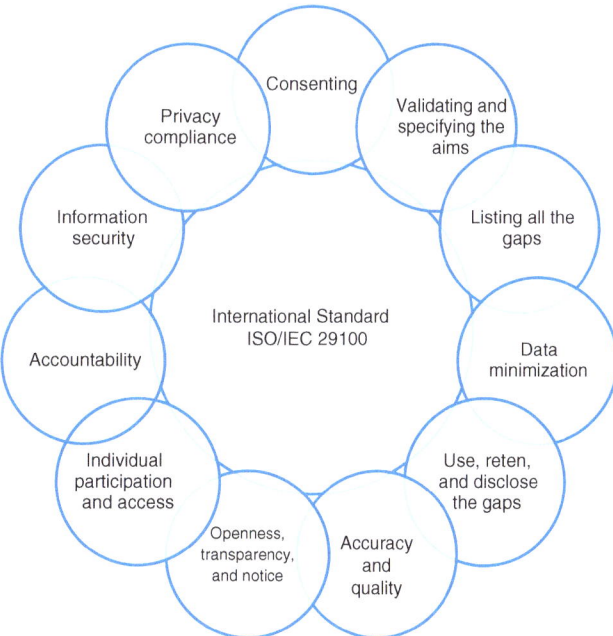

unwanted interferences and disturbances. It is closely linked, either directly or indirectly, to the ownership and control of information-sharing systems.

Given their engagement and increasing acceptance of new technologies, individuals are becoming more concerned on their private data security. Privacy concerns arise prominently during the processes of data storage, analysis, and dissemination using digital solutions such as EMRs. Therefore, it is crucial to establish mechanisms that ensure the privacy of health data stored and transmitted digitally.

The main objective of implementing privacy regulations in digital health is to achieve a balance between effectively safeguarding individuals' health-related data and enabling the required sharing of healthcare data to deliver and improve healthcare of exceptional quality. This approach aims to safeguard the health and well-being of the general public [28]. Implementing regulations that mandate reasonable safeguards to uphold the privacy of health information and impose limitations on unauthorized use and disclosure of such information across public health information systems. The right of individuals to their own data encompasses the rights to access their health records, request copies of them, transfer data in electronic format to a third party, and seek rectifications through an appeals process.

7.3.5 Privacy Principles

Generally, the "seven privacy-by-design principles" proposed by Ann Cavoukian [29], To ensure the implementation of fair information privacy protection practices during the design and implementation process, the following principles should be considered:

(i) Proactive not reactive: Emphasizing the use of technology to predict and prevent privacy threats before they occur.
(ii) Privacy as the default setting: Enforcing default privacy settings to enhance personal data security. This ensures privacy is main-

tained even if users do not actively adhere to specific privacy standards.
(iii) Privacy embedded into design: Recognizing privacy as a fundamental component or operation in any system.
(iv) Not a zero-sum game, but a positive-sum: Designing privacy in a way that achieves a "win-win" scenario, where privacy can be upheld without compromising other aspects.
(v) End-to-end security: Addressing security concerns throughout the entire lifecycle of data, from its inception to its disposal, particularly when dealing with patients' data.
(vi) Visibility and transparency: Ensuring that all stakeholders can observe and understand how information flows within the system.
(vii) Respect for user privacy: Designing user-centric solutions that actively involve both the data owner and other stakeholders to prioritize and protect user privacy.

7.3.6 Privacy Architectures

To establish robust privacy solutions, it is crucial to incorporate best practices and principles into the design phase. In general, there are four commonly employed architectures for designing information privacy systems: centralized, decentralized, third-party, and hybrid architectures. These architectures offer different approaches to address privacy concerns effectively. The architecture approaches include centralized, decentralized, third-party and hybrid approaches.

(i) *Centralized:* A centralized data storage approach involves the efficient management of data in a single location. This method offers cost-effective maintenance, but it lacks control over data usage.
(ii) *Decentralized:* A distributed data storage model allows for greater control over data security and usage. However, it comes with a higher maintenance cost.
(iii) *Third-party:* A centralized data storage type is cost-effective but carries the risk of potential data disclosure to third parties and lacks control over data usage.

(iv) *Hybrid:* The data storage type can either be centralized or distributed, leveraging the benefits of both centralized and decentralized architectures. However, the hybrid approach may present challenges in terms of management.

7.3.7   Privacy Solutions

There are various categories of privacy-preserving techniques used in protecting data privacy in any digital health systems. The commonly used are cloud-based, blockchain-based, and policy-based techniques to protect data privacy.

7.3.7.1 Cloud-Based
To address the increasing data volume generated by edge devices such as IoT, fog-based and edge-based solutions have emerged as extensions of cloud computing. These technologies distribute data processing and storage across a decentralized network of devices and fog nodes. By doing so, they enable accelerated processing and minimize latency. This decentralized approach reduces the necessity of constantly transferring data to a centralized cloud server, thereby facilitating real-time analytics, faster response times, and decreased network congestion. The utilization of fog computing and edge computing is particularly critical in applications like smart cities, industrial automation, healthcare monitoring, and autonomous systems, as they effectively tackle the challenges posed by the expanding data volume.

7.3.7.2 Blockchain-Based
As previously discussed in the section on privacy strategies, Blockchain technology is gaining significance in the realm of digital health. It is utilized to tackle privacy concerns while ensuring data accessibility.

7.3.7.3 Policy-Based
Many privacy-protecting technologies have used a privacy-by-design approach, but they fall short of meeting the needs of all stakeholders. Whereas, a privacy policy plays a significant role in the design and implementation of information privacy in digital health through addressing all the concerns raised by stakeholders.

7.3.8   How to Ensure Privacy in Digital Health?

There are different techniques of ensuring privacy of health information offered through any form of a public health informatics tools. However, there is no single effective technique suitable for all situations [30]. This section mainly focused on access Control, cryptography, anonymization and blockchain privacy preserving techniques.

7.3.8.1 Access Control
These techniques aim to limit access to only those who are legitimate to the information. The implementation of access control techniques can vary depending on the approach taken to grant permissions [31].

An example of such a technique is 'role-based access control', where authorizations are assigned on the user's predetermined role. It focuses on limiting network access based on a user's role within an organization. It grants privileges based solely on the specific responsibilities and accountabilities associated with an individual's role within the institution, as illustrated in Fig. 7.3.

Conversely, Attribute-Based Access Control (ABAC), also referred to as policy-based access control, considers attributes when assigning permissions. ABAC is utilized to protect resources, such as data, network hardware, and other assets, from unauthorized users and actions. Unauthorized users are those who lack the approved attributes specified in the institution's security policies. ABAC has evolved from the more straightforward role-based access control approach.

Components of Access Control
The primary components that influence access decisions in a system consist of subject attributes, resource attributes, action attributes, and environmental attributes.

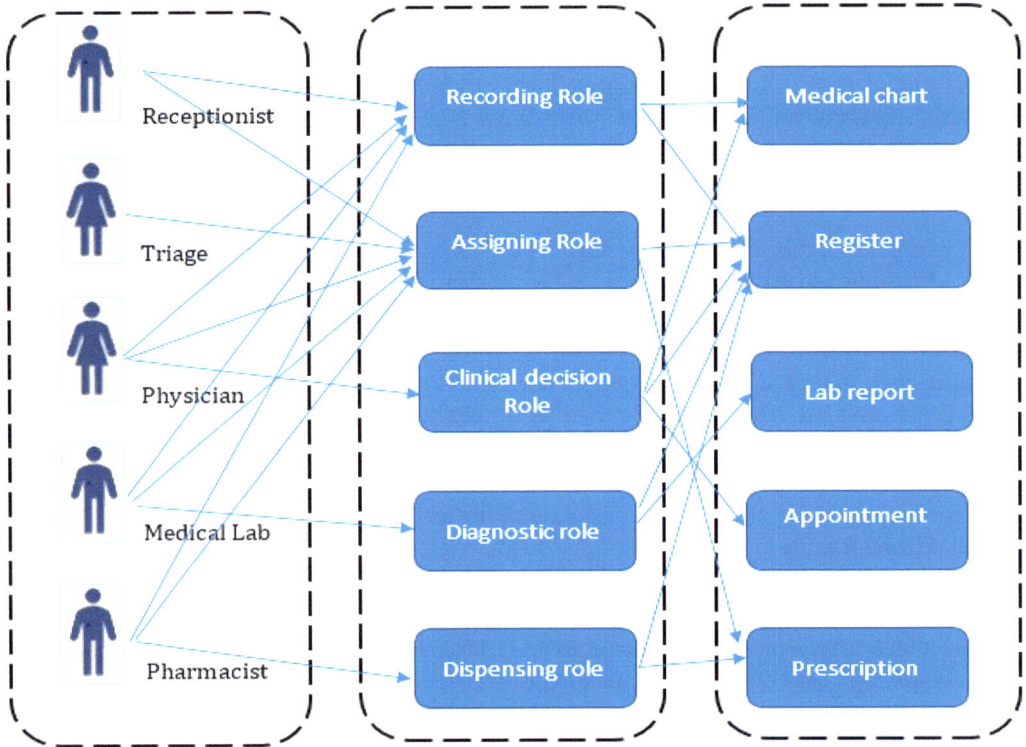

Fig. 7.3 Assigning access control using role-based access control technique

Subject Attributes

These are the characteristics associated with the user, such as their profile information (ID, job title, position, etc.). Subject attributes serve as authentication tokens during system login.

Resource Attributes

Resources refer to objects like files, applications, servers, APIs, etc. that the subject requests access to. Resource attributes provide specific details about the resources, such as a correct bank account number for accessing a bank account.

Action Attributes

Action attributes pertain to the user's activities within the system. Common action attributes include actions like "write," "read," "copy," "edit," "delete," etc. An action can have multiple attributes that describe it.

Environmental Attributes

Environmental attributes encompass contextual factors such as time and location that relate to the

access request. These attributes provide additional context for making access decisions.

Techniques of User Authentication

User authentication is the process by which a user verifies their identity to gain access to a digital health system. The most commonly employed technique for authentication is the combination of a username/identity and password. However, a privacy concern arises if an unauthorized party gains access to the user's ID and password. There are three primary techniques for user authentication, which are as follows:

Something a User Knows

This includes information that the user possesses, such as a login ID, password, or email. It relies on the user's knowledge of specific details to authenticate their identity.

Something a User Has

This involves possession of a physical item that the user carries, such as a swipe card, key, digital certificate, or access card. The user presents this item as proof of their identity.

Something That Identifies the User

This utilizes biometric characteristics unique to the individual, such as voice patterns, facial recognition, retinal patterns, or auto-fingerprints. These biological traits serve as means of identification.

7.3.8.2 Cryptography

Cryptography involves the utilization of mathematical algorithms to encode information, ensuring that only the intended recipient can decipher and read the message. Various cryptography methods are employed to safeguard privacy, including [32]:

1. *Secret Key Cryptography (SKC)*: It applies the same key for both encryption and decryption.
2. *Public Key Cryptography (PKC)*: It applies two different keys for encryption and decryption.
3. *Hash Function Cryptography (HFC)*: It generates output of fixed size from unfixed size input data.

7.3.8.3 Anonymization

Anonymization, also known as de-identification is the technique that commonly performed before undertaking distribution and analysis [32]. It is aimed to hide the identity of the individual to protect from unauthorized access. There are different techniques of data anonymization.

Masking

Data masking is a disclosure of data after modifying its values. It is done by generating a mirror image of a database through techniques such as encryption, character shuffling, or substitution of characters. For instance, a value can be replaced by symbols such as "$" or "*". In case of geographic masking [33], it follows the approach of altering the dataset in a random way to preserve the spatial location. The three geo-masking techniques include systematic swapping, truncating (rounding the coordinates), and displacing (spatial skewing/ fuzzing/perturbing/geo-scrambling or off-setting) the coordinates.

Pseudonymization

It is a technique that replaces individual identifiers with fictional identifiers, known as pseudonyms. This process involves modifying personal information in a way that renders it unidentifiable without possessing a specific secret.

Generalization

Generalization involves intentionally removing certain parts of the data to reduce its identifiability. For example, a household ID may be omitted while ensuring that other key information remains intact, aiming to remove identifiers while maintaining the accuracy of the data.

Swapping

Data swapping, also known as permutation/shuffling is about readjusting the attribute values of a dataset. For example, switching columns values can make an impact on anonymization.

Data Perturbation

By using round-numbering techniques and including random noise, data perturbation somewhat alters the original dataset. For example, using a base of five for rounding values like age.

Synthetic Data

It is artificially created information that has no connection to the case. Instead than changing or using the actual dataset, which would compromise privacy, the data is used to create fictional datasets. The techniques include development of mathematical models such as, regression, standard deviations, medians which are developed using the original dataset or using synthetic results.

7.3.8.4 Blockchain

Nakamoto [34], has initially introduced Blockchain to power Bitcoin. Currently, Blockchain [35, 36] has stretched out of the financial sector and becoming popular for facilitating decentralization and privacy in the digital health due to its multiple features like decentralization, open-source, transparency, immutability, autonomy and anonymity.

7.3.9 Maintaining Data Privacy in Resource-Limited Settings

The right to privacy is beyond regulations. Rather, a universally accepted basic human right, explicitly or implicitly, in prominent global treaties and the constitutions of numerous nations worldwide. The significance of the right to privacy is acknowledged by any democratic society.

When establishing health ICT systems, it is crucial to prioritize the protection of individual patient data. Before implementation, architects of EHRs must assess the security of the applications and associated systems. Privacy and security measures should be integrated at every stage of health ICT system development. Nevertheless, ensuring data privacy within electronic health records can be challenging and expensive, particularly in situations where multiple entities may have access to the information.

Protecting data privacy needs more attention particularly in resource-limited settings as the risk is worsen due to various complex contexts [37, 38]. There is also limited evidence how to protect data privacy, the implementation feasibility and acceptability methods in resource-limited settings [39]. One of the significant obstacles is that many developing nations are at varying stages of embracing digital technology for socioeconomic advancements, including healthcare development. The delays in progress can be attributed to a lack of global coordination in this regard. To translate commitment into action, the implementation phase needs to take place at both the national and regional levels [40].

According to a study on "EHRs and privacy protection in LMICs" [41], sharing of passwords, poor data transfer practices, unencrypted data transmission systems, low awareness on data security, lack of legal, regulatory and institutional support found to be the challenges related to EHRs in resource limited settings. As a result, loss of data, loss of trust and integrity, hacking were likely to happening.

To overcome the barriers related to data privacy, it is suggested to deploy ICT solutions, legal frameworks, sorting data by sensitivity and engaging stakeholders from the design (co-creation with clients) [41]. The reduction of data breaches can be achieved by establishing a system framework that provides a secure connection to EHR systems. Robust end-to-end encryption should be implemented to ensure the secure transfer of health data. EHR systems should incorporate strong authentication methods, such as smart health cards, tokens, one-time passwords, or biometrics, to safeguard patient confidentiality and data privacy. Therefore, all stakeholders have a responsibility to enhance data privacy in EHRs. Key actions to be taken include:

- Developing national policies and frameworks that establish standardized architectures for data protection within the digital system.
- Conducting comprehensive feasibility assessments of the technology prior to deployment.
- Ensuring that EHRs have built-in or standalone data privacy protection tools.
- Assessing readiness for scaling up the system.
- Designing the system with end-users in mind, considering social norms, behavior, and local contexts.
- Establishing guidelines for the acceptable use of the system by the implementing institution.
- Developing and implementing metrics to regularly monitor and evaluate the effectiveness of data privacy protection in digital systems

7.4 Improving Access to Health Data

Data access is a crucial element of data governance, providing foundational value and guidance for the secure and appropriate delivery of data to intended recipients while ensuring privacy and security. Data serves as the bedrock of scientific endeavors and requires proper management throughout the entire lifecycle, from collection to utilization. Various stakeholders within the healthcare system, including health facilities, public entities, and researchers, require access to health data for purposes such as planning, research, performance evaluation, and serving public interests. To facilitate research, several measures can be taken, including reducing the time it takes to access data, utilizing remote access data enclaves more frequently, and promoting awareness and establishment of guidelines for best practices in data protection. Increasing the availability of data in a meaningful way, with appropriate transparency and reproducibility, enhances the effectiveness of the scientific method and benefits society as a whole.

In the pursuit of advancing healthcare and improving health outcomes, it is crucial to enhance access to health data. However, it is equally important to strike a balance between facilitating data access and safeguarding personal information, both in the present and in future disclosures. Regulations, laws, professional codes of ethics, and best practices play a vital role in achieving this balance.

To ensure responsible use of health data while addressing security and privacy concerns, it is imperative to establish standards such as informed consent, data sharing agreements, data protection measures, de-identification techniques, and data security protocols. By implementing these regulations and ethical guidelines, individuals' privacy can be protected while enabling the responsible utilization of health data.

7.4.1   What Is Access to Health Data?

Access to health data refers to the ability of individuals, organizations, and systems to retrieve health-related data for various purposes such as research, policy-making, healthcare management, and personal health management. This health-related data encompasses a wide range of information, including medical records, public health data, health insurance claims, and more. The availability of these data sources enables informed decision-making and facilitates the use of data-driven approaches in clinical and public health practices.

Good access to health data refers to obtaining health-related data fulfilling safety, security, and respectful of privacy. Here are major characteristics of good access to health data:

- *Data should be accessible:* The essence lies in making data accessible to those who require it, precisely when they require it. This necessitates the establishment of a system that enables effortless retrieval and sharing of data. To facilitate data access, it is essential to have data sharing agreements in place.
- *Allow timely access:* Effective access to health data entails the timely availability of data to healthcare providers, researchers, and other stakeholders, enabling them to make well-informed decisions promptly.
- *Access to accurate data:* Ensuring quality access to health data involves providing accurate and reliable information. This necessitates the use of standardized methods, validated measures, and regular data quality checks.
- *Access to complete data:* To establish effective access to health data, a comprehensive approach is essential, encompassing all pertinent information. This entails incorporating multiple sources, such as medical records, laboratory results, and patient-generated data. Additionally, data sharing agreements should clearly specify the types of data that can be shared.
- *Maintaining security:* Optimal access to health data should prioritize security and safeguard against unauthorized access, use, and disclosure. This necessitates the implementation of robust data security methods, including regular access controls and monitoring measures.
- *Ethical access:* To establish proper access to health data, it is crucial to have an ethical and responsible access policy in place. This entails implementing regulations and ethical guidelines that govern the access and use of health data. Additionally, regular monitoring and evaluation systems should be established to ensure ongoing compliance and effectiveness of the access policy.

7.4.2 Controversies in Privacy and Access to Health Data

The basic tension between data access and data confidentiality is balancing the risk of breaching privacy and confidentiality with the potential utility related to the data [42].

The challenge lies in handling the highly sensitive and personal nature of health data, as there is a potential risk of unauthorized disclosure or misuse without the patient's consent. Striking a balance between the benefits of data sharing and the imperative to protect privacy is crucial. Undoubtedly, data sharing contributes to improving healthcare outcomes. However, unauthorized access and misuse of data can have severe repercussions for patients, while also eroding trust in the healthcare system. Some of the major controversies include:

- Despite security methods available, data breaching remained a problem in the healthcare industries.
- Despite data sharing improves healthcare outcomes and lead to better research and more effective treatments, but it is still with cost of compromising the risk of patient confidentiality that leads to discrimination.
- Informed consent is not always practical
- Confusions on who owns health data and who has the right to access it.
- Bias and discrimination can occur if data is not collected or analyzed in a way that is inclusive and equitable.

There are potential solutions to overcome the tension between data sharing and patient privacy. The solutions depend on the specific context. A tailored and collaborative approach is effective in addressing the possible tensions between data sharing and patient privacy. Some of the potential solutions include:

(a) Removing personal identifiers (anonymization) from health data
(b) Limiting access (controlling access) to health data to only those individuals or organizations that have a legitimate need

(c) Providing explicit consent options to patients for their health data to be used for research or other purposes
(d) Establishing clear data sharing guidelines and policies (data governance) to ensure ethical and responsible use of data.
(e) Capacity building on data sharing and its potential benefits to build trust and support

7.4.3 Why Access to Data?

The rationale behind the need of establishing a seamless system is about ensuring access to health data. Multiple foundations exist for comprehending, guaranteeing, and safeguarding access to data in shared sources such as warehouse. Accessing quality and timely data plays a crucial role in improving healthcare outcomes [43]. For instance, having access to a patient's medical history can be used for a continuum of healthcare and enable to identify potential health risks. It is the way to advance medical researches. A well-established health data infrastructure can be used for generating evidence such as identifying risk factors, track disease trends, and develop new treatments and evaluate the safety and efficacy of new drugs or medical devices. It is the way to inform public health policies and practices: The use of data to track disease outbreaks, monitor vaccination rates, and identify health disparities and to allocate resources, prioritize public health programs and empower individuals. It empower patients to take an active role in their health conditions such as lifestyle changes, monitor their health status, track their progress.

In addition, a widely and rapidly availing health data is essential to the wider global community to promote:

- New insights using innovative approaches
- Productivity and creativity through collaboration
- Prevention of unnecessary duplication of effort through efficiency/maximizing the potential impact of investments
- The value of research and program effectiveness

- Data quality through encouraging independent verification and analysis and setting data accountability systems
- Capacity building and strengthening researchers through broader access to data particularly in resource-limited countries

However, the lack of access to health data can have several negative consequences on healthcare outcomes, medical research, public health policies, and patient engagement. Hence, it is important to ensure access to health data balancing the issue of safety, security, and privacy.

7.4.4   Who Should Have Access to Health Data?

Providing access to health data is a complex issue that needs balancing purpose of data sharing and the issues of privacy and confidentiality. As health data are often highly sensitive and personal, unauthorized access to data can lead to a range of negative consequences, such as theft of identity, stigmatization and discrimination. Whereas, provision of wider and rapid access to health data is essential for safer, efficient and quality healthcare delivery. Access to accurate and complete health data helps for data-informed decision-making at all levels of the health system including clinical decisions and practices, administrative decisions, planning, monitoring and evaluation, researcher then policy, program and designing interventions and innovation and development in the health system [43]. As a result, many countries have set laws and regulations that govern access to health data in order to balance these competing needs. For instance the Health Insurance Portability and Accountability Act (HIPAA) specifies who could have access to health data.

In general, limiting the access to health data is needed only to those who have a legitimate need ensuring appropriate protection to privacy and confidentiality of the data. So that it will be able to balance the need for privacy and confidentiality with the benefits of sharing information for healthcare purposes.

7.4.5   Principles of Access to Health Data

Globally, there are principles to guide access to health data such as the global access to health data foundation supports the mission of advancing science and technology to reduce healthcare inequities and save lives [43]. The guiding principles are focused on ensuring health data are made widely and rapidly available to optimize the impact of data on global health. Some of the common guiding principles of health data access includes:

- *Respect:* Respecting individuals' and communities' identity, privacy, and confidentiality is an important ethical and moral obligation during providing access to health data.
- *Accountability:* Establishing transparent, clear, and consistent data access processes and procedures to ensure standards of quality, security, and equitable access to health data.
- *Stewardship:* Sharing responsibility to ensure quality, timely access, appropriate use, obeying standards, laws, regulations.
- *Proportionality:* Balancing expected health benefits against sponsors influences
- *Reciprocity:* Engaging individuals and communities in the process particularly from resource-limited settings to ensure mutual global health benefits.

Some of the common guiding principles also include the FAIR, CARE and TRUST principles described as follows:

7.4.5.1 The CARE Principle
There is an abundance of local-based health related dataset but indigenous Peoples' rights to access and control over their data remained limited [44]. The topic of indigenous data sovereignty gained prominence starting in the 1970s, coinciding with a resurgence of discussions surrounding indigenous knowledge, identities, and rights. This culminated in the United Nations' 2007 Declaration on the Rights of Indigenous Peoples [45]. The recognition of indigenous peoples' rights to self-

244 K. D. Gashu and H. A. Guadie

determination as political entities and the acknowledgment of indigenous control over indigenous data have been affirmed. However, the current trend towards open data and open science does not adequately address the rights and interests of indigenous peoples. The concept of Indigenous Data Sovereignty has gained relevance in the context of big data, open data, open science, and data reuse [46].

The 'CARE Principle (Collective Benefit, Authority to Control, Responsibility, and Ethics) has designed to ensure:

- *Collective benefits:* Designing and functioning the data ecosystems in way indigenous people benefited from what they deserve.
- *Authority to control:* Recognizing the rights and interests of indigenous peoples and their data controlled by their authority.
- *Responsibility:* The responsibility to share the data in a way that supports Indigenous peoples' self-determination and collective benefit.
- *Ethics:* Ensuring the primary rights and well-being of indigenous people at all stages

The CARE principle is designed to uphold indigenous data sovereignty and empower indigenous peoples by securing their rights to access, control, and have fair participation in processes related to data reuse [47, 48].

7.4.5.2 The TRUST Principle
It is for the digital repositories (Transparency, Responsibility, User focus, Sustainability and Technology use) [49].

- *Transparency:* Transparent repository services and publicly accessible
- *Responsibility:* Tasked with the responsibility of safeguarding the genuineness and completeness of data
- *User focus:* Fulfill the standards and meet user's anticipations

- *Sustainable use:* Developing and sustaining a new culture
- *Technology use:* Establishing capabilities and info-structure to facilitate a secured, sustained, and dependable use.

As ICT became pervasive, we increasingly became dependent on digital repositories; however, that must be trusted by the communities about capability of appropriately managing and provision of access the data. TRUST is ultimately aimed to make data FAIR.

7.4.5.3 The FAIR Principles
FAIR (Findability, Accessibility, Interoperability, and Reusability) is intended specifically for research data stewardship [50, 51].

- *Findability:* Indicates a clearly and unambiguously described, identified and registered or indexed dataset.
- *Accessibility:* The metadata (data description) needs to be always accessible. Clearly defining access procedure, preferably using electronically/automated ways.
- *Interoperability:* Conceptualizing and expressing the dataset and metadata with common standards
- *Reusability:* Describing the characteristics and provenance of the data to allow accessible for reuse

FAIR data increases the useful life of information, decreases related costs, and accelerates research works.

7.4.6 Techniques of Improving Access to Health Data

Improving access to health data requires a multi-faceted approach. Some of the common techniques to improve access to health data includes:

7.4.6.1 Data Standardization

Implementation of standardized data formats enables to maintain data consistency across diverse settings, systems, and organizations. This facilitates seamless data sharing and exchange, ultimately enhancing access to health data.

7.4.6.2 Implementing Health Information Exchanges

Utilizing networks is critical to facilitate data sharing among various stakeholders.

7.4.6.3 Implementing Electronic Health Records

Leveraging digital-based patient medical records that serve as a centralized repository for patient data. This enhances access to health data by facilitating timely and efficient data sharing.

7.4.6.4 Use of Patient Portals

Implementing secure online platforms that empower patients to access their health data. This enables patients to play an active role in managing their health and well-being.

7.4.6.5 Adopting Data Governance Policies

Establishing guidelines, procedures, and protocols for the management and sharing of health data. This ensures the secure and ethical access to health data by safeguarding patient privacy and maintaining confidentiality.

7.4.6.6 Providing Training for Healthcare Workers

Enhancing capacity through training and education on the practices involved in managing and sharing health data.

7.4.7   How to Control Unauthorized Access to Health Data?

Access controls are implemented to restrict the individuals who can access health data and govern their actions with the data. Multiple access control measures can be employed concurrently, including:

- The utilization of passwords, which is a commonly employed access control measure
- The adoption of two-factor authentication, such as combining a password with a fingerprint scan
- Implementation of role-based access controls, which limit access to health data based on the user's job role or function
- Employment of attribute-based access controls, which restrict access to health data based on specific attributes
- Utilization of time-based access controls, which restrict access to health data to specific times or time periods
- Application of physical access controls, which limit access to health data by controlling physical entry to the location where the data is stored

To ensure effective implementation of access control measures, it is crucial to be mindful of these common mistakes and implementing appropriate safeguards, organizations can enhance the effectiveness and security of their access control measures. Some frequently encountered errors include:

- Using weak passwords that are easily guessable or susceptible to brute-force attacks
- Neglecting to revoke access when it is no longer required, leaving unnecessary entry points open
- Granting overly broad access permissions, which can increase the risk of data breaches and unauthorized access
- Failing to conduct regular audits to verify whether authorized individuals are accessing the data and using it appropriately
- Neglecting to update access controls, such as the organization's policies, procedures, and personnel, as changes occur over time

7.4.8   Access to Health Data in Resource-Limited Settings

In general, ethical and legal challenges impose access constraints worldwide [52, 53]. The challenge becomes even more pronounced when it pertains to accessing health data in resource-limited countries. Various obstacles, including inadequate infrastructure, insufficient funding, limited technological resources, and a lack of skilled personnel, often hinder access to health data, particularly in resource-limited settings.

According to the WHO's study conducted in 35 low-and middle-income countries [54], various nations faced challenges related access to data in their health information systems. A lot of bottlenecks are directly or indirectly impeding data access platform between data supplying and demanding bodies. Some of the challenges particularly in resource-limited settings include:

- Fragmented and inadequately coordinated health information systems obstructing the data sharing processes
- Insufficient basic infrastructure, including unreliable electricity and no/limited internet connectivity are affecting the whole health information system
- Shortage of skilled manpower and low digital literacy of healthcare workers created imbalance in data supply and demand. This in turn impacts in the proper collecting, storage, managing, analyzing and utilizing health data
- Lack of the necessary policies, strategies, and regulations to safeguard data privacy and security in the process of data sharing

It's therefore, stakeholders need to invest more in health information systems and capacity building to improve access to health data in resource-limited settings. In addition, various strategies like establishing partnerships between governments, international organizations, and the private institutions to leverage resources and expertise to improve access to health data. Leveraging emerging technologies such as mHealth and telemedicine could also help to improve access to health data in resource-limited settings.

7.5 Data Security

7.5.1 Overview of Information Security

Information security encompasses the actions undertaken at both individual and organizational levels to prevent unauthorized access or utilization of information resources. In the healthcare sector, ensuring information security is crucial. Organizations place significant emphasis on the appropriate usage and authorization of employee data. It also pertains to the protocols and practices employed by businesses to safeguard information. Robust security measures must be implemented to prevent unauthorized individuals from accessing sensitive data. Information security is a vast and evolving field that encompasses various aspects, including testing, auditing, and ensuring network and infrastructure security [55, 56].

Information security, which encompasses measures to prevent unauthorized or inappropriate access to and usage of information resources, is essential at both the personal and organizational levels. In the healthcare industry, information security assumes paramount importance. Organizations prioritize safeguarding employee data by focusing on authorization and ensuring its appropriate use [57].

Information security encompasses the strategies and practices implemented by organizations to protect information. This involves establishing security measures to prevent unauthorized access to sensitive data. The field of information security is dynamic and extensive, covering various areas such as network and infrastructure security, testing, and auditing, among others [56, 58].

Within the healthcare sector, information security involves the protection of patient health records to prevent unauthorized access, use, disclosure, disruption, modification, or destruction [59, 60]. Concerns arise among patients regarding the potential impact of their private medical information on employment decisions, press coverage, or civil court proceedings. To maintain control over the disclosure of personal information and determine the timing, manner, and extent of sharing it with others, individuals, groups, and institutions have the right to privacy. Technological advancements and changes in the healthcare landscape continue to shape the ongoing and iterative development of health information security [60, 61].

During the 1960s, businesses began recognizing the importance of safeguarding their computers, leading to the rise in popularity of password protection. At that time, the primary security concerns revolved around physical safeguards and restricting access to individuals lacking adequate computer literacy, as there was no internet or extensive networks to be concerned about.

In the 1970s, the history of cybersecurity witnessed a shift towards a research agenda. As computers became increasingly interconnected and the complexity of viruses grew, information security struggled to keep pace with the continuous deluge of ingenious hacking techniques [62]. The adoption of firewalls experienced a surge in the 1990s, coinciding with the increasing availability of internet access to a wider user base. Network security concerns witnessed a significant rise by the mid-1990s, necessitating the development and deployment of firewalls and antivirus software on a large scale to safeguard the public.

In the early 2000s, governments started imposing severe penalties for hacking, aiming to protect individuals and networks. Perpetrators of hacking activities faced more straightforward judgments, including lengthy prison sentences and substantial fines. The 2010s saw some of the most significant breaches in history, attributable to the relentless advancements in technology during that period [55].

7.5.2   Why Information Security in Public Health Informatics?

Confidentiality, integrity, and availability are widely recognized as the fundamental pillars of information security. Confidentiality and privacy are closely intertwined, as the protection of privacy necessitates the preservation of information secrecy, which is achieved through the establishment of privacy policies. Preserving trust in individuals or organizations involves safeguarding the confidentiality of information, ensuring that it remains secure and undisclosed [63, 64].

Ensuring the accuracy and reliability of information is essential to prevent the dissemination of false or misleading information about individuals. Safeguarding the confidentiality and integrity of information requires protection against unauthorized access, modification, or tampering. Key procedures such as access control, authenti-

cation, and authorization play a crucial role in achieving this objective.

Access control, supported by robust authentication methods and comprehensive access privileges, serves as a deterrent against unauthorized access to data and services. Authorization, which involves determining appropriate access rights, presents both organizational and technical challenges. Decisions need to be made regarding who has the authority to grant access permissions, and mechanisms for allocating and verifying access privileges must be incorporated into the system.

Practical systems often require making compromises to address these challenges, such as finding a balance between the need-to-know principles and granting access to anything that is not explicitly forbidden. Consequently, the establishment of an access control system necessitates thoughtful consideration of compromises that effectively balance security, effectiveness, and cost.

Inadequate data security can lead to detrimental outcomes, including the loss or theft of critical information, negative customer experiences, and damage to reputation. With increasing reliance on technology, instances of data breaches, fraud, and cyber-security threats are becoming more frequent [65].

When it comes to the information security of public health surveillance [66–68], the right to privacy and confidentiality is generally recognized for all individuals, as these protections demonstrate respect for their autonomy. Both individuals and society as a whole benefit from maintaining privacy and confidentiality. Patients feel more comfortable sharing their health information with professionals when they have confidence that it will be handled appropriately. Trust is crucial in fostering a successful doctor-patient or nurse-patient relationship and enables healthcare practitioners to fulfill their responsibilities effectively. Protecting confidentiality and privacy also serves the interests of public health. The fear of personal information exposure may deter individuals from seeking professional help, leading to undiagnosed illnesses and increased transmission. Furthermore, unfortunate cases arise when sensitive health data falls into the wrong hands, resulting in prejudice, stigma, and discrimination. Privacy concerns become even more significant when information is shared outside the surveillance system. Additionally, there is a recognition of the potential harm caused by disclosing sensitive medical data, such as stigmatization or discrimination, as well as the risk of sacrificing benefits by not utilizing data effectively.

Two primary concerns often raised are the legitimacy of excluding informed consent and the risk of privacy violations during data collection and storage. Furthermore, there is apprehension about generating data that is insufficiently accurate for public health actions. Additionally, there is concern that certain groups may be left out of the data collection process and therefore not receive the benefits of surveillance.

Many challenges stem from conflicts in prioritization regarding the type of surveillance system to be employed and the potential pitfalls of poorly designed systems, such as reduced effectiveness due to inadequate consideration of critical contextual factors. Moreover, obstacles like limited funding may hinder the implementation of necessary surveillance systems, resulting in subpar or nonexistent practices.

Healthcare often relies on ethical principles such as respect for autonomy, non-maleficence, beneficence, and justice for guidance. Respecting autonomy involves granting individuals the freedom to live their lives as they choose. Beneficence entails providing beneficial treatments, while non-maleficence emphasizes the avoidance of harm to patients. Justice seeks fair distribution of resources and responsibilities.

The field of health informatics can benefit from these ethical concepts. Conflicts between the values of respect for autonomy, beneficence, and non-maleficence are frequently observed in the ethical considerations surrounding the use of computers in healthcare practices.

7.5.3 Information Security Techniques

Information security is an important aspect in healthcare settings, in general there are three major categories of security techniques [69]. Each category of security safeguarding techniques included several protection mechanisms as following Fig. 7.4.

7.5.3.1 Technical

Technical security techniques encompass a set of methods employed to authenticate users and safeguard private information and data, commonly within business settings. Once users have successfully authenticated their login credentials and data, only authorized user applications are granted the ability to read and access data and applications. This category of techniques includes data encryption, firewall protection, audit trails, access control, and virus checking. Data encryption is a protective technical measure employed to prevent unauthorized access to information. It involves scrambling the data, transforming readable "plaintext" into seemingly random and unintelligible "ciphertext"

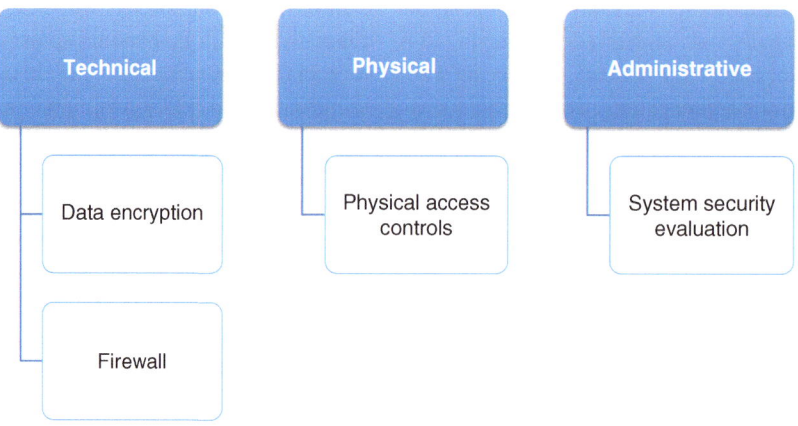

Fig. 7.4 Major security techniques applied in healthcare settings

consisting of gibberish characters. The firewall scrutinizes the incoming and outgoing traffic of a network based on a predefined set of rules. By utilizing a set of rules, the firewall effectively filters out undesirable traffic and permits only those communications deemed safe.

7.5.3.2 Physical

Physical security techniques aim to protect both the equipment housed within a room and the room itself, effectively preventing unauthorized individuals from gaining access while allowing approved individuals to enter. These techniques encompass physical access controls, designated security responsibilities, and workstation security measures. Access control is a technique or capability that enables the regulation of individuals entering a restricted area or accessing a medical record room through authentication and authorization at designated access control points. It allows for the control of who can enter and how many users can gain access.

7.5.3.3 Administrative

Administrative security techniques primarily find application in system security evaluation, disaster recovery planning, and risk analysis and management. System security testing and assessment involve evaluating and analyzing the management, operational, and technical security controls in place within a system. The purpose is to determine the effectiveness of their implementation, assess their performance as intended, and verify whether they are achieving the desired outcomes in alignment with the system's security requirements.

7.5.4 Barriers of Information Security

Information security barriers can be grouped into categories such as environmental issues, technological considerations, and operational aspects.

7.5.4.1 Environmental Factors

Privacy and security safeguards can be influenced by environmental factors, both directly and indirectly. These factors encompass an individual's surroundings, living arrangements, and social connections. In certain situations, it can become challenging to trust healthcare professionals when sharing sensitive information due to these environmental influences [70, 71].

7.5.4.2 Technological Factors

The primary challenge in this domain is the lack of interoperability among various information systems, hindering data exchange and the ability to utilize previously collected data. This issue can be attributed to several technology-related factors, including data security concerns such as limited internet and technology access, absence of digital devices, lack of data integration and sharing systems, reliance on cellular data or public Wi-Fi, and difficulties associated with digital literacy, such as inadequate knowledge and understanding of the technology being used. The inability of different information systems to communicate with each other, thereby impeding data interchange and the reuse of previously collected data, remains the most significant concern in this field [72, 73].

7.5.4.3 Operational Factors

Insufficient coordination and cooperation among stakeholders represent significant hurdles. In multi-center registries, the absence of coordinating offices or personnel leads to challenges arising from the lack of coordination between registration centers. There is limited interaction and contact between the centers as cooperation is not mandatory. Another obstacle is the absence or non-adherence to data standards, which hampers efforts to establish consistency and coordination. Additionally, issues with data collection arise when case definitions are not clearly defined, resulting in variations in cases and related data [72, 74].

7.5.5 Facilitators of Information Security

One of the most important management strategies is to finance the registry system and use of research budgets for financing, as well as planning to earn money from the results and outputs of information system. Providing counseling and training services can also help people who want to run or implement information security to carry out their work successfully [72].

7.5.6 Enhancing Information Security in Resource Limited Settings

Information security in resource-limited settings faces emerging threats, influenced by a combination of diverse and intricate factors. To enhance information security in such settings, efforts should be directed towards implementing appropriate measures.

A comprehensive evaluation of the existing health information security policies is necessary, along with the development of new policy statements. These new policy statements should not only clarify the authorized individuals within your practice who can access and oversee electronic health information but also enhance the procedures for sharing electronic health information with patients and other healthcare organizations. For instance, the policies may require the utilization of specific technologies, such as encrypting data on portable computing devices like laptops [75].

In order to mitigate potential risks to electronic health information, it is advisable to implement the updated health information security policies in your practice. This proactive step will help ensure that the security policies remain current and minimize the chances of unauthorized access, use, disclosure, disruption, modification, or destruction of electronic health information [76].

Provide training to employees on identifying potential attacks: As healthcare information technology is still in the early stages of implementation, employees may still be adjusting to its use. In order to safeguard the security of health data, it is crucial to update policies and procedures to accommodate the digitalization of patient records. However, implementing new policies alone is insufficient without providing adequate training to employees [77].

7.6 Equity in Public Health Informatics

7.6.1 What's Equity?

Equity refers to the absence of unfair and avoidable disparities among different groups of individuals, irrespective of their social, economic, demographic, geographic, or other categorizations related to inequality (such as gender, ethnicity, disability, or sexual orientation). Access to healthcare is considered a fundamental human right. Health equity is achieved when all individuals have the opportunity to achieve their full potential for health and well-being [78, 79].

People's health and health equity are influenced by a combination of factors that include the conditions of their birth, upbringing, living environment, employment, recreational activities, aging process, and biological variables. The distribution of power and resources is impacted by structural elements such as political, legal, and economic factors, as well as social norms and institutional practices. These factors are in turn shaped by the circumstances in which individuals are born, grow, live, work, play, and age [80].

Bias, stereotypes, and discrimination targeting individuals based on their sex, gender, age, race, ethnicity, disability, and other factors often contribute to worsening living conditions for affected populations. These discriminatory behaviors are deeply ingrained in institutional and systemic processes, resulting in underrepresentation or inadequate support for these groups in decision-making at various levels [81].

To achieve the progressive realization of the right to health, it is essential to systematically identify and address inequities stemming from disparities in health and living conditions. These inequities should be actively identified and eliminated as part of the ongoing process towards ensuring the right to health for all [82].

The concept of equity in public health data revolves around the equitable dissemination of health-related information among populations, ensuring equal access and benefits without discrimination based on socio-economic status, race, ethnicity, gender, or other personal characteristics. When health data is distributed in an inequitable manner, it can contribute to health disparities and worsen existing inequities in healthcare access and outcomes. Conversely, promoting equity in health data can enhance health outcomes and mitigate health disparities.

7.6.2 Why Equity in Public Health Informatics?

Equity in public health informatics is vital to address disparities in service provision arising from various factors. Innovative and interdisciplinary approaches such as e-Health interventions can play a crucial role in mitigating racial and ethnic inequities. e-Health systems have the potential to overcome barriers to healthcare access caused by transportation limitations, caregiving responsibilities, financial constraints, and time constraints related to work. Furthermore, by improving patient engagement and the quality of communication between patients and healthcare providers, e-Health approaches can integrate patient-generated health data to enable remote monitoring of chronic conditions, expand healthcare accessibility, enhance continuity of care, and facilitate more effective and personalized care for different patient populations.

To address and manage specific diseases in racial and ethnic minorities, leveraging new technologies in informatics, data utilization, and patient engagement within continuous learning health systems proves to be effective tools. These advancements offer valuable means for combating and preventing diseases, as well as promoting ongoing education and improvement in healthcare outcomes for minority populations.

Health informatics and digital transformation within learning health systems present novel avenues to generate groundbreaking research findings, thereby addressing one of the gaps in achieving health equity. These advancements create opportunities to leverage data and technology in innovative ways, leading to transformative discoveries that can contribute significantly to reducing health inequities [83–87].

7.6.3 Opportunities to Reduce Inequity by Using PHI in LMIC

Digital health innovations are revolutionizing healthcare by granting medical professionals access to physiological measurements and empowering individuals to engage in mobile diagnostic examinations. With the progression of healthcare digitalization, patients are gaining more control over gathering essential health data and delivering clinically relevant information to healthcare providers. This significant change has led to the emergence of a wide array of novel digital tech, such as smartphones, microchip platforms, home-care devices, cloud-computing, AI among others. The advancements of digital tech enables a rapid patient diagnosis, as well as the prediction of future health patterns and disease trends [88–90].

The driving force behind e-Health could be understood from the different standpoints. One of the perceptions could be the care-seeker's ability to seek and play an active role in managing their own health by utilizing new digital health tools and accessing information that helps to inform personal healthcare decisions and activities. Secondly, healthcare professionals require e-Health technologies that helps to improve professional and organizational efficiency, quality of healthcare, and optimize healthcare delivery. It is also crucial to reduce healthcare inequity, as digital technologies facilitate inclusive services through providing different opinions for disadvantaged and marginalized communities. By doing so, we can collectively identify the most effective solutions that address the needs and perspectives of both patients and healthcare professionals [91].

All stakeholders engaged in healthcare delivery, including patients, healthcare providers, and institutions, are dedicated to initiating a process of digital transformation. Ensuring health equity should be a paramount concern at every level, from the development of new technologies to active participation in evidence generation. The current initiatives, which should be strongly supported by clinicians, their patients, and medical professional organizations, hold significant importance. In general, effective communication regarding the potential of technologies that can enhance access and bridge the digital health gap for all groups is crucial [92, 93].

7.6.4 Challenges of Equity Related to PHI in Resource-Limited Settings

Confidentiality and privacy concerns arise in relation to de-identified data stratified by equity, especially when considering its potential public release. It is important to make information about health equity accessible to the public for several reasons. Firstly, health equity plays a crucial role in determining overall health outcomes. Secondly, civil society has the power to influence public policy, which directly affects individuals' access to quality healthcare. Despite these considerations, careful attention must be given to address concerns surrounding the confidentiality and privacy of de-identified data when considering its dissemination [94, 95]. Particular people or households may be recognizable if data is disaggregated for relatively small populations, such as those living in a village, and feel as though their privacy rights have been violated. As a result, while developing health information systems, it is important to expressly plan for the public dissemination of equity-oriented health information [96].

Achieving equity in public health informatics (PHI) within resource-limited settings presents distinct challenges arising from multiple factors, including limited resources, insufficient infrastructure, and socio-economic disparities. The following are key challenges associated with equity in PHI within resource-limited settings:

- Access to technology, such as computers and smartphones, may be limited, which can make it difficult for individuals to access and use health information systems. This can exacerbate existing health disparities and limit individuals' ability to receive timely and appropriate healthcare services.
- Limited health literacy, which can make it difficult for them to understand and use health

information. This may lead to incorrect or incomplete health information, which can negatively impact health outcomes.
- Individuals may speak different languages or dialects, which can make it difficult to share and access health information. This can lead to miscommunication and misunderstandings, which can negatively impact health outcomes.
- Limited financial and human resources to support the development and implementation of health information systems. This can make it difficult to develop and implement systems that are accessible and inclusive of all individuals and populations.

7.7 Accountability in Public Health Informatics

7.7.1 What Is Accountability?

Accountability refers to the concept of holding an individual responsible for ensuring the security and control of tools, materials, and data. This individual is held answerable to the relevant authorities in the event of loss or improper use of these items [97].

In the context of healthcare, fostering a culture of accountability involves creating an environment where all members, including doctors, nurses, administrators, and patients, feel comfortable openly discussing errors and concerns. By holding each other accountable, healthcare organizations can collaborate to identify areas for improvement and implement measures to prevent the recurrence of errors [98].

Gaining knowledge, taking action, and assuming responsibility are essential stages in the process. Assemblages of accountability in public health serve as prime illustrations of bio politics, as they delineate the individuals or entities that must possess specific knowledge and act upon it for the benefit or control of others [98, 99].

In the modern era, discussions surrounding accountability revolve around concepts such as "open government" and "transparency through digitization." Accountability encompasses the belief that individuals must assume responsibility for their decisions and provide justifications for them. Generally, being able to defend one's actions leads to positive outcomes or rewards. Conversely, when unable to sufficiently explain a mistake or misconduct, there are consequences that follow [100].

Accountability holds immense significance in the realm of healthcare, as it contributes to the delivery of high-quality patient care, upholding ethical standards, and fostering advancements in health outcomes. Within the healthcare industry, health information systems play a pivotal role in establishing accountability. These systems offer essential tools and procedures that enable organizations to monitor, assess, and take ownership of their actions. This article examines the concept of accountability in healthcare, explores various accountability models, and emphasizes the crucial role of robust health information systems in promoting transparency and accountability [98].

Health information systems serve as the backbone of strong health systems, providing the necessary infrastructure and mechanisms for accountability. They allow healthcare managers, policymakers, and individual service providers to access timely and accurate data for planning, resource allocation, and monitoring health services. HIS enables the evaluation of compliance with accountability domains, facilitates performance assessment, and supports the dissemination of evaluation findings [101].

7.7.2 Why Accountability in Public Health Informatics?

Establishing an accountability system in public health informatics is of significant importance to ensure the ethical and responsible design, implementation, and utilization of public health information systems and technologies. Accountability ensures transparency, dependability, and trustworthiness in these systems, which are essential for maintaining public trust and promoting health equity. Overall, implementing accountability in public health informatics contributes to the improvement of population health outcomes and the reduction of health disparities. By having

transparent, reliable, and trustworthy information systems and technology, public health efforts are enhanced. Additionally, an accountability system protects legal and ethical concerns, such as individuals' privacy rights, once it is well established. It also ensures that stakeholders' needs and perspectives are taken into consideration for health system improvements. Ultimately, an accountability system maintains public trust and confidence in public health systems and technologies, while also achieving health equity and improving population health outcomes.

7.7.3 Accountability Principles in Public Health Informatics

The principles of accountability in healthcare are based on the ethical principles of autonomy, beneficence, non-maleficence, and justice. Accountability requires a commitment to ethical principles and a willingness to prioritize the privacy, security, and well-being of patients over other considerations. Some key principles of accountability includes:

7.7.3.1 Transparency
Transparency is a fundamental aspect of accountability, which involves openly sharing policies and procedures related to the collection, storage, and utilization of public health data. Additionally, it requires providing patients with clear information regarding their rights and available choices for managing their own health data.

7.7.3.2 Responsibility
Responsibility is a key principle of accountability in public health informatics (PHI). It guarantees that public health data is collected, stored, and used in a responsible and ethical manner. Furthermore, it holds individuals or organizations accountable in the event of privacy or security breaches associated with the handling of such data.

7.7.3.3 Confidentiality
Confidentiality is a vital aspect of ensuring the privacy and security of public health data. It mandates that such data be kept confidential and pro-

tected from unauthorized access. Disclosure of health data should only occur with the explicit consent of the patient or as legally mandated by applicable laws or regulations.

7.7.3.4 Accuracy

It is essential to ensure the accuracy and completeness of public health data, and measures should be taken to rectify any identified errors or inaccuracies.

7.7.3.5 Accessibility

Accessibility guarantees that public health data is readily available to authorized individuals, including patients. It is important to provide patients with timely access to their own health data, allowing them to retrieve and review the information pertaining to their health.

7.7.3.6 Respect for Autonomy

Respecting patients' autonomy is a fundamental principle of accountability in public health informatics. It involves providing patients with comprehensive information regarding their health data and empowering them to make informed decisions about the usage and handling of their personal health information.

7.7.3.7 Continuous Improvement

Continuous improvement serves as a fundamental principle of accountability in public health informatics. It entails the ongoing monitoring and evaluation of policies and procedures related to the management of health data. Necessary changes are made to enhance effectiveness and ensure adherence to ethical and legal standards.

7.7.4 Data Accountability Frameworks

Frameworks for data accountability offer an organized way to guarantee that health data is gathered, maintained, and utilized in an ethical and responsible way. The components of data accountability frameworks are as follows:

7.7.4.1 Developing Data Governance

In order to manage health data, including its collection, storage, sharing, and use, policies, processes, and structures must be established. This entails creating data quality guidelines, assigning roles and duties, and setting up data access controls.

7.7.4.2 Ensuring Data Privacy and Security

Protecting health information from unauthorized use, access, or disclosure as well as making sure that data is sent and stored securely are all part of assuring data privacy and security. This entails putting in place organizational and technical security measures including encryption, access limits, and recurring security audits.

7.7.4.3 Maintaining Data Quality

Ensuring that health data is precise, comprehensive, consistent, and satisfies stakeholder needs is part of maintaining data quality.

This entails putting data quality metrics in place, doing data validation tests, and tracking and reporting on data quality.

7.7.4.4 Ensuring Data Sharing and Interoperability

Assuring secure and consistent sharing and exchange of health data between various systems and organizations is a crucial aspect of assuring data sharing and interoperability. It entails creating contracts for data sharing, approving interoperability guidelines, and putting safe data exchange procedures in place.

7.7.4.5 Engaging Stakeholders

Involving patients, healthcare professionals, and other stakeholders in the creation and execution of data accountability frameworks is crucial. It is essential to address their needs and concerns by providing education and training on data management and privacy. Additionally, seeking feedback on data management policies and practices is necessary to ensure their active participation and contribution.

7.7.5   Opportunities and Challenges of Accountability in PHI

As there are challenges, there are also potential opportunities public health informatics in resource limited settings [102–104]. Limited resources, infrastructure, and technical capacity are potentially hindering the development of robust systems. Limited funding, outdated or inadequate infrastructure, and a lack of technical expertise can impede the implementation and effectiveness of data management systems.

The advancements in digital technologies and enhanced connectivity present opportunities for overcoming these challenges. The rapid progress in technology has resulted in more affordable and accessible solutions, simplifying the establishment and maintenance of robust systems. For instance, cloud computing enables scalable and cost-effective storage and processing of large volumes of data, while advancements in network infrastructure have expanded internet access, even in remote areas. Additionally, the widespread availability of mobile devices and internet connectivity has opened doors for data collection, sharing, and analysis. This increased connectivity allows for real-time data monitoring, remote consultations, and the implementation of digital health interventions. It also fosters collaboration and knowledge-sharing among healthcare professionals and researchers.

7.8   Data Integrity

Integrity encompasses the qualities of honesty, ethics, and trustworthiness. Preserving data integrity is crucial to effectively utilize health data for informed decision-making, enhanced health outcomes, and patient safety. Achieving data integrity necessitates a combination of technical, organizational, and cultural elements. This includes implementing suitable data collection and management procedures, conducting data quality checks, employing data security and privacy measures, and fostering a culture of ethical and responsible data usage. By prioritizing data integrity, healthcare organizations can establish trust among patients, healthcare professionals, and other stakeholders, ensuring the effective and responsible utilization of health data to improve health outcomes [23].

This section aimed to address the definition of data integrity; the growing challenges of data and corruption and infodemics; the rationale of data integrity; principles related to data integrity and the challenges and opportunities of data integrity and way outs in resource-limited settings.

7.8.1   What Is Data Integrity?

Data integrity pertains to the extent to which data exhibit qualities such as completeness, consistency, accuracy, trustworthiness, and reliability. It ensures that these characteristics are preserved throughout the entire data life cycle [105]. Data integrity involves the proper and secure collection and maintenance of data to ensure the preservation of their originality, accuracy, reliability, and trustworthiness. When data have integrity, it means that the system used to generate them is safeguarded from intentional bias or manipulation. It involves mitigating the potential risks of data corruption, misinformation, and disinformation associated with health data/information.

Integrity in documentation refers to the overall accuracy of the entire medical file. This encompasses conducting document validity audits during the process of filing reimbursement claims, ensuring proper patient identification, validating authorship, managing changes, and conducting record repairs when necessary. Maintaining data integrity entails ensuring that the data remains accurate and consistent throughout its entire life cycle [106–108].

Issues with data integrity have a significant impact on the utilization of medical data for quality improvement, public health initiatives, and research. These problems also result in intangible social costs and undermine public trust in government systems. Data integrity concerns affect both manual and automated decision-making processes. It is essential to prioritize data integrity for both paper-based (manual) and electronic data, addressing not only technical aspects but also human factors. Taking a proactive approach to address data integrity problems is preferable to being solely compliant. To ensure data integrity within such systems, authentication levels, access control, and decision-making processes should be clearly defined and implemented. Data integrity problems can arise due to overreliance on human practices, inadequate control and validation of automated systems, and insufficient evaluation and maintenance of original data and records. Moreover, common causes of data integrity errors include human errors, non-compliant operational processes, data transmission issues, software glitches, tampered hardware, and compromises in physical device security [109].

7.8.2 Data Corruption in the Health System

Health data corruption is about intentional/unintentional modification, deletion, or destruction of health-related data by unauthorized person.

Intentionally it can be occurred using malicious actions inside or outside the organization by hacking, cyberattacks, or theft of data. It could also happen through manipulation of data manually for their personal benefits. For instance, people could purposely inflate/deflate the figures for personal welfare such as seeking political appointments.

Unintentional corruption is a human error such as accidental deletion of data or incorrect data entry that can naturally occur due to technical and system malfunctions.

Data corruption, regardless of its causes, can have serious consequences, such as compromised patient safety, quality of care and treatments. It can also lead to losses of resources, and reputational damage for the institutions [106–108].

7.8.3 Misinformation and Disinformation

Infodemics such as misinformation and disinformation are becoming a public health threat due to the new order of digital communication that created a reckless and wide open access to health information. Misinformation is a false created with no intention of causing harm but deliberately intended to deceive [110–112]. It is also considered as information that contradicts the scientific community's epistemic consensus on a phenomenon [113]. According to this definition, what is considered true and false changes all the time as new evidence emerges and approaches and procedures improve through time. Disinformation also consists of biased or misleading information, manipulated narratives or facts, and propaganda.

It has been observed that many social media platforms played a crucial role in facilitating the rapid and widespread dissemination of information. The characteristics of misinformation and disinformation encompass amplifying fear and panic, misconstruing scientific knowledge, fostering opinion polarization, and other similar phenomena [114].

As an example, during the Munich Security Conference, the Director-General of the World Health Organization (WHO) emphasized that the battle against COVID-19 extended beyond just combating the epidemic itself; it also involved addressing an "infodemic" Despite the best efforts of global health organizations such as the WHO to manage and contain the COVID-19 outbreak, the rapid dissemination of misinformation through social media platforms created a significant public health menace [115].

A study in Northwest Ethiopia [116], indicated that five of ten community members were misinformed on the COVID-19 vaccine. Social media platforms were the main source of misinformation. Uncontrolled spread of misinformation through social media platforms is currently a challenge not only in health but also in all socioeconomic and political spaces all over the world.

Addressing challenges related to infodemics, misinformation, and disinformation in the health system can be tackled through several measures. These include the development and implementation of legal policies, raising awareness among the public, improving the quality of content in mass media, and enhancing digital and health literacy. In order to address the issue of misinformation, it is necessary to utilize mainstream media as a means of distributing accurate information about the COVID-19 vaccine. Mainstream media is subject to more control and regulation compared to social media platforms. It is also crucial to encourage the community to obtain health-related information from official social media pages of health agencies and mass media sources. Above all, it needs to set a responsible use of social media and accountability systems that regulate any act of infodemics, misinformation, and disinformation in public health [116].

7.8.4 Why Integrity in Public Health Informatics?

Data integrity plays a vital role in health information systems by ensuring that data is collected in a proper manner and remains accurate, complete, and consistent. Inaccurate or incomplete data can lead to misleading clinical and administrative decisions and practices. Moreover, it can have detrimental effects on research endeavors and compromise public health interventions. Maintaining data integrity requires implementing robust data storage and cybersecurity measures. Health data should be stored in secure databases with restricted access granted only to the authorized individuals. It is crucial to establish appropriate security measures to safeguard against unauthorized access, data breaches, and cyber threats.

Data integrity is of utmost importance for health systems to efficiently utilize health data in decision-making, research, and patient care. The presence of accurate, complete, and consistent data empowers health systems to identify health trends, monitor disease outbreaks, allocate resources effectively, and evaluate the effectiveness of interventions. Therefore, it is vital for health systems to give high priority to data integrity in their operations and establish the required infrastructure, policies, and procedures to uphold it.

In order to uphold data integrity, health systems should adhere to standardized data collection methods, implement procedures for data quality assurance and quality control, and adopt effective data management practices. It is crucial to provide training for healthcare workers on

accurate data collection techniques, and data entry should undergo double-checking to minimize errors. Regular data quality checks and audits must be performed to identify and rectify any errors or inconsistencies in the data [105–108].

7.8.5 The Principles of Data Integrity

According to the Medicines & Healthcare products Regulatory Agency [105], to ensure good data integrity in healthcare systems, there are certain principles that should be followed:

- Foster a culture of responsibility within institutions to ensure data completeness, consistency, and accuracy across all forms, including paper and electronic formats
- Establish an environment that enables effective data integrity controls, with due respect given to people, systems, and facilities, ensuring a suitable working environment
- Endorse data governance policies at the highest levels of the organization
- Implement a documented system designed to provide an acceptable level of control based on the risks associated with data integrity, supported by appropriate rationale
- Maintain appropriate levels of control within systems, while implementing broader data governance measures that facilitate periodic audits to identify potential data integrity failures
- Allocate resources and effort in proportion to the risk and impact that a data integrity failure could have on patients or the environment
- Transitioning between automated/computerized systems and paper-based/manual systems does not eliminate the need for proper data integrity controls
- When data integrity weaknesses are identified, take corrective and preventive actions across all relevant activities and systems, avoiding isolated fixes
- Notify regulatory authorities appropriately when significant data integrity incidents are identified

- Data governance measures should ensure that data remains complete, consistent, enduring, and accessible throughout its entire lifecycle

7.8.6 Data Integrity in Resource-Limited Settings: Barriers and Opportunities

In low- and middle-income countries, there exist diverse hurdles in maintaining the integrity of health data. These barriers are intricate and interconnected, encompassing several significant challenges. In low- and middle-income countries, there are notable limitations in terms of financial and human resources available to support the development and implementation of robust data management systems. This insufficiency can pose challenges in ensuring data integrity. Additionally, healthcare professionals and relevant personnel in LMICs may lack adequate training and opportunities for capacity building in effectively managing health data. This knowledge gap can result in errors, inconsistencies, and incomplete data. Furthermore, inadequate infrastructure, including unreliable electricity and internet connectivity, can present obstacles in collecting, storing, and managing health data within LMICs. These limitations hamper the smooth flow of data and can impede data management efforts. Moreover, weak governance and regulatory frameworks exist, which can make it challenging to enforce data privacy and security policies, as well as maintain data quality standards. This lack of a strong governance structure can further compromise the integrity of health data in LMICs.

LMICs still have opportunities to uphold data integrity within their health systems. Embracing newer, advanced technologies instead of relying on traditional ones presents a cost-effective and efficient opportunity to maintain health data integrity. Engaging stakeholders in the development and implementation of data management systems is another opportunity that yields positive results, ensuring accessibility, inclusivity, and responsiveness to the diverse needs of populations. Community engagement plays a crucial role in fostering trust and enhancing data quality. Collaborative platforms with international organizations offer significant opportunities to share resources, expertise, and best practices, thereby improving capacity and the reliability of health data. By prioritizing health equity in their data management systems, there is an opportunity to reduce disparities in health outcomes. Additionally, focusing on interoperability, which enables different systems to exchange and communicate data, can enhance the accuracy, completeness, and consistency of health data.

7.8.7 How to Ensure Data Integrity?

Ensure data integrity requires appropriate quality and risk management systems, scientific principles and good documentation practices [105–108]. There are several actions to maintain data integrity in health care system in day-to-day practices. Some of the actions include attribution, clarity and legibility, contemporaneous and accuracy.

7.8.7.1 Attribution
Attribution refers to each piece of patient's data should clearly and precisely indicate the observer's identity, the date of recording, and the patient to whom it pertains. This information must be distinct and accurate for every instance of patient data. Adding attribution is essential to improving data integrity. The process of assigning a source or origin to data enhances data integrity by promoting accountability and transparency. By guaranteeing that data can be linked to its source or originator, attribution makes it possible to verify, validate, and evaluate its quality. It contributes to establishing the validity and consistency of data, facilitating improved research, analysis, and decision-making. Data integrity is enhanced and confidence in the correctness, consistency, and completeness of the information is fostered with appropriate attribution.

7.8.7.2 Clarity and Legibility
It is about patients/client's health records need to be easily readable, straightforward to understand,

and securely stored. Data that is easily under-standable and clear lowers the possibility of mis-understandings or errors in comprehending. Data that is readable and clear improves comprehen-sion and guarantees that the intended information is correctly recorded and conveyed. Data analysis and interpretation are also made easier with improved clarity and readability. It makes it pos-sible for administrators, researchers, and medical experts to draw insightful conclusions and decide wisely based on precise and intelligible data. Additionally, data that is readable and transparent fosters productive stakeholder engagement and communication. People from different depart-ments and disciplines may readily discuss, exam-ine, and comprehend information when it is presented in an easy-to-read style.

7.8.7.3 Contemporaneous
It is about recording patient notes and data in real-time, contemporaneously, as they are observed during consultations, tests, or opera-tions. Since contemporaneous recording fosters precision, thoroughness, timeliness, transpar-ency, and dependability, it is essential for pre-serving data integrity. Instantaneous data capture minimizes mistakes, guarantees the availability of important information, and upholds the reli-ability and integrity of the recorded information.

7.8.7.4 Accuracy
Health-related data/information ought to be pre-cise, devoid of inaccuracies, and compliant with the most recent industry regulations and stan-dards. Precise information is the cornerstone of trustworthy data, valid insights, and self-assured decision-making, all of which enhance the data's overall quality and credibility.

Furthermore, in resource-limited settings, there are strategies that can be adopted to promote health data integrity. One such strategy is the standardiza-tion of data collection processes, which ensures the accuracy, completeness, and consistency of data. This involves developing standardized data collection forms and procedures and providing training to healthcare professionals and relevant personnel on accurate data collection and record-ing techniques. In resource-limited settings, utiliz-

ing open-source software can be a cost-effective and adaptable solution for data management. Open-source software can be customized to suit specific settings and can be used on various hard-ware platforms, providing flexibility and afford-ability. Regular data quality checks are essential to identify and rectify errors, inconsistencies, and missing data. These checks should be conducted regularly and integrated into data management workflows to maintain data integrity.

Safeguarding the privacy and security of health data is paramount. Implementing data encryption, access controls, and training health-care professionals and relevant personnel on data privacy and security best practices are crucial steps in ensuring data integrity. Engaging stake-holders in the design and implementation of data management systems is vital to ensure accessibil-ity, inclusivity, and responsiveness to diverse populations. This includes involving community leaders, patients, and other stakeholders in the development of data management policies and procedures. By following these strategies, resource-limited settings can enhance health data integrity, leading to improved data quality, better decision-making, and ultimately, enhanced healthcare outcomes.

References

1. Assembly UNG, Puybaret E. Universal declaration of human rights. Inter-American Institute for Human Rights; 1999.
2. Have H, Jean M. The UNESCO universal declara-tion on bioethics and human rights: background, principles and application. UNESCO Publishing; 2009.
3. United States. National Commission for the Protection of Human Subjects of Biomedical and Behavioral Research. The Belmont report: ethical principles and guidelines for the protection of human subjects of research. Creative Media Partners; 2018.
4. Annas GJ, Grodin M. The Nazi Doctors and the Nuremberg code: human rights in human experi-mentation. Oxford University Press; 1992.
5. Grodin M, Glantz LH. Children as research subjects: science, ethics, and law. Oxford University Press; 1994.
6. Di Mattia P. Ethics. In: Kirch W, editor. Encyclopedia of public health. Dordrecht: Springer Netherlands; 2008. p. 371–83.

7. Louden RB. Kant's virtue ethics. Philosophy. 1986;61(238):473–89.
8. Hursthouse R. Virtue ethics and human nature. Hume Stud. 1999;25(1):67–82.
9. Mingers J, Walsham G. Toward ethical information systems: the contribution of discourse ethics. MIS Q. 2010;34:833–54.
10. LaFollette H. The practice of ethics. Wiley-Blackwell; 2006.
11. Bioethics. In: Kirch W, editor. Encyclopedia of public health. Dordrecht: Springer Netherlands. 2008. p. 65.
12. Beauchamp TL, Childress JF. Principles of biomedical ethics. Edicoes Loyola; 1994.
13. Autonomy. In: Kirch W, editor. Encyclopedia of public health. Dordrecht: Springer Netherlands. 2008. p. 56.
14. Jahn WT. The 4 basic ethical principles that apply to forensic activities are respect for autonomy, beneficence, nonmaleficence, and justice. J Chiropr Med. 2011;10(3):225–6.
15. Beneficence. In: Kirch W, editor. Encyclopedia of public health. Dordrecht: Springer Netherlands. 2008. p. 60–61.
16. Non-maleficence. In: Kirch W, editor. Encyclopedia of public health. Dordrecht: Springer Netherlands. 2008. p. 993.
17. Di Mattia P. Ethical principles ethical principles. In: Kirch W, editor. Encyclopedia of public health. Dordrecht: Springer Netherlands; 2008. p. 364–7.
18. Gotterbarn D, Miller K, Rogerson S. Software engineering code of ethics. Commun ACM. 1997;40(11):110–8.
19. Jokinen A, Stolt M, Suhonen R. Ethical issues related to eHealth: an integrative review. Nurs Ethics. 2021;28(2):253–71.
20. Yüksel B, Küpçü A, Özkasap Ö. Research issues for privacy and security of electronic health services. Futur Gener Comput Syst. 2017;68:1–13.
21. Rippen H, Risk A. e-Health code of ethics (May 24). J Med Internet Res. 2000;2(2):e9.
22. Rippen H, Risk A. e-Health ethics draft code (Feb 18). J Med Internet Res. 2000;2(1):e2.
23. Nissenbaum H. Privacy in context. Stanford University Press; 2009.
24. Fried C. Privacy. Yale Law J. 1968;77(3):475–93.
25. Westin AF. Privacy and freedom. Wash Lee Law Rev. 1968;25(1):166.
26. Bornschein R, Schmidt L, Maier E. The effect of consumers' perceived power and risk in digital information privacy: the example of cookie notices. J Public Policy Mark. 2020;39(2):135–54.
27. Altman I, Gover W. Privacy: definitions and properties. In: The environment and social behavior: privacy, personal space, territory, crowding. Monterey: Brooks/Cole; 1975. p. 10–31.
28. Anderson DR. Health and Human Services Standards for Privacy of Individually Identifiable Health Information. US Att'ys Bull. 2002;50:16.
29. Cavoukian A. Privacy by design: the 7 foundational principles, vol. 5. Information and Privacy Commissioner of Ontario, Canada; 2009.
30. Fang W, et al. A survey of big data security and privacy preserving. IETE Tech Rev. 2017;34(5):544–60.
31. Kruse CS, et al. Security techniques for the electronic health records. J Med Syst. 2017;41:1–9.
32. El Ouazzani Z, El Bakkali H. A classification of non-cryptographic anonymization techniques ensuring privacy in big data. Int J Commun Netw Inform Secur. 2020;12(1):142–52.
33. Allshouse WB, et al. Geomasking sensitive health data and privacy protection: an evaluation using an E911 database. Geocarto Int. 2010;25(6):443–52.
34. Nakamoto, Satoshi, Bitcoin: A Peer-to-Peer Electronic Cash System (August 21, 2008). Available at SSRN: http://dx.doi.org/10.2139/ssrn.3440802.
35. Preethi D, Khare N, Tripathy B. Security and privacy issues in blockchain technology. In: Blockchain technology and the internet of things. Apple Academic Press; 2020. p. 245–63.
36. Johari R, et al. BLOSOM: blockchain technology for security of medical records. ICT Express. 2022;8(1):56–60.
37. Tomlinson M, et al. The use of mobile phones as a data collection tool: a report from a household survey in South Africa. BMC Med Inform Decis Mak. 2009;9(1):1–8.
38. Lester RT, Gelmon L, Plummer FA. Cell phones: tightening the communication gap in resource-limited antiretroviral programmes? AIDS. 2006;20(17):2242–4.
39. Zurovac D, Talisuna AO, Snow RW. Mobile phone text messaging: tool for malaria control in Africa. PLoS Med. 2012;9(2):e1001176.
40. Basu S. E-government and developing countries: an overview. Int Rev Law Comput Technol. 2004;18(1):109–32.
41. Wambugu S. EHRs and privacy: protection in LMICs. Global Digital Health Forum Presentations, Digital Square. 2016. https://lib.digitalsquare.io/handle/123456789/77283. Accessed 26 May 2023.
42. Winkler WE. Overview of record linkage and current research directions. Technical report, Bureau of the Census. 2006.
43. Global health data acces principles. http://www.gatesfoundation.org/global-health/Documents/data-access-principles.pdf. Accessed 30 May 2023.
44. OCAP. First Nations Information Governance Centre. The First Nations principles of OCAP. https://fnigc.ca/ocap-training/. Accessed 26 May 2023.
45. UN General Assembly. United Nations declaration on the rights of indigenous peoples: resolution/adopted by the General Assembly, 2 October 2007, A/RES/61/295. https://www.refworld.org/docid/471355a82.html. Accessed 26 May 2023.
46. Carroll SR, Rodriguez-Lonebear D, Martinez A. Indigenous data governance: strategies from United States Native Nations. Data Sci J. 2019;18:31.

47. Castellano MB. Ethics of Aboriginal research. Int J Indig Health. 2004;1(1):98–114.

48. Carroll SR, et al. The CARE principles for indigenous data governance. Data Sci J. 2020;19:43.

49. Lin D, et al. The TRUST principles for digital repositories. Sci Data. 2020;7(1):144.

50. Carroll SR, et al. Operationalizing the CARE and FAIR principles for Indigenous data futures. Sci Data. 2021;8(1):108.

51. Wilkinson MD, et al. The FAIR guiding principles for scientific data management and stewardship. Sci Data. 2016;3(1):1–9.

52. Barrows RC Jr, Clayton PD. Privacy, confidentiality, and electronic medical records. J Am Med Inform Assoc. 1996;3(2):139–48.

53. Fernández-Alemán JL, et al. Security and privacy in electronic health records: a systematic literature review. J Biomed Inform. 2013;46(3):541–62.

54. World Health Organization. Monitoring the building blocks of health systems: a handbook of indicators and their measurement strategies. World Health Organization; 2010.

55. Jofre M, et al. Cybersecurity and privacy risk assessment of point-of-care systems in healthcare—a use case approach. Appl Sci. 2021;11(15):6699.

56. Ashenden D. Information security management: a human challenge? Inf Secur Tech Rep. 2008;13:195–201.

57. Flowerday S, Tuyikeze T. Information security policy development and implementation: the what, how and who. Comput Secur. 2016;61:169–83.

58. Soomro ZA, Shah MH, Ahmed J. Information security management needs more holistic approach: a literature review. Int J Inf Manag. 2016;36(2):215–25.

59. Hajrahimi N, Dehaghani SMH, Sheikhtaheri A. Health information security: a case study of three selected medical centers in iran. Acta Inform Med. 2013;21(1):42.

60. Ferreira A, et al. Grounding information security in healthcare. Int J Med Inform. 2010;79(4):268–83.

61. Page BB. Exploring organizational culture for information security in healthcare organizations: a literature review. In: 2017 Portland International Conference on Management of Engineering and Technology (PICMET). IEEE; 2017.

62. Haux R. Health information systems—past, present, future. Int J Med Inform. 2006;75(3–4):268–81.

63. Posthumus S, von Solms R. A framework for the governance of information security. Comput Secur. 2004;23(8):638–46.

64. Crotty BH, Mostaghimi A. Confidentiality in the digital age. BMJ. 2014;348:g2943.

65. Samy GN, Ahmad R, Ismail Z. Security threats categories in healthcare information systems. Health Informatics J. 2010;16(3):201–9.

66. Iwaya LH, et al. mhealth: a privacy threat analysis for public health surveillance systems. In: 2018 IEEE 31st International Symposium on Computer-Based Medical Systems (CBMS). IEEE; 2018.

67. Dehling T, Sunyaev A. Secure provision of patient-centered health information technology services in public networks—leveraging security and privacy features provided by the German nationwide health information technology infrastructure. Electron Mark. 2014;24:89–99.

68. Aldis W. Health security as a public health concept: a critical analysis. Health Policy Plan. 2008;23(6):369–75.

69. Kruse CS, et al. Security techniques for the electronic health records. J Med Syst. 2017;41(8):127.

70. Coventry, L. et al. Cyber-Risk in healthcare: Exploring facilitators and barriers to secure behaviour. In: Moallem, A. (eds) HCI for Cybersecurity, Privacy and Trust. HCII 2020. Lecture Notes in Computer Science. 2020, vol 12210. Springer, Cham. https://doi.org/10.1007/978-3-030-50309-3_8.

71. Raina MacIntyre C, et al. Converging and emerging threats to health security. Environ Syst Decis. 2018;38(2):198–207.

72. Eden KB, et al. Barriers and facilitators to exchanging health information: a systematic review. Int J Med Inform. 2016;88:44–51.

73. Lin C, Lin I-C, Roan J. Barriers to physicians' adoption of healthcare information technology: an empirical study on multiple hospitals. J Med Syst. 2012;36:1965–77.

74. Dönmez E, et al. Readiness for health information technology is associated to information security in healthcare institutions. Acta Inform Med. 2020;28(4):265–71.

75. Söderström E, Åhlfeldt RM, Eriksson N. Standards for information security and processes in healthcare. J Syst Inf Technol. 2009;11(3):295–308.

76. Bhuyan SS, et al. Transforming healthcare cybersecurity from reactive to proactive: current status and future recommendations. J Med Syst. 2020;44:1–9.

77. Renaud K, Goucher W. Health service employees and information security policies: an uneasy partnership? Inf Manag Comput Secur. 2012;20(4):296–311.

78. Lane H, et al. Equity in healthcare resource allocation decision making: a systematic review. Soc Sci Med. 2017;175:11–27.

79. Thomas SL, Wakerman J, Humphreys JS. Ensuring equity of access to primary health care in rural and remote Australia—what core services should be locally available? Int J Equity Health. 2015;14:111.

80. Richard L, et al. Equity of access to primary healthcare for vulnerable populations: the IMPACT international online survey of innovations. Int J Equity Health. 2016;15(1):64.

81. Stangl AL, et al. The health stigma and discrimination framework: a global, crosscutting framework to inform research, intervention development, and policy on health-related stigmas. BMC Med. 2019;17(1):31.

82. Penman-Aguilar A, et al. Measurement of health disparities, health inequities, and social determinants of health to support the advancement of health equity. J

Public Health Manag Pract. 2016;22 Suppl 1(Suppl 1):S33–42.

83. Brown S-A, et al. The pursuit of health equity in digital transformation, health informatics, and the cardiovascular learning healthcare system. Am Heart J Plus Cardiol Res Pract. 2022;17:100160.

84. Brewer LC, Fortuna KL. Back to the future: achieving health equity through health informatics and digital health. JMIR Mhealth Uhealth. 2020;8(1):e14512.

85. Rodriguez JA, Clark CR, Bates DW. Digital health equity as a necessity in the 21st century cures act era. JAMA. 2020;323(23):2381–2.

86. Veinot TC, Ancker JS, Bakken S. Health informatics and health equity: improving our reach and impact. J Am Med Inform Assoc. 2019;26(8–9):689–95.

87. Bambas L. Integrating equity into health information systems: a human rights approach to health and information. PLoS Med. 2005;2(4):e102.

88. Hernandez MF, Rodriguez F. Health techequity: opportunities for digital health innovations to improve equity and diversity in cardiovascular care. Curr Cardiovasc Risk Rep. 2023;17(1):1–20.

89. Kaihlanen A-M, et al. Towards digital health equity—a qualitative study of the challenges experienced by vulnerable groups in using digital health services in the COVID-19 era. BMC Health Serv Res. 2022;22(1):188.

90. Crowe-Cumella H, et al. Editorial: digital health equity. Front Digit Health. 2023;5:1184847.

91. Rodriguez JA, et al. Digital healthcare equity in primary care: implementing an integrated digital health navigator. J Am Med Inform Assoc. 2023;30(5):965–70.

92. Marmot M, Allen JJ. Social determinants of health equity. Am J Public Health. 2014;104 Suppl 4(Suppl 4):S517–9.

93. Jensen N, Kelly AH. Health equity and health system strengthening—Time for a WHO re-think. Glob Public Health. 2022;17(3):377–90.

94. Lyles CR, Wachter RM, Sarkar U. Focusing on digital health equity. JAMA. 2021;326(18):1795–6.

95. Richardson S, et al. A framework for digital health equity. NPJ Digit Med. 2022;5(1):119.

96. Cruz TM, Smith SA. Health equity beyond data: health care worker perceptions of race, ethnicity, and language data collection in electronic health records. Med Care. 2021;59(5):379–85.

97. Brinkerhoff DW. Accountability and health systems: toward conceptual clarity and policy relevance. Health Policy Plan. 2004;19(6):371–9.

98. Magnan S, et al. Achieving accountability for health and health care. Minn Med. 2012;95(11):37–9.

99. Forster AJ, van Walraven C. The use of quality indicators to promote accountability in health care: the good, the bad, and the ugly. Open Med. 2012;6(2):e75–9.

100. Derick W Brinkerhoff, Accountability and health systems: toward conceptual clarity and policy relevance,

Health Policy and Planning. 2004;19(6):371–9. https://doi.org/10.1093/heapol/czh052.

101. Nolen LB, et al. Strengthening health information systems to address health equity challenges. Bull World Health Organ. 2005;83(8):597–603.

102. Gilson L, Lehmann U, Schneider H. Practicing governance towards equity in health systems: LMIC perspectives and experience. Int J Equity Health. 2017;16(1):171.

103. Habli I, Lawton T, Porter Z. Artificial intelligence in health care: accountability and safety. Bull World Health Organ. 2020;98(4):251–6.

104. Lee TD, Park H, Lee J. Collaborative accountability for sustainable public health: a Korean perspective on the effective use of ICT-based health risk communication. Gov Inf Q. 2019;36(2):226–36.

105. MHRA. Data integrity guidance and definitions. London: Medicines and Healthcare Products Regulatory Agency; 2018.

106. Zarour M, Alenezi M. Ensuring data integrity of healthcare information in the era of digital health. Healthc Technol Lett. 2021;8(3):66–77.

107. Tijani B, et al. Improving data integrity in public health: a case study of an outbreak management system in Nigeria. Glob Health Sci Pract. 2021;9(Suppl 2):S226–33.

108. Silverstone DE, Lim MC. Ensuring information integrity in the electronic health record: the crisis and the challenge. Ophthalmology. 2014;121(2):435–7.

109. Group AW. Managing the integrity of patient identity in health information exchange (2014 update). J AHIMA. 2014;85(5):60–5.

110. Wardle C, Derakhshan H. Information disorder: toward an interdisciplinary framework for research and policymaking. Council of Europe Strasbourg; 2017.

111. Kluge HHP, Azzopardi-Muscat N, Novillo-Ortiz D. Leveraging digital transformation for better health in Europe. Bull World Health Organ. 2022;100(12):751–751A.

112. Wardle C, Singerman E. Too little, too late: social media companies' failure to tackle vaccine misinformation poses a real threat. BMJ. 2021;372:n26.

113. Swire-Thompson B, Lazer D. Public health and online misinformation: challenges and recommendations. Annu Rev Public Health. 2020;41:433–51.

114. Borges do Nascimento IJ, et al. Infodemics and health misinformation: a systematic review of reviews. Bull World Health Organ. 2022;100(9):544–61.

115. WHO. WHO COVID-19 infodemic. 2022. https://www.who.int/news/item/02-02-2021-who-public-health-research-agenda-for-managing-infodemics.

116. Jember MZ, et al. Misinformation on COVID-19 vaccine and its associated factors among residents in Gondar, Ethiopia, 2022. Biomed Res Int. 2024;2024:9947720.

Index

K. D. Gashu et al. (eds.), *Public Health Informatics*, Sustainable Development Goals Series, https://doi.org/10.1007/978-3-031-71118-3